BEFORE AN EMERGENCY – BECOME FAMILIAR WITH THIS GUIDEBOOK! In the U.S., according to the requirements of the U.S. Department of Labor's Occupational Safety and Health Administration (OSHA, 29 CFR 1910.120), and regulations issued by the U.S. Environmental Protection Agency (EPA, 40 CFR Part 311), first responders must be trained regarding the use of this guidebook.

RESIST RUSHING IN !
APPROACH INCIDENT FROM UPWIND
STAY CLEAR OF ALL SPILLS, VAPORS, FUMES, SMOKE AND SUSPICIOUS SOURCES

HOW TO USE THIS GUIDEBOOK DURING AN INCIDENT INVOLVING DANGEROUS GOODS

STEP ONE: IDENTIFY THE MATERIAL. USE **ANY** OF THE FOLLOWING:

- **IDENTIFICATION NUMBER (4-DIGIT ID) FROM** A PLACARD, ORANGE PANEL, SHIPPING PAPER OR PACKAGE (after UN/NA)
- **NAME OF THE MATERIAL FROM** A SHIPPING DOCUMENT OR PACKAGE

STEP TWO: IDENTIFY 3-DIGIT GUIDE NUMBER USE:

- ID NUMBER INDEX in yellow-bordered pages or
- NAME OF MATERIAL INDEX in blue-bordered pages

Guide number supplemented with the letter "**P**" indicates that the material may undergo violent polymerization if subjected to heat or contamination.

INDEX ENTRIES HIGHLIGHTED IN GREEN are TIH (Toxic Inhalation Hazard) material, a chemical warfare agent or a Dangerous Water Reactive Material (produces toxic gas upon contact with water). IDENTIFY ID NUMBER AND NAME OF MATERIAL IN TABLE 1 – INITIAL ISOLATION AND PROTECTIVE ACTION DISTANCES (the green-bordered pages). **IF NECESSARY, BEGIN PROTECTIVE ACTIONS IMMEDIATELY** (see Protective Actions page 296). If no protective action required, use the information jointly with the 3-digit guide.

STEP THREE: TURN TO THE NUMBERED GUIDE (the orange-bordered pages) READ CAREFULLY.

USE GUIDE 112 FOR ALL EXPLOSIVES EXCEPT FOR EXPLOSIVES 1.4 (EXPLOSIVES C) WHERE GUIDE 114 IS TO BE CONSULTED.

NOTE: IF ABOVE STEPS CANNOT BE COMPLETED AND PLACARD IS VISIBLE: Turn to pages 16-17; use 3-digit guide next to placard; PROCEED TO NUMBERED GUIDE (orange-bordered pages). If shipping document is available, call emergency response telephone number listed. If document or emergency response telephone is not available, IMMEDIATELY CALL the appropriate **emergency response agency listed in the back of this guidebook**. Provide as much information as possible, such as the name of the carrier (trucking company or railroad) and vehicle number. **IF A REFERENCE TO A GUIDE CANNOT BE FOUND AND THIS INCIDENT IS BELIEVED TO INVOLVE DANGEROUS GOODS**, TURN TO **GUIDE 111** NOW, AND USE IT UNTIL ADDITIONAL INFORMATION BECOMES AVAILABLE.

AS A LAST RESORT: IF ONLY THE CONTAINER CAN BE IDENTIFIED, CONSULT THE TABLE OF RAIL CAR AND ROAD TRAILER IDENTIFICATION CHART (pages18-19). REMEMBER THAT THE INFORMATION ASSOCIATED WITH THESE CONTAINERS IS FOR WORST CASE SCENARIOS.

The 2008 Emergency Response Guidebook (ERG2008) was developed jointly by Transport Canada (TC), the U.S. Department of Transportation (DOT), the Secretariat of Transport and Communications of Mexico (SCT) and with the collaboration of CIQUIME (Centro de Información Química para Emergencias) of Argentina, for use by fire fighters, police, and other emergency services personnel who may be the first to arrive at the scene of a transportation incident involving dangerous goods. **It is primarily a guide to aid first responders in quickly identifying the specific or generic hazards of the material(s) involved in the incident, and protecting themselves and the general public during the initial response phase of the incident.** For the purposes of this guidebook, the "initial response phase" is that period following arrival at the scene of an incident during which the presence and/or identification of dangerous goods is confirmed, protective actions and area securement are initiated, and assistance of qualified personnel is requested. It is not intended to provide information on the physical or chemical properties of dangerous goods.

This guidebook will assist responders in making initial decisions upon arriving at the scene of a dangerous goods incident. It should not be considered as a substitute for emergency response training, knowledge or sound judgment. ERG2008 does not address all possible circumstances that may be associated with a dangerous goods incident. It is primarily designed for use at a dangerous goods incident occurring on a highway or railroad. Be mindful that there may be limited value in its application at fixed facility locations.

ERG2008 incorporates dangerous goods lists from the most recent United Nations Recommendations as well as from other international and national regulations. Explosives are not listed individually by either proper shipping name or ID Number. They do, however, appear under the general heading "Explosives" on the first page of the ID Number index (yellow-bordered pages) and alphabetically in the Name of Material index (blue-bordered pages). Also, the letter **"P"** following the guide number in the yellow-bordered and blue-bordered pages identifies those materials which present a polymerization hazard under certain conditions, for example: Acrolein, stabilized   **131P**.

First responders at the scene of a dangerous goods incident should seek additional specific information about any material in question as soon as possible. The information received by contacting the appropriate emergency response agency, by calling the emergency response telephone number on the shipping document, or by consulting the information on or accompanying the shipping document, may be more specific and accurate than this guidebook in providing guidance for the materials involved.

<u>BEFORE AN EMERGENCY</u> – **BECOME FAMILIAR WITH THIS GUIDEBOOK!** In the U.S., according to the requirements of the U.S. Department of Labor's Occupational Safety and Health Administration (OSHA, 29 CFR 1910.120), and regulations issued by the U.S. Environmental Protection Agency (EPA, 40 CFR Part 311), first responders must be trained regarding the use of this guidebook.

1-Yellow-bordered pages: Index list of dangerous goods in numerical order of ID number. This section quickly identifies the guide to be consulted from the ID Number of the material involved. This list displays the 4-digit ID number of the material followed by its assigned emergency response guide and the material name.

For example:	ID No.	GUIDE No.	Name of Material
	1090	127	Acetone

2-Blue-bordered pages: Index list of dangerous goods in alphabetical order of material name. This section quickly identifies the guide to be consulted from the name of the material involved. This list displays the name of the material followed by its assigned emergency response guide and 4-digit ID number.

For example:	Name of Material	GUIDE No.	ID No.
	Sulfuric acid	137	1830

3-Orange-bordered pages: This section is the most important section of the guidebook because it is where all safety recommendations are provided. It comprises a total of 62 individual guides, presented in a two-page format. Each guide provides safety recommendations and emergency response information to protect yourself and the public. The left hand page provides safety related information whereas the right hand page provides emergency response guidance and activities for fire situations, spill or leak incidents and first aid. Each guide is designed to cover a group of materials which possess similar chemical and toxicological characteristics.

The guide title identifies the general hazards of the dangerous goods covered.

For example: **GUIDE 124** - Gases-Toxic and/or Corrosive-Oxidizing.

Each guide is divided into three main sections: the first section describes **potential hazards** that the material may display in terms of fire/explosion and health effects upon exposure. The highest potential is listed first. The emergency responder should consult this section first. This allows the responder to make decisions regarding the protection of the emergency response team as well as the surrounding population.

The second section outlines suggested **public safety** measures based on the situation at hand. It provides general information regarding immediate isolation of the incident site, recommended type of protective clothing and respiratory protection. Suggested evacuation distances are listed for small and large spills and for fire situations (fragmentation hazard). It also directs the reader to consult the tables listing Toxic Inhalation Hazard (TIH) materials, chemical warfare agents and water-reactive materials (green-bordered pages) when the material is highlighted in the yellow-bordered and blue-bordered pages.

The third section covers **emergency response** actions, including first aid. It outlines special precautions for incidents which involve fire, spill or chemical exposure. Several recommendations are listed under each part which will further assist in the decision making process. The information on first aid is general guidance prior to seeking medical care.

4-Green-bordered pages: This section contains two tables. Table 1 lists, by ID number order, TIH materials, including certain chemical warfare agents, and water-reactive materials which produce toxic gases upon contact with water. This table provides two different types of recommended safe distances which are "Initial isolation distances" and "Protective action distances." The materials are highlighted in green for easy identification in both numeric (yellow-bordered pages) and alphabetic (blue-bordered pages) lists of the guidebook. This table provides distances for both small (approximately 200 liters or less for liquids and 300 kilograms or less for solids when spilled in water) and large spills (more than 200 liters for liquids and more than 300 kilograms for solids when spilled in water) for all highlighted materials. The list is further subdivided into daytime and nighttime situations. This is necessary due to varying atmospheric conditions which greatly affect the size of the hazardous area. The distances change from daytime to nighttime due to different mixing and dispersion conditions in the air. During the night, the air is generally calmer and this causes the material to disperse less and therefore create a toxic zone which is greater than would usually occur during the day. During the day, a more active atmosphere will cause a greater dispersion of the material resulting in a lower concentration of the material in the surrounding air. The actual area where toxic levels are reached will be smaller (due to increased dispersion). In fact, it is the quantity or concentration of the material vapor that poses problems not its mere presence. Table 2 lists, by ID number order, materials which produce large amounts of Toxic Inhalation Hazard (TIH) gases when spilled in water and identifies the TIH gases produced. These Water Reactive materials are easily identified in Table 1 as their name is immediately followed by (when spilled in water). Note, however, if this material is NOT spilled in water, Table 1 and Table 2 do not apply and safety distances will be found within the appropriate orange guide.

The "Initial Isolation Distance" is a distance within which all persons should be considered for evacuation in all directions from the actual spill/leak source. It is a distance (radius) which defines a circle (Initial Isolation Zone) within which persons may be exposed to dangerous concentrations upwind of the source and may be exposed to life threatening concentrations downwind of the source. For example, in the case of Compressed gas, toxic, n.o.s., ID No. 1955, Inhalation Hazard Zone A, the isolation distance for small spills is 100 meters, therefore, representing an evacuation circle of 200 meters in diameter.

For the same material, the "Protective Action Distance" for a small spill is 0.5 kilometers for a daytime incident and 2.1 kilometers for a nighttime incident, these distances represent a downwind distance from the spill/leak source within which Protective Actions could be implemented. Protective Actions are those steps taken to preserve the health and safety of emergency responders and the public. People in this area could be evacuated and/or sheltered in-place. For more information, consult pages 293 to 299.

What is a TIH? It is a gas or volatile liquid which is known to be so toxic to humans as to pose a hazard to health during transportation, or in the absence of adequate data on human

toxicity, is presumed to be toxic to humans because when tested on laboratory animals it has a Lethal Concentration 50 (LC50) value of not more than 5000 ppm.

It is important to note that even though the term zone is used, the hazard zones do not represent any actual area or distance. The assignment of the zones is strictly a function of their Lethal Concentration 50 (LC50); for example, TIH Zone A is more toxic than Zone D. All distances which are listed in the green-bordered pages are calculated by the use of mathematical models for each TIH material. For the assignment of hazard zones refer to the glossary.

ISOLATION AND EVACUATION DISTANCES

Isolation or evacuation distances are shown in the guides (orange-bordered pages) and in the Table 1 - Initial Isolation and Protective Action Distances (green-bordered pages). This may confuse users not thoroughly familiar with ERG2008.

It is important to note that some guides refer only to non-TIH materials (36 guides), some refer to both TIH and non-TIH materials (21 guides) and some (5 guides) refer only to TIH or Water-reactive materials (WRM). A guide refers to both TIH and non-TIH materials (for example see GUIDE 131) when the following sentence appears under the title EVACUATION-Spill: "See Table 1 - Initial Isolation and Protective Action Distances for highlighted materials. For non-highlighted materials, increase, in the downwind direction, as necessary, the isolation distance shown under 'PUBLIC SAFETY.'" A guide refers only to TIH or WRM materials (for example see GUIDE 124) when the following sentence appears under the title EVACUATION-Spill: "See Table 1 - Initial Isolation and Protective Action Distances". If the previous sentences do not appear in a guide, then this particular guide refers only to non-TIH materials (for example see GUIDE 128).

In order to identify appropriate isolation and protective action distances, use the following:

If you are dealing with a **TIH/WRM/Chemical warfare** material (highlighted entries in the index lists), the isolation and evacuation distances are found directly in the green-bordered pages. The guides (orange-bordered pages) also remind the user to refer to the green-bordered pages for evacuation specific information involving highlighted materials.

If you are dealing with a **non-TIH material but the guide refers to both TIH and non-TIH materials**, an immediate isolation distance is provided under the heading PUBLIC SAFETY as a precautionary measure to prevent injuries. It applies to the non-TIH materials only. In addition, for evacuation purposes, the guide informs the user under the title EVACUATION-Spill to increase, for non-highlighted materials, in the downwind direction, if necessary, the immediate isolation distance listed under "PUBLIC SAFETY". For example, GUIDE 131 – Flammable Liquids-Toxic, instructs the user to: "As an immediate precautionary measure, isolate spill or leak area for at least 50 meters (150 feet) in all directions." In case of a large spill, the isolation area could be expanded from 50 meters to a distance deemed as safe by the On-scene commander and emergency responders.

If you are dealing with a **non-TIH material and the guide refers only to non-TIH materials**, the immediate isolation and evacuation distances are specified as actual distances in the guide (orange-bordered pages) and are not referenced in the green-bordered pages.

SAFETY PRECAUTIONS

APPROACH CAUTIOUSLY FROM UPWIND. If wind direction allows, consider approaching the incident from uphill. Resist the urge to rush in; others cannot be helped until the situation has been fully assessed.

SECURE THE SCENE. Without entering the immediate hazard area, isolate the area and assure the safety of people and the environment, keep people away from the scene and outside the safety perimeter. Allow enough room to move and remove your own equipment.

IDENTIFY THE HAZARDS. Placards, container labels, shipping documents, material safety data sheets, Rail Car and Road Trailer Identification Charts, and/or knowledgeable persons on the scene are valuable information sources. Evaluate all available information and consult the recommended guide to reduce immediate risks. **Additional information, provided by the shipper or obtained from another authoritative source, may change some of the emphasis or details found in the guide.** Remember, the guide provides only the most important and worst case scenario information for the initial response in relation to a family or class of dangerous goods. As more material-specific information becomes available, the response should be tailored to the situation.

ASSESS THE SITUATION. Consider the following:
- Is there a fire, a spill or a leak?
- What are the weather conditions?
- What is the terrain like?
- Who/what is at risk: people, property or the environment?
- What actions should be taken: Is an evacuation necessary? Is diking necessary? What resources (human and equipment) are required and are readily available?
- What can be done immediately?

OBTAIN HELP. Advise your headquarters to notify responsible agencies and call for assistance from qualified personnel.

DECIDE ON SITE ENTRY. Any efforts made to rescue persons, protect property or the environment must be weighed against the possibility that you could become part of the problem. Enter the area only when wearing appropriate protective gear (see PROTECTIVE CLOTHING, page 348).

RESPOND. Respond in an appropriate manner. Establish a command post and lines of communication. Rescue casualties where possible and evacuate if necessary. Maintain control of the site. Continually reassess the situation and modify the response accordingly. The first duty is to consider the safety of people in the immediate area, including your own.

ABOVE ALL. Do not walk into or touch spilled material. Avoid inhalation of fumes, smoke and vapors, even if no dangerous goods are known to be involved. Do not assume that gases or vapors are harmless because of lack of a smell—odorless gases or vapors may be harmful. Use **CAUTION** when handling empty containers because they may still present hazards until they are cleaned and purged of all residues.

WHO TO CALL FOR ASSISTANCE

Upon arrival at the scene, a first responder is expected to recognize the presence of dangerous goods, protect oneself and the public, secure the area, and call for the assistance of trained personnel as soon as conditions permit. Follow the steps outlined in your organization's standard operating procedures and/or local emergency response plan for obtaining qualified assistance. Generally, the notification sequence and requests for technical information beyond what is available in this guidebook should occur in the following order:

1. ORGANIZATION/AGENCY

Notify your organization/agency. This will set in motion a series of events based upon the information provided. Actions may range from dispatching additional trained personnel to the scene to activating the local emergency response plan. Ensure that local fire and police departments have been notified.

2. EMERGENCY RESPONSE TELEPHONE NUMBER

Locate and call the telephone number listed on the shipping document. The person answering the phone at the listed emergency response number must be knowledgeable of the materials and mitigation actions to be taken, or must have immediate access to a person who has the required knowledge.

3. NATIONAL ASSISTANCE

Contact the appropriate emergency response agency listed on the inside back cover of this guidebook when the emergency response telephone number is not available from the shipping papers. Upon receipt of a call describing the nature of the incident, the agency will provide immediate advice on handling the early stages of the incident. The agency will also contact the shipper or manufacturer of the material for more detailed information and request on-scene assistance when necessary.

Collect and provide as much of the following information as can safely be obtained to your chain-of-command and specialists contacted for technical guidance:

Your name, call back telephone number, FAX number
Location and nature of problem (spill, fire, etc.)
Name and identification number of material(s) involved
Shipper/consignee/point of origin
Carrier name, rail car or truck number
Container type and size
Quantity of material transported/released
Local conditions (weather, terrain, proximity to schools, hospitals, waterways, etc.)
Injuries and exposures
Local emergency services that have been notified

CANADA

1. CANUTEC

CANUTEC is the **Canadian Transport Emergency Centre** operated by the Transport Dangerous Goods Directorate of Transport Canada.

CANUTEC provides a national bilingual (French and English) advisory service and is staffed by professional scientists experienced and trained in interpreting technical information and providing emergency response advice.

In an emergency, CANUTEC may be called collect at
613-996-6666 (24 hours)
***666 cellular (Press Star 666, Canada only)**

In a non-emergency situation, please call the information line at 613-992-4624 (24 hours).

2. PROVINCIAL AGENCIES

Although technical information and emergency response assistance can be obtained from **CANUTEC,** there are federal and provincial regulations requiring the reporting of dangerous goods incidents to certain authorities.

The following list of provincial agencies is supplied for your convenience.

Province	Emergency Authority and/or Telephone Number
Alberta	Local Police and Provincial Authorities 1-800-272-9600* or 780-422-9600
British Columbia	Local Police and Provincial Authorities 1-800-663-3456
Manitoba	Provincial Authority 204-945-4888 and Local Police or fire brigade, as appropriate
New Brunswick	Local Police or 1-800-565-1633** or 902-426-6030
Newfoundland and Labrador	Local Police and 709-772-2083
Northwest Territories	867-920-8130
Nova Scotia	Local Police or 1-800-565-1633** or 902-426-6030
Nunavut Territory	Local Police and 1-800-693-1666 or 867-979-6262
Ontario	Local Police
Prince Edward Island	Local Police or 1-800-565-1633** or 902-426-6030
Quebec	Local Police
Saskatchewan	Local Police or 1-800-667-7525
Yukon Territory	867-667-7244

* This number is not accessible from outside Alberta.
** This number is not accessible from outside of New Brunswick, Nova Scotia or Prince Edward Island.

NOTE:

1. The appropriate federal agency must be notified in the case of rail, air or marine incidents.

2. The nearest police department must be notified in the case of lost, stolen or misplaced explosives, radioactive materials or infectious substances.

3. **CANUTEC must** be notified in the case of:

   a. lost, stolen or misplaced infectious substances;
   b. an incident involving infectious substances;
   c. an accidental release from a cylinder that has suffered a catastrophic failure;
   d. an incident where the shipping documents display **CANUTEC's** telephone number 613-996-6666 as the emergency telephone number; or
   e. a dangerous goods incident in which a railway vehicle, a ship, an aircraft, an aerodrome or an air cargo facility is involved.

UNITED STATES

1. **CHEMTREC®**, a 24-hour emergency response communication service, can be reached as follows:

CALL **CHEMTREC®** (24 hours)
1-800-424-9300
(Toll-free in the U.S., Canada, and the U.S. Virgin Islands)
For calls originating elsewhere:
703-527-3887 (Collect calls are accepted)

2. **CHEMTEL, INC.**, a 24-hour emergency response communication service, can be reached as follows:

CALL **CHEMTEL, INC.** (24 hours)
1-888-255-3924
(Toll-free in the U.S., Canada, Puerto Rico and the U.S. Virgin Islands)
For calls originating elsewhere:
813-248-0585 (Collect calls are accepted)

3. **INFOTRAC**, a 24-hour emergency response communication service, can be reached as follows:

CALL **INFOTRAC** (24 hours)
1-800-535-5053
(Toll-free in the U.S., Canada, and the U.S. Virgin Islands)
For calls originating elsewhere:
352-323-3500 (Collect calls are accepted)

4. **3E COMPANY**, a 24-hour emergency response communication service, can be reached as follows:

CALL **3E COMPANY** (24 hours)
1-800-451-8346
(Toll-free in the U.S., Canada, and the U.S. Virgin Islands)
For calls originating elsewhere:
760-602-8703 (Collect calls are accepted)

The emergency response information services shown above have requested to be listed as providers of emergency response information and have agreed to provide emergency response information to all callers. They maintain periodically updated lists of state and Federal radiation authorities who provide information and technical assistance on handling incidents involving radioactive materials.

5. **MILITARY SHIPMENTS**

For assistance at incidents involving materials being shipped by, for, or to the Department of Defense (DOD), call one of the following numbers (24 hours):

703-697-0218 (call collect) (U.S. Army Operations Center) for incidents involving explosives and ammunition.

1-800-851-8061 (toll-free in the U.S.) (Defense Logistics Agency) for incidents involving dangerous goods other than explosives and ammunition.

6. **NATIONWIDE POISON CONTROL CENTER** (United States Only)

Emergency and information calls are answered by the nearest Poison Center (24 hours):

1-800-222-1222 (toll-free in the U.S.).

The above numbers are for **emergencies** only.

NATIONAL RESPONSE CENTER (NRC)

The NRC, which is operated by the U.S. Coast Guard, receives reports required when dangerous goods and hazardous substances are spilled. After receiving notification of an incident, the NRC will immediately notify the appropriate Federal On-Scene Coordinator and concerned Federal agencies. Federal law requires that anyone who releases into the environment a reportable quantity of a hazardous substance (including oil when water is, or may be affected) or a material identified as a marine pollutant, must **immediately** notify the NRC. When in doubt as to whether the amount released equals the required reporting levels for these materials, the NRC should be notified.

CALL **NRC** (24 hours)
1-800-424-8802
(Toll-free in the U.S., Canada, and the U.S. Virgin Islands)
202-267-2675 in the District of Columbia

Calling the emergency response telephone number, CHEMTREC®, CHEMTEL, INC., INFOTRAC or 3E COMPANY, does not constitute compliance with regulatory requirements to call the NRC.

MEXICO

1. **SETIQ** (Emergency Transportation System for the Chemical Industry), a service of the National Association of Chemical Industries (ANIQ), can be reached as follows:

CALL **SETIQ** (24 hours)
01-800-00-214-00 in the Mexican Republic
For calls originating in Mexico City and the Metropolitan Area
5559-1588
For calls originating elsewhere, call
+52-55-5559-1588

2. **CENACOM**, the National Center for Communications of the Civil Protection Agency, can be reached as follows:

CALL **CENACOM** (24 hours)
01-800-00-413-00 in the Mexican Republic
For calls originating in Mexico City and the Metropolitan Area
5128-0000 exts. 11470, 11471, 11472, 11473, 11474, 11475, 11476 and 11477
For calls originating elsewhere, call
+52-55-5128-0000 exts. 11470, 11471, 11472, 11474, 11475 and 11476

ARGENTINA

1. **CIQUIME** (Chemistry Information Center for Emergencies) a 24-hour emergency response information service, can be reached as follows:

CALL **CIQUIME** (24 hours)
0-800-222-2933 in the Republic of Argentina

For calls originating elsewhere, call
+54-11-4613-1100

BRAZIL

1. **PRÓ-QUÍMICA** a 24-hour emergency response information service, can be reached as follows:

CALL **PRÓ-QUÍMICA** (24 hours)
0-800-118270 in the Federal Republic of Brazil

For calls originating elsewhere, call
+55-11-232-1144

COLOMBIA

1. **CISPROQUIM** a 24-hour emergency response information service, can be reached as follows:

CALL **CISPROQUIM** (24 hours)
01-800-091-6012 in Colombia
For calls originating in Bogotá, Colombia call
288-6012
For calls originating elsewhere, call
+57-1-288-6012

HAZARD CLASSIFICATION SYSTEM

The hazard class of dangerous goods is indicated either by its class (or division) number or name. Placards are used to identify the class or division of a material. The hazard class or division number must be displayed in the lower corner of a placard and is required for both primary and subsidiary hazard classes and divisions, if applicable. For other than Class 7 or the OXYGEN placard, text indicating a hazard (for example, "CORROSIVE") is not required. Text is shown only in the U.S. The hazard class or division number and subsidiary hazard classes or division numbers placed in parentheses (when applicable), must appear on the shipping document after each proper shipping name.

Class 1 - Explosives

Division 1.1	Explosives with a mass explosion hazard
Division 1.2	Explosives with a projection hazard
Division 1.3	Explosives with predominantly a fire hazard
Division 1.4	Explosives with no significant blast hazard
Division 1.5	Very insensitive explosives with a mass explosion hazard
Division 1.6	Extremely insensitive articles

Class 2 - Gases

Division 2.1	Flammable gases
Division 2.2	Non-flammable, non-toxic* gases
Division 2.3	Toxic* gases

Class 3 - Flammable liquids (and Combustible liquids [U.S.])

Class 4 - Flammable solids; Spontaneously combustible materials; and Dangerous when wet materials/Water-reactive substances

Division 4.1	Flammable solids
Division 4.2	Spontaneously combustible materials
Division 4.3	Water-reactive substances/Dangerous when wet materials

Class 5 - Oxidizing substances and Organic peroxides

Division 5.1	Oxidizing substances
Division 5.2	Organic peroxides

Class 6 - Toxic* substances and Infectious substances

Division 6.1	Toxic*substances
Division 6.2	Infectious substances

Class 7 - Radioactive materials

Class 8 - Corrosive substances

Class 9 - Miscellaneous hazardous materials/Products, Substances or Organisms

* The words "poison" or "poisonous" are synonymous with the word "toxic".

INTRODUCTION TO THE TABLE OF PLACARDS

USE THIS TABLE ONLY IF YOU HAVE NOT BEEN ABLE TO IDENTIFY THE MATERIAL(S) IN TRANSPORT BY ID NUMBER OR SHIPPING NAME

The next two pages display the placards used on transport vehicles carrying dangerous goods. As you approach a reported or suspected dangerous goods incident involving a placarded vehicle:

1. **Approach the incident cautiously from upwind to a point from which you can safely identify and/or read the placard or orange panel information.** If wind direction allows, consider approaching the incident from uphill. Use binoculars, if available.

2. **Match the vehicle placard(s) with one of the placards displayed on the next two pages.**

3. **Consult the numbered guide associated with the sample placard. Use that information for now.** For example, a FLAMMABLE (Class 3) placard leads to GUIDE **127**. A CORROSIVE (Class 8) placard leads to GUIDE **153**. If multiple placards point to more than one guide, initially use the most conservative guide (i.e., the guide requiring the greatest degree of protective actions).

4. **Remember that the guides associated with the placards provide the most significant risk and/or hazard information.**

5. **When specific information,** such as ID number or shipping name, **becomes available, the more specific guide recommended for that material must be consulted.**

6. **If GUIDE 111 is being used because only the DANGER/DANGEROUS placard is displayed or the nature of the spilled, leaking, or burning material is not known, as soon as possible, get more specific information concerning the material(s) involved.**

7. **Asterisks (*) on orange placards represent explosives "Compatibility Group" letters; refer to the Glossary (page 357).**

8. **Double asterisks (**) on orange placards represent the division of the explosive.**

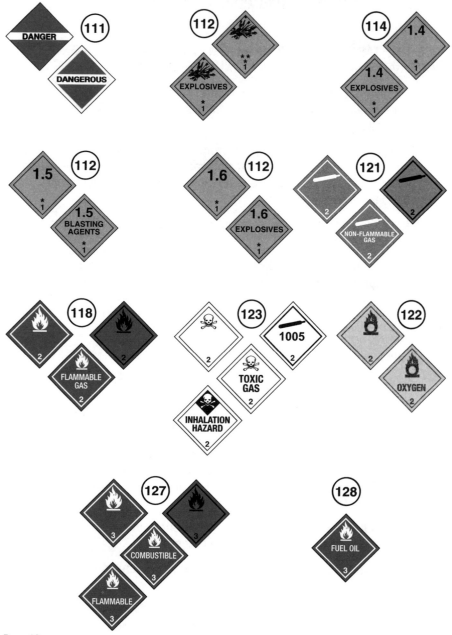

RESPONSE GUIDE TO USE ON-SCENE
USING THE SHIPPING DOCUMENT, NUMBERED PLACARD, OR ORANGE PANEL NUMBER

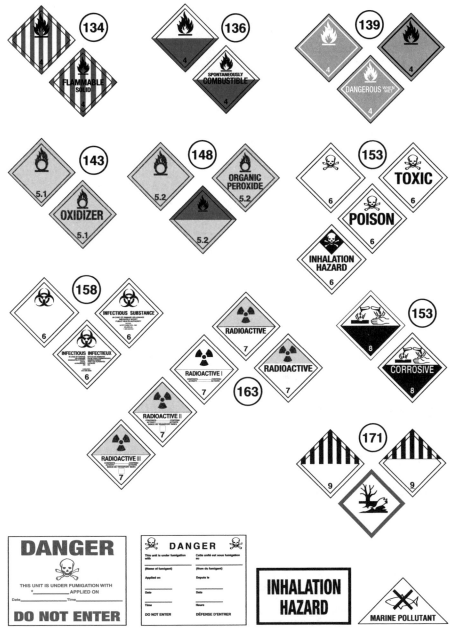

RAIL CAR IDENTIFICATION CHART*

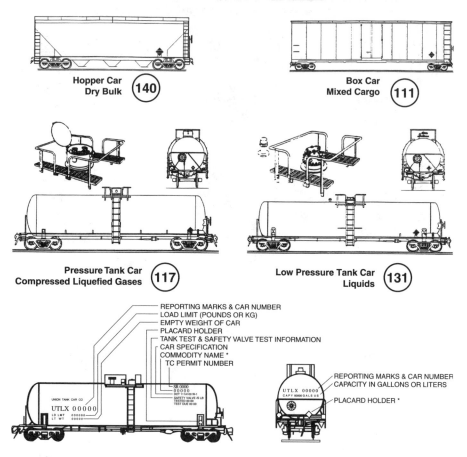

CAUTION: Emergency response personnel must be aware that rail tank cars vary widely in construction, fittings and purpose. Tank cars could transport products that may be solids, liquids or gases. The products may be under pressure. It is essential that products be identified by consulting shipping documents or train consist or contacting dispatch centers before emergency response is initiated.

The information stenciled on the sides or ends of tank cars, as illustrated above, may be used to identify the product utilizing:

a.   the commodity name shown; or

b.   the other information shown, especially reporting marks and car number which, when supplied to a dispatch center, will facilitate the identification of the product.

*   **The recommended guides should be considered as last resort if the material cannot be identified by any other means**.

ROAD TRAILER IDENTIFICATION CHART*

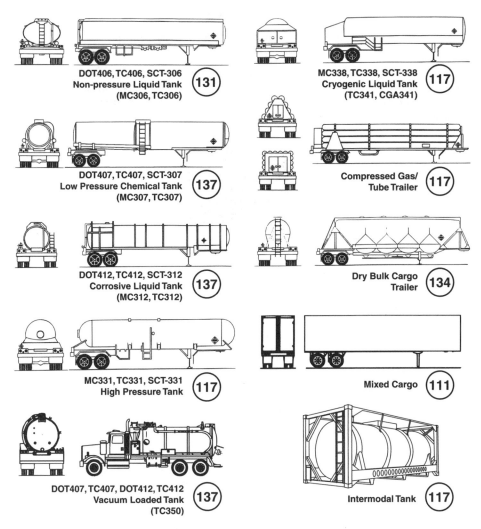

DOT406, TC406, SCT-306
Non-pressure Liquid Tank (131)
(MC306, TC306)

DOT407, TC407, SCT-307
Low Pressure Chemical Tank (137)
(MC307, TC307)

DOT412, TC412, SCT-312
Corrosive Liquid Tank (137)
(MC312, TC312)

MC331, TC331, SCT-331
High Pressure Tank (117)

DOT407, TC407, DOT412, TC412
Vacuum Loaded Tank (137)
(TC350)

MC338, TC338, SCT-338
Cryogenic Liquid Tank (117)
(TC341, CGA341)

Compressed Gas/
Tube Trailer (117)

Dry Bulk Cargo
Trailer (134)

Mixed Cargo (111)

Intermodal Tank (117)

CAUTION: This chart depicts only the most general shapes of road trailers. Emergency response personnel must be aware that there are many variations of road trailers, not illustrated above, that are used for shipping chemical products. The suggested guides are for the most hazardous products that may be transported in these trailer types.

* **The recommended guides should be considered as last resort if the material cannot be identified by any other means.**

HAZARD IDENTIFICATION CODES
DISPLAYED ON SOME INTERMODAL CONTAINERS

Hazard identification codes, referred to as "hazard identification numbers" (also referred to as the Kemler Code) under European and some South American regulations, may be found in the top half of an orange panel on some intermodal bulk containers. The 4-digit identification number is in the bottom half of the orange panel.

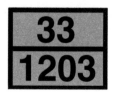

The hazard identification code in the top half of the orange panel consists of two or three digits. In general, the digits indicate the following hazards:

2 - EMISSION OF GAS DUE TO PRESSURE OR CHEMICAL REACTION

3 - FLAMMABILITY OF LIQUIDS (VAPORS) AND GASES OR SELF-HEATING LIQUID

4 - FLAMMABILITY OF SOLIDS OR SELF-HEATING SOLID

5 - OXIDIZING (FIRE-INTENSIFYING) EFFECT

6 - TOXICITY OR RISK OF INFECTION

7 - RADIOACTIVITY

8 - CORROSIVITY

9 - MISCELLANEOUS DANGEROUS SUBSTANCE

- Doubling of a digit indicates an intensification of that particular hazard (i.e. 33, 66, 88).

- Where the hazard associated with a material can be adequately indicated by a single digit, the digit is followed by a zero (i.e. 30, 40, 50).

- A hazard identification code prefixed by the letter "X" indicates that the material will react dangerously with water (i.e. X88).

- When 9 appears as a 2nd or 3rd digit, this may present a risk of spontaneous violent reaction.

HAZARD IDENTIFICATION CODES
DISPLAYED ON SOME INTERMODAL CONTAINERS

The hazard identification codes listed below have the following meanings:

20	Asphyxiant gas
22	Refrigerated liquefied gas, asphyxiant
223	Refrigerated liquefied gas, flammable
225	Refrigerated liquefied gas, oxidizing (fire-intensifying)
23	Flammable gas
236	Flammable gas, toxic
239	Flammable gas which can spontaneously lead to violent reaction
25	Oxidizing (fire-intensifying) gas
26	Toxic gas
263	Toxic gas, flammable
265	Toxic gas, oxidizing (fire-intensifying)
266	Highly toxic gas
268	Toxic gas, corrosive
30	Flammable liquid
323	Flammable liquid which reacts with water, emitting flammable gas
X323	Flammable liquid which reacts dangerously with water, emitting flammable gas
33	Highly flammable liquid
333	Pyrophoric liquid
X333	Pyrophoric liquid which reacts dangerously with water
336	Highly flammable liquid, toxic
338	Highly flammable liquid, corrosive
X338	Highly flammable liquid, corrosive, which reacts dangerously with water
339	Highly flammable liquid which can spontaneously lead to violent reaction
36	Flammable liquid, toxic, or self-heating liquid, toxic
362	Flammable liquid, toxic, which reacts with water, emitting flammable gas
X362	Flammable liquid, toxic, which reacts dangerously with water, emitting flammable gas
368	Flammable liquid, toxic, corrosive
38	Flammable liquid, corrosive or self-heating liquid, corrosive
382	Flammable liquid, corrosive, which reacts with water, emitting flammable gas
X382	Flammable liquid, corrosive, which reacts dangerously with water, emitting flammable gas
39	Flammable liquid which can spontaneously lead to violent reaction
40	Flammable solid, or self-reactive material, or self-heating material
423	Solid which reacts with water, emitting flammable gas

HAZARD IDENTIFICATION CODES
DISPLAYED ON SOME INTERMODAL CONTAINERS

X423	Flammable solid which reacts dangerously with water, emitting flammable gas
43	Spontaneously flammable (pyrophoric) solid
44	Flammable solid, in the molten state at an elevated temperature
446	Flammable solid, toxic, in the molten state at an elevated temperature
46	Flammable solid, toxic, or self-heating solid, toxic
462	Toxic solid which reacts with water, emitting flammable gas
X462	Solid which reacts dangerously with water, emitting toxic gas
48	Flammable or self-heating solid, corrosive
482	Corrosive solid which reacts with water, emitting flammable gas
X482	Solid which reacts dangerously with water, emitting corrosive gas

50	Oxidizing (fire-intensifying) substance
539	Flammable organic peroxide
55	Strongly oxidizing (fire-intensifying) substance
556	Strongly oxidizing (fire-intensifying) substance, toxic
558	Strongly oxidizing (fire-intensifying) substance, corrosive
559	Strongly oxidizing (fire-intensifying) substance which can spontaneously lead to violent reaction
56	Oxidizing (fire-intensifying) substance, toxic
568	Oxidizing (fire-intensifying) substance, toxic, corrosive
58	Oxidizing (fire-intensifying) substance, corrosive
59	Oxidizing (fire intensifying) substance which can spontaneously lead to violent reaction

60	Toxic material
606	Infectious substance
623	Toxic liquid which reacts with water, emitting flammable gas
63	Toxic liquid, flammable
638	Toxic liquid, flammable, corrosive
639	Toxic liquid, flammable, which can spontaneously lead to violent reaction
64	Toxic solid, flammable or self-heating
642	Toxic solid which reacts with water, emitting flammable gas
65	Toxic material, oxidizing (fire-intensifying)
66	Highly toxic material
663	Highly toxic liquid, flammable
664	Highly toxic solid, flammable or self-heating
665	Highly toxic material, oxidizing (fire-intensifying)
668	Highly toxic material, corrosive

HAZARD IDENTIFICATION CODES
DISPLAYED ON SOME INTERMODAL CONTAINERS

669	Highly toxic material which can spontaneously lead to violent reaction
68	Toxic material, corrosive
69	Toxic material which can spontaneously lead to violent reaction

70	Radioactive material
72	Radioactive gas
723	Radioactive gas, flammable
73	Radioactive liquid, flammable
74	Radioactive solid, flammable
75	Radioactive material, oxidizing (fire-intensifying)
76	Radioactive material, toxic
78	Radioactive material, corrosive

80	Corrosive material
X80	Corrosive material which reacts dangerously with water
823	Corrosive liquid which reacts with water, emitting flammable gas
83	Corrosive liquid, flammable
X83	Corrosive liquid, flammable, which reacts dangerously with water
839	Corrosive liquid, flammable, which can spontaneously lead to violent reaction
X839	Corrosive liquid, flammable, which can spontaneously lead to violent reaction and which reacts dangerously with water
84	Corrosive solid, flammable or self-heating
842	Corrosive solid which reacts with water, emitting flammable gas
85	Corrosive material, oxidizing (fire-intensifying)
856	Corrosive material, oxidizing (fire-intensifying) and toxic
86	Corrosive material, toxic
88	Highly corrosive material
X88	Highly corrosive material which reacts dangerously with water
883	Highly corrosive liquid, flammable
884	Highly corrosive solid, flammable or self-heating
885	Highly corrosive material, oxidizing (fire-intensifying)
886	Highly corrosive material, toxic
X886	Highly corrosive material, toxic, which reacts dangerously with water
89	Corrosive material which can spontaneously lead to violent reaction

90	Miscellaneous dangerous substance; environmentally hazardous substance
99	Miscellaneous dangerous substance transported at elevated temperature

PIPELINE TRANSPORTATION

Hazardous materials are transported in North America through millions of miles of underground pipelines. Products commonly transported through these pipeline systems include natural gas, crude oil, gasoline, diesel fuel, and jet fuel. Although the pipelines are buried, there are aboveground structures and signs indicating the presence of underground pipelines.

Liquid Pipelines

Surface indications of a liquid pipeline leak can include:

- Liquids bubbling from the ground
- "Oil slick" on flowing or standing water
- Flames that appear to be coming from the ground
- Vapor clouds

Structures – Storage Tanks, Valves, Pump Stations, Aerial Patrol Markers

Signs – Will often appear at road, railroad, and water crossings. Signs may also be posted at property boundaries. The signs will include the operator's name, product transported, and an emergency phone number for the operator. Warning, Caution, or Danger will appear on the signs.

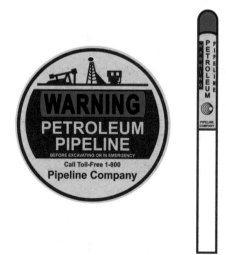

Gas Pipelines

Surface indications of a gas pipeline leak can include:
- Hissing, roaring, or blowing sound
- Dirt or water being blown in the air
- Continuous bubbling in wet or flooded areas
- Flames that appear to be coming from the ground
- Dead or brown vegetation in an otherwise green field
- In winter, melted snow over the pipeline

Gas **Transmission** pipelines are large-diameter, steel lines transporting flammable, toxic, or corrosive gas at very high pressure.

Structures – Compressor Station Buildings, Valves, Metering Stations, and Aerial Patrol Markers

Signs – Will often appear at road, railroad, and water crossings. Signs may also be posted at property boundaries. The signs will include the operator's name, product transported, and an emergency phone number for the operator. Warning, Caution, or Danger will appear on the signs.

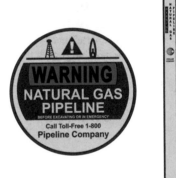

Natural gas **Distribution** pipelines are typically smaller-diameter, lower-pressure pipelines and may be steel, plastic, or cast iron. Natural gas is delivered directly to customers through distribution pipelines.

Regulator stations, customer meters & regulators, and valve box covers are generally the only aboveground indications of gas distribution pipelines.

Should you notice a leak or a spill, remember to only approach from upwind and uphill, identify the emergency telephone number for the company and then call that number as well as 911. Be cautious concerning the risks of asphyxiation, flammability as well as the danger of a potential explosion.

If you know the material involved, identify the three-digit guide number by looking up the name in the alphabetical list (blue-bordered pages) and then by using the three-digit guide number, consult the recommendations outlined in the recommended guide.

Note: If an entry is highlighted in green in either the yellow-bordered or blue-bordered pages AND THERE IS NO FIRE, go directly to Table 1 - Initial Isolation and Protective Action Distances (green bordered pages) and look up the ID number and name of material to obtain initial isolation and protective action distances. IF THERE IS A FIRE, or IF A FIRE IS INVOLVED, ALSO CONSULT the assigned guide (orange-bordered pages) and apply as appropriate the evacuation information shown under PUBLIC SAFETY. Please remember that, if the name in Table 1 is shown with (when spilled in water), and the material has not been spilled in water, Table 1 does not apply and safety distances can be found within the appropriate guide.

ID No.	Guide No.	Name of Material
——	112	Ammonium nitrate-fuel oil mixtures
——	158	Biological agents
——	112	Blasting agent, n.o.s.
——	112	Explosive A
——	112	Explosive B
——	114	Explosive C
——	112	Explosives, division 1.1, 1.2, 1.3, 1.5 or 1.6
——	114	Explosives, division 1.4
——	153	Toxins
1001	116	Acetylene
1001	116	Acetylene, dissolved
1002	122	Air, compressed
1003	122	Air, refrigerated liquid (cryogenic liquid)
1003	122	Air, refrigerated liquid (cryogenic liquid), non-pressurized
1005	125	Ammonia, anhydrous
1005	125	Anhydrous ammonia
1006	121	Argon
1006	121	Argon, compressed
1008	125	Boron trifluoride
1008	125	Boron trifluoride, compressed
1009	126	Bromotrifluoromethane
1009	126	Refrigerant gas R-13B1
1010	116P	Butadienes, stabilized
1010	116P	Butadienes and hydrocarbon mixture, stabilized
1011	115	Butane
1011	115	Butane mixture
1012	115	Butylene
1013	120	Carbon dioxide
1013	120	Carbon dioxide, compressed
1014	122	Carbon dioxide and Oxygen mixture
1014	122	Carbon dioxide and Oxygen mixture, compressed
1014	122	Oxygen and Carbon dioxide mixture
1014	122	Oxygen and Carbon dioxide mixture, compressed
1015	126	Carbon dioxide and Nitrous oxide mixture
1015	126	Nitrous oxide and Carbon dioxide mixture
1016	119	Carbon monoxide
1016	119	Carbon monoxide, compressed
1017	124	Chlorine
1018	126	Chlorodifluoromethane
1018	126	Refrigerant gas R-22
1020	126	Chloropentafluoroethane
1020	126	Refrigerant gas R-115
1021	126	1-Chloro-1,2,2,2-tetrafluoroethane
1021	126	Chlorotetrafluoroethane
1021	126	Refrigerant gas R-124
1022	126	Chlorotrifluoromethane
1022	126	Refrigerant gas R-13
1023	119	Coal gas
1023	119	Coal gas, compressed
1026	119	Cyanogen
1026	119	Cyanogen gas
1027	115	Cyclopropane
1028	126	Dichlorodifluoromethane
1028	126	Refrigerant gas R-12
1029	126	Dichlorofluoromethane
1029	126	Refrigerant gas R-21

ID No.	Guide No.	Name of Material	ID No.	Guide No.	Name of Material
1030	115	1,1-Difluoroethane	1046	121	Helium
1030	115	Difluoroethane	1046	121	Helium, compressed
1030	115	Refrigerant gas R-152a	1048	125	Hydrogen bromide, anhydrous
1032	118	Dimethylamine, anhydrous	1049	115	Hydrogen
1033	115	Dimethyl ether	1049	115	Hydrogen, compressed
1035	115	Ethane	1050	125	Hydrogen chloride, anhydrous
1035	115	Ethane, compressed	1051	117	AC
1036	118	Ethylamine	1051	117	Hydrocyanic acid, aqueous solutions, with more than 20% Hydrogen cyanide
1037	115	Ethyl chloride			
1038	115	Ethylene, refrigerated liquid (cryogenic liquid)	1051	117	Hydrogen cyanide, anhydrous, stabilized
1039	115	Ethyl methyl ether	1051	117	Hydrogen cyanide, stabilized
1039	115	Methyl ethyl ether	1052	125	Hydrogen fluoride, anhydrous
1040	119P	Ethylene oxide	1053	117	Hydrogen sulfide
1040	119P	Ethylene oxide with Nitrogen	1053	117	Hydrogen sulphide
1041	115	Carbon dioxide and Ethylene oxide mixture, with more than 9% but not more than 87% Ethylene oxide	1055	115	Isobutylene
			1056	121	Krypton
			1056	121	Krypton, compressed
1041	115	Carbon dioxide and Ethylene oxide mixtures, with more than 6% Ethylene oxide	1057	115	Lighter refills (cigarettes) (flammable gas)
			1057	115	Lighters (cigarettes) (flammable gas)
1041	115	Ethylene oxide and Carbon dioxide mixture, with more than 9% but not more than 87% Ethylene oxide	1058	120	Liquefied gases, non-flammable, charged with Nitrogen, Carbon dioxide or Air
1041	115	Ethylene oxide and Carbon dioxide mixtures, with more than 6 % Ethylene oxide	1060	116P	Methylacetylene and Propadiene mixture, stabilized
1043	125	Fertilizer, ammoniating solution, with free Ammonia	1060	116P	Propadiene and Methylacetylene mixture, stabilized
1044	126	Fire extinguishers with compressed gas	1061	118	Methylamine, anhydrous
1044	126	Fire extinguishers with liquefied gas	1062	123	Methyl bromide
1045	124	Fluorine	1063	115	Methyl chloride
1045	124	Fluorine, compressed			

ID No.	Guide No.	Name of Material	ID No.	Guide No.	Name of Material
1063	115	Refrigerant gas R-40	1077	115	Propylene
1064	117	Methyl mercaptan	1078	126	Dispersant gas, n.o.s.
1065	121	Neon	1078	126	Refrigerant gas, n.o.s.
1065	121	Neon, compressed	1079	125	Sulfur dioxide
1066	121	Nitrogen	1079	125	Sulphur dioxide
1066	121	Nitrogen, compressed	1080	126	Sulfur hexafluoride
1067	124	Dinitrogen tetroxide	1080	126	Sulphur hexafluoride
1067	124	Nitrogen dioxide	1081	116P	Tetrafluoroethylene, stabilized
1069	125	Nitrosyl chloride	1082	119P	Trifluorochloroethylene, stabilized
1070	122	Nitrous oxide			
1070	122	Nitrous oxide, compressed	1083	118	Trimethylamine, anhydrous
1071	119	Oil gas	1085	116P	Vinyl bromide, stabilized
1071	119	Oil gas, compressed	1086	116P	Vinyl chloride, stabilized
1072	122	Oxygen	1087	116P	Vinyl methyl ether, stabilized
1072	122	Oxygen, compressed	1088	127	Acetal
1073	122	Oxygen, refrigerated liquid (cryogenic liquid)	1089	129	Acetaldehyde
			1090	127	Acetone
1075	115	Butane	1091	127	Acetone oils
1075	115	Butane mixture	1092	131P	Acrolein, stabilized
1075	115	Butylene	1093	131P	Acrylonitrile, stabilized
1075	115	Isobutane	1098	131	Allyl alcohol
1075	115	Isobutane mixture	1099	131	Allyl bromide
1075	115	Isobutylene	1100	131	Allyl chloride
1075	115	Liquefied petroleum gas	1104	129	Amyl acetates
1075	115	LPG	1105	129	Amyl alcohols
1075	115	Petroleum gases, liquefied	1105	129	Pentanols
1075	115	Propane	1106	132	Amylamines
1075	115	Propane mixture	1107	129	Amyl chloride
1075	115	Propylene	1108	128	n-Amylene
1076	125	CG	1108	128	1-Pentene
1076	125	Diphosgene	1109	129	Amyl formates
1076	125	DP	1110	127	n-Amyl methyl ketone
1076	125	Phosgene	1110	127	Amyl methyl ketone

ID No.	Guide No.	Name of Material	ID No.	Guide No.	Name of Material
1110	127	Methyl amyl ketone	1150	130P	1,2-Dichloroethylene
1111	130	Amyl mercaptan	1150	130P	Dichloroethylene
1112	140	Amyl nitrate	1152	130	Dichloropentanes
1113	129	Amyl nitrite	1153	127	Ethylene glycol diethyl ether
1114	130	Benzene	1154	132	Diethylamine
1120	129	Butanols	1155	127	Diethyl ether
1123	129	Butyl acetates	1155	127	Ethyl ether
1125	132	n-Butylamine	1156	127	Diethyl ketone
1126	130	1-Bromobutane	1157	128	Diisobutyl ketone
1126	130	n-Butyl bromide	1158	132	Diisopropylamine
1127	130	Butyl chloride	1159	127	Diisopropyl ether
1127	130	Chlorobutanes	1160	132	Dimethylamine, aqueous solution
1128	129	n-Butyl formate	1160	132	Dimethylamine, solution
1129	129	Butyraldehyde	1161	129	Dimethyl carbonate
1130	128	Camphor oil	1162	155	Dimethyldichlorosilane
1131	131	Carbon bisulfide	1163	131	1,1-Dimethylhydrazine
1131	131	Carbon bisulphide	1163	131	Dimethylhydrazine, unsymmetrical
1131	131	Carbon disulfide	1164	130	Dimethyl sulfide
1131	131	Carbon disulphide	1164	130	Dimethyl sulphide
1133	128	Adhesives (flammable)	1165	127	Dioxane
1134	130	Chlorobenzene	1166	127	Dioxolane
1135	131	Ethylene chlorohydrin	1167	128P	Divinyl ether, stabilized
1136	128	Coal tar distillates, flammable	1169	127	Extracts, aromatic, liquid
1139	127	Coating solution	1170	127	Ethanol
1143	131P	Crotonaldehyde	1170	127	Ethanol, solution
1143	131P	Crotonaldehyde, stabilized	1170	127	Ethyl alcohol
1144	128	Crotonylene	1170	127	Ethyl alcohol, solution
1145	128	Cyclohexane	1171	127	Ethylene glycol monoethyl ether
1146	128	Cyclopentane	1172	129	Ethylene glycol monoethyl ether acetate
1147	130	Decahydronaphthalene	1173	129	Ethyl acetate
1148	129	Diacetone alcohol	1175	130	Ethylbenzene
1149	128	Butyl ethers			
1149	128	Dibutyl ethers			

ID No.	Guide No.	Name of Material	ID No.	Guide No.	Name of Material
1176	129	Ethyl borate	1202	128	Diesel fuel
1177	130	2-Ethylbutyl acetate	1202	128	Fuel oil
1177	130	Ethylbutyl acetate	1202	128	Fuel oil, no. 1,2,4,5,6
1178	130	2-Ethylbutyraldehyde	1202	128	Gas oil
1179	127	Ethyl butyl ether	1202	128	Heating oil, light
1180	130	Ethyl butyrate	1203	128	Gasohol
1181	155	Ethyl chloroacetate	1203	128	Gasoline
1182	155	Ethyl chloroformate	1203	128	Motor spirit
1183	139	Ethyldichlorosilane	1203	128	Petrol
1184	131	Ethylene dichloride	1204	127	Nitroglycerin, solution in alcohol, with not more than 1% Nitroglycerin
1185	131P	Ethyleneimine, stabilized			
1188	127	Ethylene glycol monomethyl ether	1206	128	Heptanes
1189	129	Ethylene glycol monomethyl ether acetate	1207	130	Hexaldehyde
			1208	128	Hexanes
1190	129	Ethyl formate	1208	128	Neohexane
1191	129	Ethylhexaldehydes	1210	129	Ink, printer's, flammable
1191	129	Octyl aldehydes	1210	129	Printing ink, flammable
1192	129	Ethyl lactate	1210	129	Printing ink related material
1193	127	Ethyl methyl ketone	1212	129	Isobutanol
1193	127	Methyl ethyl ketone	1212	129	Isobutyl alcohol
1194	131	Ethyl nitrite, solution	1213	129	Isobutyl acetate
1195	129	Ethyl propionate	1214	132	Isobutylamine
1196	155	Ethyltrichlorosilane	1216	128	Isooctenes
1197	127	Extracts, flavoring, liquid	1218	130P	Isoprene, stabilized
1197	127	Extracts, flavouring, liquid	1219	129	Isopropanol
1198	132	Formaldehyde, solution, flammable	1219	129	Isopropyl alcohol
			1220	129	Isopropyl acetate
1198	132	Formaldehyde, solutions (Formalin)	1221	132	Isopropylamine
			1222	130	Isopropyl nitrate
1199	132P	Furaldehydes	1223	128	Kerosene
1199	132P	Furfural	1224	127	Ketones, liquid, n.o.s.
1199	132P	Furfuraldehydes			
1201	127	Fusel oil			

ID No.	Guide No.	Name of Material	ID No.	Guide No.	Name of Material
1226	128	Lighters for cigars, cigarettes (flammable liquid)	1262	128	Isooctane
			1262	128	Octanes
1228	131	Mercaptan mixture, liquid, flammable, poisonous, n.o.s.	1263	128	Paint (flammable)
			1263	128	Paint related material (flammable)
1228	131	Mercaptan mixture, liquid, flammable, toxic, n.o.s.	1264	129	Paraldehyde
1228	131	Mercaptans, liquid, flammable, poisonous, n.o.s.	1265	128	Isopentane
			1265	128	n-Pentane
1228	131	Mercaptans, liquid, flammable, toxic, n.o.s.	1265	128	Pentanes
1229	129	Mesityl oxide	1266	127	Perfumery products, with flammable solvents
1230	131	Methanol	1267	128	Petroleum crude oil
1230	131	Methyl alcohol	1268	128	Petroleum distillates, n.o.s.
1231	129	Methyl acetate	1268	128	Petroleum products, n.o.s.
1233	130	Methylamyl acetate	1270	128	Oil, petroleum
1234	127	Methylal	1270	128	Petroleum oil
1235	132	Methylamine, aqueous solution	1272	129	Pine oil
1237	129	Methyl butyrate	1274	129	n-Propanol
1238	155	Methyl chloroformate	1274	129	normal Propyl alcohol
1239	131	Methyl chloromethyl ether	1274	129	Propyl alcohol, normal
1242	139	Methyldichlorosilane	1275	129	Propionaldehyde
1243	129	Methyl formate	1276	129	n-Propyl acetate
1244	131	Methylhydrazine	1277	132	Monopropylamine
1245	127	Methyl isobutyl ketone	1277	132	Propylamine
1246	127P	Methyl isopropenyl ketone, stabilized	1278	129	1-Chloropropane
			1278	129	Propyl chloride
1247	129P	Methyl methacrylate monomer, stabilized	1279	130	1,2-Dichloropropane
			1279	130	Dichloropropane
1248	129	Methyl propionate	1279	130	Propylene dichloride
1249	127	Methyl propyl ketone	1280	127P	Propylene oxide
1250	155	Methyltrichlorosilane	1281	129	Propyl formates
1251	131P	Methyl vinyl ketone, stabilized	1282	129	Pyridine
1259	131	Nickel carbonyl	1286	127	Rosin oil
1261	129	Nitromethane			

ID No.	Guide No.	Name of Material	ID No.	Guide No.	Name of Material
1287	127	Rubber solution	1314	133	Calcium resinate, fused
1288	128	Shale oil	1318	133	Cobalt resinate, precipitated
1289	132	Sodium methylate, solution in alcohol	1320	113	Dinitrophenol, wetted with not less than 15% water
1292	129	Ethyl silicate	1321	113	Dinitrophenolates, wetted with not less than 15% water
1292	129	Tetraethyl silicate	1322	113	Dinitroresorcinol, wetted with not less than 15% water
1293	127	Tinctures, medicinal			
1294	130	Toluene	1323	170	Ferrocerium
1295	139	Trichlorosilane	1324	133	Films, nitrocellulose base
1296	132	Triethylamine	1325	133	Flammable solid, n.o.s.
1297	132	Trimethylamine, aqueous solution	1325	133	Flammable solid, organic, n.o.s.
			1325	133	Fusee (rail or highway)
1298	155	Trimethylchlorosilane	1325	133	Medicines, flammable, solid, n.o.s.
1299	128	Turpentine			
1300	128	Turpentine substitute	1326	170	Hafnium powder, wetted with not less than 25% water
1301	129P	Vinyl acetate, stabilized			
1302	127P	Vinyl ethyl ether, stabilized	1327	133	Bhusa, wet, damp or contaminated with oil
1303	130P	Vinylidene chloride, stabilized	1327	133	Hay, wet, damp or contaminated with oil
1304	127P	Vinyl isobutyl ether, stabilized	1327	133	Straw, wet, damp or contaminated with oil
1305	155P	Vinyltrichlorosilane			
1305	155P	Vinyltrichlorosilane, stabilized	1328	133	Hexamethylenetetramine
1306	129	Wood preservatives, liquid	1328	133	Hexamine
1307	130	Xylenes	1330	133	Manganese resinate
1308	170	Zirconium metal, liquid suspension	1331	133	Matches, "strike anywhere"
			1332	133	Metaldehyde
1308	170	Zirconium suspended in a flammable liquid	1333	170	Cerium, slabs, ingots or rods
			1334	133	Naphthalene, crude
1308	170	Zirconium suspended in a liquid (flammable)	1334	133	Naphthalene, refined
1309	170	Aluminum powder, coated	1336	113	Nitroguanidine (Picrite), wetted with not less than 20% water
1310	113	Ammonium picrate, wetted with not less than 10% water	1336	113	Nitroguanidine, wetted with not less than 20% water
1312	133	Borneol			
1313	133	Calcium resinate			

ID No.	Guide No.	Name of Material	ID No.	Guide No.	Name of Material
1336	113	Picrite, wetted	1345	133	Rubber scrap, powdered or granulated
1337	113	Nitrostarch, wetted with not less than 20% water	1345	133	Rubber shoddy, powdered or granulated
1337	113	Nitrostarch, wetted with not less than 30% solvent	1346	170	Silicon powder, amorphous
1338	133	Phosphorus, amorphous	1347	113	Silver picrate, wetted with not less than 30% water
1338	133	Phosphorus, amorphous, red	1348	113	Sodium dinitro-o-cresolate, wetted with not less than 15% water
1338	133	Red phosphorus			
1338	133	Red phosphorus, amorphous	1348	113	Sodium dinitro-ortho-cresolate, wetted
1339	139	Phosphorus heptasulfide, free from yellow and white Phosphorus	1349	113	Sodium picramate, wetted with not less than 20% water
1339	139	Phosphorus heptasulphide, free from yellow and white Phosphorus	1350	133	Sulfur
			1350	133	Sulphur
1340	139	Phosphorus pentasulfide, free from yellow and white Phosphorus	1352	170	Titanium powder, wetted with not less than 25% water
1340	139	Phosphorus pentasulphide, free from yellow and white Phosphorus	1353	133	Fabrics impregnated with weakly nitrated Nitrocellulose, n.o.s.
1341	139	Phosphorus sesquisulfide, free from yellow and white Phosphorus	1353	133	Fibers impregnated with weakly nitrated Nitrocellulose, n.o.s.
1341	139	Phosphorus sesquisulphide, free from yellow and white Phosphorus	1353	133	Fibres impregnated with weakly nitrated Nitrocellulose, n.o.s.
			1353	133	Toe puffs, nitrocellulose base
1343	139	Phosphorus trisulfide, free from yellow and white Phosphorus	1354	113	Trinitrobenzene, wetted with not less than 30% water
1343	139	Phosphorus trisulphide, free from yellow and white Phosphorus	1355	113	Trinitrobenzoic acid, wetted with not less than 30% water
1344	113	Picric acid, wet, with not less than 10% water	1356	113	TNT, wetted with not less than 30% water
1344	113	Picric acid, wetted with not less than 30% water	1356	113	Trinitrotoluene, wetted with not less than 30% water
1344	113	Trinitrophenol, wetted with not less than 30% water	1357	113	Urea nitrate, wetted with not less than 20% water
			1358	170	Zirconium metal, powder, wet

ID No.	Guide No.	Name of Material
1358	170	Zirconium powder, wetted with not less than 25% water
1360	139	Calcium phosphide
1361	133	Carbon, animal or vegetable origin
1361	133	Charcoal
1362	133	Carbon, activated
1363	135	Copra
1364	133	Cotton waste, oily
1365	133	Cotton
1365	133	Cotton, wet
1366	135	Diethylzinc
1369	135	p-Nitrosodimethylaniline
1370	135	Dimethylzinc
1372	133	Fiber, animal or vegetable, n.o.s., burnt, wet or damp
1372	133	Fibers, animal or vegetable, burnt, wet or damp
1372	133	Fibres, animal or vegetable, burnt, wet or damp
1373	133	Fabrics, animal or vegetable or synthetic, n.o.s. with oil
1373	133	Fibers, animal or vegetable or synthetic, n.o.s. with oil
1373	133	Fibres, animal or vegetable or synthetic, n.o.s. with oil
1374	133	Fish meal, unstabilized
1374	133	Fish scrap, unstabilized
1376	135	Iron oxide, spent
1376	135	Iron sponge, spent
1378	170	Metal catalyst, wetted
1379	133	Paper, unsaturated oil treated
1380	135	Pentaborane
1381	136	Phosphorus, white, dry or under water or in solution
1381	136	Phosphorus, yellow, dry or under water or in solution
1381	136	White phosphorus, dry
1381	136	White phosphorus, in solution
1381	136	White phosphorus, under water
1381	136	Yellow phosphorus, dry
1381	136	Yellow phosphorus, in solution
1381	136	Yellow phosphorus, under water
1382	135	Potassium sulfide, anhydrous
1382	135	Potassium sulfide, with less than 30% water of crystallization
1382	135	Potassium sulfide, with less than 30% water of hydration
1382	135	Potassium sulphide, anhydrous
1382	135	Potassium sulphide, with less than 30% water of crystallization
1382	135	Potassium sulphide, with less than 30% water of hydration
1383	135	Aluminum powder, pyrophoric
1383	135	Pyrophoric alloy, n.o.s.
1383	135	Pyrophoric metal, n.o.s.
1384	135	Sodium dithionite
1384	135	Sodium hydrosulfite
1384	135	Sodium hydrosulphite
1385	135	Sodium sulfide, anhydrous
1385	135	Sodium sulfide, with less than 30% water of crystallization
1385	135	Sodium sulphide, anhydrous
1385	135	Sodium sulphide, with less than 30% water of crystallization
1386	135	Seed cake, with more than 1.5% oil and not more than 11% moisture
1387	133	Wool waste, wet

ID No.	Guide No.	Name of Material	ID No.	Guide No.	Name of Material
1389	**138**	Alkali metal amalgam	1412	**139**	Lithium amide
1389	**138**	Alkali metal amalgam, liquid	1413	**138**	Lithium borohydride
1389	**138**	Alkali metal amalgam, solid	1414	**138**	Lithium hydride
1390	**139**	Alkali metal amides	1415	**138**	Lithium
1391	**138**	Alkali metal dispersion	1417	**138**	Lithium silicon
1391	**138**	Alkaline earth metal dispersion	1418	**138**	Magnesium alloys powder
1392	**138**	Alkaline earth metal amalgam	1418	**138**	Magnesium powder
1392	**138**	Alkaline earth metal amalgam, liquid	1419	**139**	Magnesium aluminum phosphide
1393	**138**	Alkaline earth metal alloy, n.o.s.	1420	**138**	Potassium, metal alloys
1394	**138**	Aluminum carbide	1420	**138**	Potassium, metal alloys, liquid
1395	**139**	Aluminum ferrosilicon powder	1421	**138**	Alkali metal alloy, liquid, n.o.s.
1396	**138**	Aluminum powder, uncoated	1422	**138**	Potassium sodium alloys
1397	**139**	Aluminum phosphide	1422	**138**	Potassium sodium alloys, liquid
1398	**138**	Aluminum silicon powder, uncoated	1422	**138**	Sodium potassium alloys
1400	**138**	Barium	1422	**138**	Sodium potassium alloys, liquid
1401	**138**	Calcium	1423	**138**	Rubidium
1402	**138**	Calcium carbide	1423	**138**	Rubidium metal
1403	**138**	Calcium cyanamide, with more than 0.1% Calcium carbide	1426	**138**	Sodium borohydride
1404	**138**	Calcium hydride	1427	**138**	Sodium hydride
1405	**138**	Calcium silicide	1428	**138**	Sodium
1406	**138**	Calcium silicon	1431	**138**	Sodium methylate
1407	**138**	Caesium	1431	**138**	Sodium methylate, dry
1407	**138**	Cesium	1432	**139**	Sodium phosphide
1408	**139**	Ferrosilicon	1433	**139**	Stannic phosphides
1409	**138**	Hydrides, metal, n.o.s.	1435	**138**	Zinc ashes
1409	**138**	Metal hydrides, water-reactive, n.o.s.	1435	**138**	Zinc dross
1410	**138**	Lithium aluminum hydride	1435	**138**	Zinc residue
1411	**138**	Lithium aluminum hydride, ethereal	1435	**138**	Zinc skimmings
			1436	**138**	Zinc dust
			1436	**138**	Zinc powder
			1437	**138**	Zirconium hydride
			1438	**140**	Aluminum nitrate
			1439	**141**	Ammonium dichromate

ID No.	Guide No.	Name of Material	ID No.	Guide No.	Name of Material
1442	143	Ammonium perchlorate	1466	140	Ferric nitrate
1444	140	Ammonium persulfate	1467	143	Guanidine nitrate
1444	140	Ammonium persulphate	1469	141	Lead nitrate
1445	141	Barium chlorate	1470	141	Lead perchlorate
1445	141	Barium chlorate, solid	1470	141	Lead perchlorate, solid
1446	141	Barium nitrate	1470	141	Lead perchlorate, solution
1447	141	Barium perchlorate	1471	140	Lithium hypochlorite, dry
1447	141	Barium perchlorate, solid	1471	140	Lithium hypochlorite mixture
1448	141	Barium permanganate	1471	140	Lithium hypochlorite mixtures, dry
1449	141	Barium peroxide			
1450	141	Bromates, inorganic, n.o.s.	1472	143	Lithium peroxide
1451	140	Caesium nitrate	1473	140	Magnesium bromate
1451	140	Cesium nitrate	1474	140	Magnesium nitrate
1452	140	Calcium chlorate	1475	140	Magnesium perchlorate
1453	140	Calcium chlorite	1476	140	Magnesium peroxide
1454	140	Calcium nitrate	1477	140	Nitrates, inorganic, n.o.s.
1455	140	Calcium perchlorate	1479	140	Oxidizing solid, n.o.s.
1456	140	Calcium permanganate	1481	140	Perchlorates, inorganic, n.o.s.
1457	140	Calcium peroxide	1482	140	Permanganates, inorganic, n.o.s.
1458	140	Borate and Chlorate mixtures			
1458	140	Chlorate and Borate mixtures	1483	140	Peroxides, inorganic, n.o.s.
1459	140	Chlorate and Magnesium chloride mixture	1484	140	Potassium bromate
			1485	140	Potassium chlorate
1459	140	Chlorate and Magnesium chloride mixture, solid	1486	140	Potassium nitrate
			1487	140	Potassium nitrate and Sodium nitrite mixture
1459	140	Magnesium chloride and Chlorate mixture	1487	140	Sodium nitrite and Potassium nitrate mixture
1459	140	Magnesium chloride and Chlorate mixture, solid	1488	140	Potassium nitrite
1461	140	Chlorates, inorganic, n.o.s.	1489	140	Potassium perchlorate
1462	143	Chlorites, inorganic, n.o.s.	1490	140	Potassium permanganate
1463	141	Chromic acid, solid	1491	144	Potassium peroxide
1463	141	Chromium trioxide, anhydrous	1492	140	Potassium persulfate
1465	140	Didymium nitrate	1492	140	Potassium persulphate

ID No.	Guide No.	Name of Material
1493	**140**	Silver nitrate
1494	**141**	Sodium bromate
1495	**140**	Sodium chlorate
1496	**143**	Sodium chlorite
1498	**140**	Sodium nitrate
1499	**140**	Potassium nitrate and Sodium nitrate mixture
1499	**140**	Sodium nitrate and Potassium nitrate mixture
1500	**140**	Sodium nitrite
1502	**140**	Sodium perchlorate
1503	**140**	Sodium permanganate
1504	**144**	Sodium peroxide
1505	**140**	Sodium persulfate
1505	**140**	Sodium persulphate
1506	**143**	Strontium chlorate
1506	**143**	Strontium chlorate, solid
1506	**143**	Strontium chlorate, solution
1507	**140**	Strontium nitrate
1508	**140**	Strontium perchlorate
1509	**143**	Strontium peroxide
1510	**143**	Tetranitromethane
1511	**140**	Urea hydrogen peroxide
1512	**140**	Zinc ammonium nitrite
1513	**140**	Zinc chlorate
1514	**140**	Zinc nitrate
1515	**140**	Zinc permanganate
1516	**143**	Zinc peroxide
1517	**113**	Zirconium picramate, wetted with not less than 20% water
1541	**155**	Acetone cyanohydrin, stabilized
1544	**151**	Alkaloids, solid, n.o.s. (poisonous)
1544	**151**	Alkaloid salts, solid, n.o.s. (poisonous)
1545	**155**	Allyl isothiocyanate, stabilized
1546	**151**	Ammonium arsenate
1547	**153**	Aniline
1548	**153**	Aniline hydrochloride
1549	**157**	Antimony compound, inorganic, n.o.s.
1549	**157**	Antimony compound, inorganic, solid, n.o.s.
1549	**157**	Antimony tribromide, solid
1549	**157**	Antimony tribromide, solution
1549	**157**	Antimony trifluoride, solid
1549	**157**	Antimony trifluoride, solution
1550	**151**	Antimony lactate
1551	**151**	Antimony potassium tartrate
1553	**154**	Arsenic acid, liquid
1554	**154**	Arsenic acid, solid
1555	**151**	Arsenic bromide
1556	**152**	Arsenic compound, liquid, n.o.s.
1556	**152**	Arsenic compound, liquid, n.o.s., inorganic
1556	**152**	MD
1556	**152**	Methyldichloroarsine
1556	**152**	PD
1557	**152**	Arsenic compound, solid, n.o.s.
1557	**152**	Arsenic compound, solid, n.o.s., inorganic
1557	**152**	Arsenic sulfide
1557	**152**	Arsenic sulphide
1557	**152**	Arsenic trisulfide
1557	**152**	Arsenic trisulphide
1558	**152**	Arsenic
1559	**151**	Arsenic pentoxide

ID No.	Guide No.	Name of Material
1560	157	Arsenic chloride
1560	157	Arsenic trichloride
1561	151	Arsenic trioxide
1562	152	Arsenical dust
1564	154	Barium compound, n.o.s.
1565	157	Barium cyanide
1566	154	Beryllium compound, n.o.s.
1567	134	Beryllium powder
1569	131	Bromoacetone
1570	152	Brucine
1571	113	Barium azide, wetted with not less than 50% water
1572	151	Cacodylic acid
1573	151	Calcium arsenate
1574	151	Calcium arsenate and Calcium arsenite mixture, solid
1574	151	Calcium arsenite, solid
1574	151	Calcium arsenite and Calcium arsenate mixture, solid
1575	157	Calcium cyanide
1577	153	Chlorodinitrobenzenes
1577	153	Chlorodinitrobenzenes, liquid
1577	153	Chlorodinitrobenzenes, solid
1577	153	Dinitrochlorobenzenes
1578	152	Chloronitrobenzenes
1578	152	Chloronitrobenzenes, liquid
1578	152	Chloronitrobenzenes, solid
1579	153	4-Chloro-o-toluidine hydrochloride
1579	153	4-Chloro-o-toluidine hydrochloride, solid
1580	154	Chloropicrin
1581	123	Chloropicrin and Methyl bromide mixture
1581	123	Methyl bromide and Chloropicrin mixture
1582	119	Chloropicrin and Methyl chloride mixture
1582	119	Methyl chloride and Chloropicrin mixture
1583	154	Chloropicrin mixture, n.o.s.
1585	151	Copper acetoarsenite
1586	151	Copper arsenite
1587	151	Copper cyanide
1588	157	Cyanides, inorganic, n.o.s.
1588	157	Cyanides, inorganic, solid, n.o.s.
1589	125	CK
1589	125	Cyanogen chloride, stabilized
1590	153	Dichloroanilines
1590	153	Dichloroanilines, liquid
1590	153	Dichloroanilines, solid
1591	152	o-Dichlorobenzene
1593	160	Dichloromethane
1593	160	Methylene chloride
1594	152	Diethyl sulfate
1594	152	Diethyl sulphate
1595	156	Dimethyl sulfate
1595	156	Dimethyl sulphate
1596	153	Dinitroanilines
1597	152	Dinitrobenzenes
1597	152	Dinitrobenzenes, liquid
1597	152	Dinitrobenzenes, solid
1598	153	Dinitro-o-cresol
1599	153	Dinitrophenol, solution
1600	152	Dinitrotoluenes, molten
1601	151	Disinfectant, solid, poisonous, n.o.s.
1601	151	Disinfectant, solid, toxic, n.o.s.

ID No.	Guide No.	Name of Material	ID No.	Guide No.	Name of Material
1601	151	Disinfectants, solid, n.o.s. (poisonous)	1622	151	Magnesium arsenate
1602	151	Dye, liquid, poisonous, n.o.s.	1623	151	Mercuric arsenate
1602	151	Dye, liquid, toxic, n.o.s.	1624	154	Mercuric chloride
1602	151	Dye intermediate, liquid, poisonous, n.o.s.	1625	141	Mercuric nitrate
1602	151	Dye intermediate, liquid, toxic, n.o.s.	1626	157	Mercuric potassium cyanide
1603	155	Ethyl bromoacetate	1627	141	Mercurous nitrate
1604	132	Ethylenediamine	1629	151	Mercury acetate
1605	154	Ethylene dibromide	1630	151	Mercury ammonium chloride
1606	151	Ferric arsenate	1631	154	Mercury benzoate
1607	151	Ferric arsenite	1634	154	Mercuric bromide
1608	151	Ferrous arsenate	1634	154	Mercurous bromide
1610	159	Halogenated irritating liquid, n.o.s.	1634	154	Mercury bromides
1611	151	Hexaethyl tetraphosphate	1636	154	Mercuric cyanide
1611	151	Hexaethyl tetraphosphate, liquid	1636	154	Mercury cyanide
1611	151	Hexaethyl tetraphosphate, solid	1637	151	Mercury gluconate
1612	123	Hexaethyl tetraphosphate and compressed gas mixture	1638	151	Mercury iodide
1613	154	Hydrocyanic acid, aqueous solution, with less than 5% Hydrogen cyanide	1639	151	Mercury nucleate
			1640	151	Mercury oleate
			1641	151	Mercury oxide
1613	154	Hydrocyanic acid, aqueous solution, with not more than 20% Hydrogen cyanide	1642	151	Mercuric oxycyanide
			1642	151	Mercury oxycyanide, desensitized
1613	154	Hydrogen cyanide, aqueous solution, with not more than 20% Hydrogen cyanide	1643	151	Mercury potassium iodide
			1644	151	Mercury salicylate
1614	152	Hydrogen cyanide, stabilized (absorbed)	1645	151	Mercuric sulfate
			1645	151	Mercuric sulphate
1616	151	Lead acetate	1645	151	Mercury sulfate
1617	151	Lead arsenates	1645	151	Mercury sulphate
1618	151	Lead arsenites	1646	151	Mercury thiocyanate
1620	151	Lead cyanide	1647	151	Ethylene dibromide and Methyl bromide mixture, liquid
1621	151	London purple	1647	151	Methyl bromide and Ethylene dibromide mixture, liquid
			1648	127	Acetonitrile

ID No.	Guide No.	Name of Material
1648	127	Methyl cyanide
1649	131	Motor fuel anti-knock mixture
1649	131	Tetraethyl lead, liquid
1650	153	beta-Naphthylamine
1650	153	beta-Naphthylamine, solid
1650	153	Naphthylamine (beta)
1650	153	Naphthylamine (beta), solid
1651	153	Naphthylthiourea
1652	153	Naphthylurea
1653	151	Nickel cyanide
1654	151	Nicotine
1655	151	Nicotine compound, solid, n.o.s.
1655	151	Nicotine preparation, solid, n.o.s.
1656	151	Nicotine hydrochloride
1656	151	Nicotine hydrochloride, liquid
1656	151	Nicotine hydrochloride, solid
1656	151	Nicotine hydrochloride, solution
1657	151	Nicotine salicylate
1658	151	Nicotine sulfate, solid
1658	151	Nicotine sulfate, solution
1658	151	Nicotine sulphate, solid
1658	151	Nicotine sulphate, solution
1659	151	Nicotine tartrate
1660	124	Nitric oxide
1660	124	Nitric oxide, compressed
1661	153	Nitroanilines
1662	152	Nitrobenzene
1663	153	Nitrophenols
1664	152	Nitrotoluenes
1664	152	Nitrotoluenes, liquid
1664	152	Nitrotoluenes, solid
1665	152	Nitroxylenes
1665	152	Nitroxylenes, liquid
1665	152	Nitroxylenes, solid
1669	151	Pentachloroethane
1670	157	Perchloromethyl mercaptan
1671	153	Phenol, solid
1672	151	Phenylcarbylamine chloride
1673	153	Phenylenediamines
1674	151	Phenylmercuric acetate
1677	151	Potassium arsenate
1678	154	Potassium arsenite
1679	157	Potassium cuprocyanide
1680	157	Potassium cyanide
1680	157	Potassium cyanide, solid
1683	151	Silver arsenite
1684	151	Silver cyanide
1685	151	Sodium arsenate
1686	154	Sodium arsenite, aqueous solution
1687	153	Sodium azide
1688	152	Sodium cacodylate
1689	157	Sodium cyanide
1689	157	Sodium cyanide, solid
1690	154	Sodium fluoride
1690	154	Sodium fluoride, solid
1691	151	Strontium arsenite
1692	151	Strychnine
1692	151	Strychnine salts
1693	159	Tear gas devices
1693	159	Tear gas substance, liquid, n.o.s.
1693	159	Tear gas substance, solid, n.o.s.
1694	159	Bromobenzyl cyanides
1694	159	Bromobenzyl cyanides, liquid
1694	159	Bromobenzyl cyanides, solid
1694	159	CA

ID No.	Guide No.	Name of Material
1695	**131**	Chloroacetone, stabilized
1697	**153**	Chloroacetophenone
1697	**153**	Chloroacetophenone, liquid
1697	**153**	Chloroacetophenone, solid
1697	**153**	CN
1698	**154**	Adamsite
1698	**154**	Diphenylamine chloroarsine
1698	**154**	DM
1699	**151**	DA
1699	**151**	Diphenylchloroarsine
1699	**151**	Diphenylchloroarsine, liquid
1699	**151**	Diphenylchloroarsine, solid
1700	**159**	Tear gas candles
1700	**159**	Tear gas grenades
1701	**152**	Xylyl bromide
1701	**152**	Xylyl bromide, liquid
1702	**151**	1,1,2,2-Tetrachloroethane
1702	**151**	Tetrachloroethane
1704	**153**	Tetraethyl dithiopyrophosphate
1704	**153**	Tetraethyl dithiopyrophosphate, mixture, dry or liquid
1707	**151**	Thallium compound, n.o.s.
1707	**151**	Thallium sulfate, solid
1707	**151**	Thallium sulphate, solid
1708	**153**	Toluidines
1708	**153**	Toluidines, liquid
1708	**153**	Toluidines, solid
1709	**151**	2,4-Toluenediamine
1709	**151**	2,4-Toluylenediamine
1709	**151**	2,4-Toluylenediamine, solid
1710	**160**	Trichloroethylene
1711	**153**	Xylidines
1711	**153**	Xylidines, liquid
1711	**153**	Xylidines, solid
1712	**151**	Zinc arsenate
1712	**151**	Zinc arsenate and Zinc arsenite mixture
1712	**151**	Zinc arsenite
1712	**151**	Zinc arsenite and Zinc arsenate mixture
1713	**151**	Zinc cyanide
1714	**139**	Zinc phosphide
1715	**137**	Acetic anhydride
1716	**156**	Acetyl bromide
1717	**155**	Acetyl chloride
1718	**153**	Acid butyl phosphate
1718	**153**	Butyl acid phosphate
1719	**154**	Caustic alkali liquid, n.o.s.
1722	**155**	Allyl chlorocarbonate
1722	**155**	Allyl chloroformate
1723	**132**	Allyl iodide
1724	**155**	Allyltrichlorosilane, stabilized
1725	**137**	Aluminum bromide, anhydrous
1726	**137**	Aluminum chloride, anhydrous
1727	**154**	Ammonium bifluoride, solid
1727	**154**	Ammonium hydrogendifluoride, solid
1727	**154**	Ammonium hydrogen fluoride, solid
1728	**155**	Amyltrichlorosilane
1729	**156**	Anisoyl chloride
1730	**157**	Antimony pentachloride, liquid
1731	**157**	Antimony pentachloride, solution
1732	**157**	Antimony pentafluoride
1733	**157**	Antimony trichloride
1733	**157**	Antimony trichloride, liquid

ID No.	Guide No.	Name of Material
1733	157	Antimony trichloride, solid
1733	157	Antimony trichloride, solution
1736	137	Benzoyl chloride
1737	156	Benzyl bromide
1738	156	Benzyl chloride
1739	137	Benzyl chloroformate
1740	154	Hydrogendifluorides, n.o.s.
1740	154	Hydrogendifluorides, solid, n.o.s.
1741	125	Boron trichloride
1742	157	Boron trifluoride acetic acid complex
1742	157	Boron trifluoride acetic acid complex, liquid
1743	157	Boron trifluoride propionic acid complex
1743	157	Boron trifluoride propionic acid complex, liquid
1744	154	Bromine
1744	154	Bromine, solution
1744	154	Bromine, solution (Inhalation Hazard Zone A)
1744	154	Bromine, solution (Inhalation Hazard Zone B)
1745	144	Bromine pentafluoride
1746	144	Bromine trifluoride
1747	155	Butyltrichlorosilane
1748	140	Calcium hypochlorite, dry
1748	140	Calcium hypochlorite mixture, dry, with more than 39% available Chlorine (8.8% available Oxygen)
1749	124	Chlorine trifluoride
1750	153	Chloroacetic acid, liquid
1750	153	Chloroacetic acid, solution
1751	153	Chloroacetic acid, solid
1752	156	Chloroacetyl chloride
1753	156	Chlorophenyltrichlorosilane
1754	137	Chlorosulfonic acid
1754	137	Chlorosulfonic acid and Sulfur trioxide mixture
1754	137	Chlorosulphonic acid
1754	137	Chlorosulphonic acid and Sulphur trioxide mixture
1754	137	Sulfur trioxide and Chlorosulfonic acid mixture
1754	137	Sulphur trioxide and Chlorosulphonic acid mixture
1755	154	Chromic acid, solution
1756	154	Chromic fluoride, solid
1757	154	Chromic fluoride, solution
1758	137	Chromium oxychloride
1759	154	Corrosive solid, n.o.s.
1759	154	Ferrous chloride, solid
1759	154	Medicines, corrosive, solid, n.o.s.
1760	154	Chemical kit
1760	154	Compound, cleaning liquid (corrosive)
1760	154	Compound, tree or weed killing, liquid (corrosive)
1760	154	Corrosive liquid, n.o.s.
1760	154	Ferrous chloride, solution
1760	154	Medicines, corrosive, liquid, n.o.s.
1760	154	Titanium sulfate, solution
1760	154	Titanium sulphate, solution
1761	154	Cupriethylenediamine, solution
1762	156	Cyclohexenyltrichlorosilane
1763	156	Cyclohexyltrichlorosilane
1764	153	Dichloroacetic acid

ID No.	Guide No.	Name of Material
1765	156	Dichloroacetyl chloride
1766	156	Dichlorophenyltrichlorosilane
1767	155	Diethyldichlorosilane
1768	154	Difluorophosphoric acid, anhydrous
1769	156	Diphenyldichlorosilane
1770	153	Diphenylmethyl bromide
1771	156	Dodecyltrichlorosilane
1773	157	Ferric chloride
1773	157	Ferric chloride, anhydrous
1774	154	Fire extinguisher charges, corrosive liquid
1775	154	Fluoboric acid
1775	154	Fluoroboric acid
1776	154	Fluorophosphoric acid, anhydrous
1777	137	Fluorosulfonic acid
1777	137	Fluorosulphonic acid
1778	154	Fluorosilicic acid
1778	154	Fluosilicic acid
1778	154	Hydrofluorosilicic acid
1779	153	Formic acid
1779	153	Formic acid, with more than 85% acid
1780	156	Fumaryl chloride
1781	156	Hexadecyltrichlorosilane
1782	154	Hexafluorophosphoric acid
1783	153	Hexamethylenediamine, solution
1784	156	Hexyltrichlorosilane
1786	157	Hydrofluoric acid and Sulfuric acid mixture
1786	157	Hydrofluoric acid and Sulphuric acid mixture
1786	157	Sulfuric acid and Hydrofluoric acid mixture
1786	157	Sulphuric acid and Hydrofluoric acid mixture
1787	154	Hydriodic acid
1787	154	Hydriodic acid, solution
1788	154	Hydrobromic acid
1788	154	Hydrobromic acid, solution
1789	157	Hydrochloric acid
1789	157	Hydrochloric acid, solution
1789	157	Muriatic acid
1790	157	Hydrofluoric acid
1790	157	Hydrofluoric acid, solution
1791	154	Hypochlorite solution
1791	154	Hypochlorite solution, with more than 5% available Chlorine
1792	157	Iodine monochloride
1793	153	Isopropyl acid phosphate
1794	154	Lead sulfate, with more than 3% free acid
1794	154	Lead sulphate, with more than 3% free acid
1796	157	Nitrating acid mixture
1798	157	Aqua regia
1798	157	Nitrohydrochloric acid
1799	156	Nonyltrichlorosilane
1800	156	Octadecyltrichlorosilane
1801	156	Octyltrichlorosilane
1802	140	Perchloric acid, with not more than 50% acid
1803	153	Phenolsulfonic acid, liquid
1803	153	Phenolsulphonic acid, liquid
1804	156	Phenyltrichlorosilane
1805	154	Phosphoric acid

ID No.	Guide No.	Name of Material	ID No.	Guide No.	Name of Material
1805	154	Phosphoric acid, liquid	1823	154	Sodium hydroxide, granular
1805	154	Phosphoric acid, solid	1823	154	Sodium hydroxide, solid
1805	154	Phosphoric acid, solution	1824	154	Caustic soda, solution
1806	137	Phosphorus pentachloride	1824	154	Sodium hydroxide, solution
1807	137	Phosphorus pentoxide	1825	157	Sodium monoxide
1808	137	Phosphorus tribromide	1826	157	Nitrating acid mixture, spent
1809	137	Phosphorus trichloride	1827	137	Stannic chloride, anhydrous
1810	137	Phosphorus oxychloride	1827	137	Tin tetrachloride
1811	154	Potassium hydrogendifluoride	1828	137	Sulfur chlorides
1811	154	Potassium hydrogen difluoride, solid	1828	137	Sulphur chlorides
			1829	137	Sulfur trioxide, inhibited
1812	154	Potassium fluoride	1829	137	Sulfur trioxide, stabilized
1812	154	Potassium fluoride, solid	1829	137	Sulfur trioxide, uninhibited
1813	154	Caustic potash, dry, solid	1829	137	Sulphur trioxide, inhibited
1813	154	Potassium hydroxide, dry, solid	1829	137	Sulphur trioxide, stabilized
1813	154	Potassium hydroxide, flake	1829	137	Sulphur trioxide, uninhibited
1813	154	Potassium hydroxide, solid	1830	137	Sulfuric acid
1814	154	Caustic potash, liquid	1830	137	Sulfuric acid, with more than 51% acid
1814	154	Caustic potash, solution			
1814	154	Potassium hydroxide, solution	1830	137	Sulphuric acid
1815	132	Propionyl chloride	1830	137	Sulphuric acid, with more than 51% acid
1816	155	Propyltrichlorosilane			
1817	137	Pyrosulfuryl chloride	1831	137	Sulfuric acid, fuming
1817	137	Pyrosulphuryl chloride	1831	137	Sulfuric acid, fuming, with less than 30% free Sulfur trioxide
1818	157	Silicon tetrachloride			
1819	154	Sodium aluminate, solution	1831	137	Sulfuric acid, fuming, with not less than 30% free Sulfur trioxide
1823	154	Caustic soda, bead			
1823	154	Caustic soda, flake	1831	137	Sulphuric acid, fuming
1823	154	Caustic soda, granular	1831	137	Sulphuric acid, fuming, with less than 30% free Sulphur trioxide
1823	154	Caustic soda, solid			
1823	154	Sodium hydroxide, bead	1831	137	Sulphuric acid, fuming, with not less than 30% free Sulphur trioxide
1823	154	Sodium hydroxide, dry			
1823	154	Sodium hydroxide, flake	1832	137	Sulfuric acid, spent

ID No.	Guide No.	Name of Material
1832	137	Sulphuric acid, spent
1833	154	Sulfurous acid
1833	154	Sulphurous acid
1834	137	Sulfuryl chloride
1834	137	Sulphuryl chloride
1835	153	Tetramethylammonium hydroxide
1835	153	Tetramethylammonium hydroxide, solution
1836	137	Thionyl chloride
1837	157	Thiophosphoryl chloride
1838	137	Titanium tetrachloride
1839	153	Trichloroacetic acid
1840	154	Zinc chloride, solution
1841	171	Acetaldehyde ammonia
1843	141	Ammonium dinitro-o-cresolate
1843	141	Ammonium dinitro-o-cresolate, solid
1845	120	Carbon dioxide, solid
1845	120	Dry ice
1846	151	Carbon tetrachloride
1847	153	Potassium sulfide, hydrated, with not less than 30% water of crystallization
1847	153	Potassium sulfide, hydrated, with not less than 30% water of hydration
1847	153	Potassium sulphide, hydrated, with not less than 30% water of crystallization
1847	153	Potassium sulphide, hydrated, with not less than 30% water of hydration
1848	132	Propionic acid
1848	132	Propionic acid, with not less than 10% and less than 90% acid
1849	153	Sodium sulfide, hydrated, with not less than 30% water
1849	153	Sodium sulphide, hydrated, with not less than 30% water
1851	151	Medicine, liquid, poisonous, n.o.s.
1851	151	Medicine, liquid, toxic, n.o.s.
1854	135	Barium alloys, pyrophoric
1855	135	Calcium, metal and alloys, pyrophoric
1855	135	Calcium, pyrophoric
1855	135	Calcium alloys, pyrophoric
1856	133	Rags, oily
1857	133	Textile waste, wet
1858	126	Hexafluoropropylene
1858	126	Refrigerant gas R-1216
1859	125	Silicon tetrafluoride
1859	125	Silicon tetrafluoride, compressed
1860	116P	Vinyl fluoride, stabilized
1862	130	Ethyl crotonate
1863	128	Fuel, aviation, turbine engine
1865	131	n-Propyl nitrate
1866	127	Resin solution
1868	134	Decaborane
1869	138	Magnesium
1869	138	Magnesium, in pellets, turnings or ribbons
1869	138	Magnesium alloys, with more than 50% Magnesium, in pellets, turnings or ribbons
1870	138	Potassium borohydride
1871	170	Titanium hydride
1872	141	Lead dioxide
1873	143	Perchloric acid, with more than 50% but not more than 72% acid

ID No.	Guide No.	Name of Material	ID No.	Guide No.	Name of Material
1884	157	Barium oxide	1912	115	Methyl chloride and Methylene chloride mixture
1885	153	Benzidine			
1886	156	Benzylidene chloride	1912	115	Methylene chloride and Methyl chloride mixture
1887	160	Bromochloromethane			
1888	151	Chloroform	1913	120	Neon, refrigerated liquid (cryogenic liquid)
1889	157	Cyanogen bromide			
1891	131	Ethyl bromide	1914	130	Butyl propionates
1892	151	ED	1915	127	Cyclohexanone
1892	151	Ethyldichloroarsine	1916	152	2,2'-Dichlorodiethyl ether
1894	151	Phenylmercuric hydroxide	1916	152	Dichloroethyl ether
1895	151	Phenylmercuric nitrate	1917	129P	Ethyl acrylate, stabilized
1897	160	Perchloroethylene	1918	130	Cumene
1897	160	Tetrachloroethylene	1918	130	Isopropylbenzene
1898	156	Acetyl iodide	1919	129P	Methyl acrylate, stabilized
1902	153	Diisooctyl acid phosphate	1920	128	Nonanes
1903	153	Disinfectant, liquid, corrosive, n.o.s.	1921	131P	Propyleneimine, stabilized
			1922	132	Pyrrolidine
1903	153	Disinfectants, corrosive, liquid, n.o.s.	1923	135	Calcium dithionite
			1923	135	Calcium hydrosulfite
1905	154	Selenic acid	1923	135	Calcium hydrosulphite
1906	153	Acid, sludge	1928	135	Methyl magnesium bromide in Ethyl ether
1906	153	Sludge acid			
1907	154	Soda lime, with more than 4% Sodium hydroxide	1929	135	Potassium dithionite
			1929	135	Potassium hydrosulfite
1908	154	Chlorite solution	1929	135	Potassium hydrosulphite
1908	154	Chlorite solution, with more than 5% available Chlorine	1931	171	Zinc dithionite
			1931	171	Zinc hydrosulfite
1908	154	Sodium chlorite, solution, with more than 5% available Chlorine	1931	171	Zinc hydrosulphite
			1932	135	Zirconium scrap
1910	157	Calcium oxide	1935	157	Cyanide solution, n.o.s.
1911	119	Diborane	1938	156	Bromoacetic acid
1911	119	Diborane, compressed	1938	156	Bromoacetic acid, solution
1911	119	Diborane mixtures	1939	137	Phosphorus oxybromide
			1939	137	Phosphorus oxybromide, solid

ID No.	Guide No.	Name of Material
1940	153	Thioglycolic acid
1941	171	Dibromodifluoromethane
1942	140	Ammonium nitrate, with not more than 0.2% combustible substances
1944	133	Matches, safety
1945	133	Matches, wax "vesta"
1950	126	Aerosol dispensers
1950	126	Aerosols
1951	120	Argon, refrigerated liquid (cryogenic liquid)
1952	126	Carbon dioxide and Ethylene oxide mixtures, with not more than 6% Ethylene oxide
1952	126	Carbon dioxide and Ethylene oxide mixtures, with not more than 9% Ethylene oxide
1952	126	Ethylene oxide and Carbon dioxide mixtures, with not more than 6% Ethylene oxide
1952	126	Ethylene oxide and Carbon dioxide mixtures, with not more than 9% Ethylene oxide
1953	119	Compressed gas, flammable, poisonous, n.o.s. (Inhalation Hazard Zone A)
1953	119	Compressed gas, flammable, poisonous, n.o.s. (Inhalation Hazard Zone B)
1953	119	Compressed gas, flammable, poisonous, n.o.s. (Inhalation Hazard Zone C)
1953	119	Compressed gas, flammable, poisonous, n.o.s. (Inhalation Hazard Zone D)
1953	119	Compressed gas, flammable, toxic, n.o.s. (Inhalation Hazard Zone A)
1953	119	Compressed gas, flammable, toxic, n.o.s. (Inhalation Hazard Zone B)
1953	119	Compressed gas, flammable, toxic, n.o.s. (Inhalation Hazard Zone C)
1953	119	Compressed gas, flammable, toxic, n.o.s. (Inhalation Hazard Zone D)
1953	119	Compressed gas, poisonous, flammable, n.o.s.
1953	119	Compressed gas, poisonous, flammable, n.o.s. (Inhalation Hazard Zone A)
1953	119	Compressed gas, poisonous, flammable, n.o.s. (Inhalation Hazard Zone B)
1953	119	Compressed gas, poisonous, flammable, n.o.s. (Inhalation Hazard Zone C)
1953	119	Compressed gas, poisonous, flammable, n.o.s. (Inhalation Hazard Zone D)
1953	119	Compressed gas, toxic, flammable, n.o.s.
1953	119	Compressed gas, toxic, flammable, n.o.s. (Inhalation Hazard Zone A)
1953	119	Compressed gas, toxic, flammable, n.o.s. (Inhalation Hazard Zone B)
1953	119	Compressed gas, toxic, flammable, n.o.s. (Inhalation Hazard Zone C)
1953	119	Compressed gas, toxic, flammable, n.o.s. (Inhalation Hazard Zone D)
1954	115	Compressed gas, flammable, n.o.s.
1954	115	Dispersant gas, n.o.s. (flammable)

ID No.	Guide No.	Name of Material
1954	115	Insecticide gas, flammable, n.o.s.
1954	115	Refrigerant gas, n.o.s. (flammable)
1954	115	Refrigerating machines, containing flammable, non-poisonous, non-corrosive, liquefied gas
1955	123	Compressed gas, poisonous, n.o.s.
1955	123	Compressed gas, poisonous, n.o.s. (Inhalation Hazard Zone A)
1955	123	Compressed gas, poisonous, n.o.s. (Inhalation Hazard Zone B)
1955	123	Compressed gas, poisonous, n.o.s. (Inhalation Hazard Zone C)
1955	123	Compressed gas, poisonous, n.o.s. (Inhalation Hazard Zone D)
1955	123	Compressed gas, toxic, n.o.s.
1955	123	Compressed gas, toxic, n.o.s. (Inhalation Hazard Zone A)
1955	123	Compressed gas, toxic, n.o.s. (Inhalation Hazard Zone B)
1955	123	Compressed gas, toxic, n.o.s. (Inhalation Hazard Zone C)
1955	123	Compressed gas, toxic, n.o.s. (Inhalation Hazard Zone D)
1955	123	Organic phosphate compound mixed with compressed gas
1955	123	Organic phosphate mixed with compressed gas
1955	123	Organic phosphorus compound mixed with compressed gas
1956	126	Accumulators, pressurized, pneumatic or hydraulic
1956	126	Compressed gas, n.o.s.
1956	126	Hexafluoropropylene oxide
1957	115	Deuterium
1957	115	Deuterium, compressed
1958	126	1,2-Dichloro-1,1,2,2-tetrafluoroethane
1958	126	Dichlorotetrafluoroethane
1958	126	Refrigerant gas R-114
1959	116P	1,1-Difluoroethylene
1959	116P	Refrigerant gas R-1132a
1960	115	Engine starting fluid
1961	115	Ethane, refrigerated liquid
1961	115	Ethane-Propane mixture, refrigerated liquid
1961	115	Propane-Ethane mixture, refrigerated liquid
1962	116P	Ethylene
1962	116P	Ethylene, compressed
1963	120	Helium, refrigerated liquid (cryogenic liquid)
1964	115	Hydrocarbon gas, compressed, n.o.s.
1964	115	Hydrocarbon gas mixture, compressed, n.o.s.
1965	115	Hydrocarbon gas, liquefied, n.o.s.
1965	115	Hydrocarbon gas mixture, liquefied, n.o.s.
1966	115	Hydrogen, refrigerated liquid (cryogenic liquid)
1967	123	Insecticide gas, poisonous, n.o.s.
1967	123	Insecticide gas, toxic, n.o.s.
1967	123	Parathion and compressed gas mixture
1968	126	Insecticide gas, n.o.s.

ID No.	Guide No.	Name of Material	ID No.	Guide No.	Name of Material
1969	115	Isobutane	1976	126	Octafluorocyclobutane
1969	115	Isobutane mixture	1976	126	Refrigerant gas RC-318
1970	120	Krypton, refrigerated liquid (cryogenic liquid)	1977	120	Nitrogen, refrigerated liquid (cryogenic liquid)
1971	115	Methane	1978	115	Propane
1971	115	Methane, compressed	1978	115	Propane mixture
1971	115	Natural gas, compressed	1979	121	Rare gases mixture
1972	115	Liquefied natural gas (cryogenic liquid)	1979	121	Rare gases mixture, compressed
1972	115	LNG (cryogenic liquid)	1980	121	Oxygen and Rare gases mixture
1972	115	Methane, refrigerated liquid (cryogenic liquid)	1980	121	Oxygen and Rare gases mixture, compressed
1972	115	Natural gas, refrigerated liquid (cryogenic liquid)	1980	121	Rare gases and Oxygen mixture
1973	126	Chlorodifluoromethane and Chloropentafluoroethane mixture	1980	121	Rare gases and Oxygen mixture, compressed
1973	126	Chloropentafluoroethane and Chlorodifluoromethane mixture	1981	121	Nitrogen and Rare gases mixture
1973	126	Refrigerant gas R-502	1981	121	Nitrogen and Rare gases mixture, compressed
1974	126	Bromochlorodifluoromethane	1981	121	Rare gases and Nitrogen mixture
1974	126	Chlorodifluorobromomethane	1981	121	Rare gases and Nitrogen mixture, compressed
1974	126	Refrigerant gas R-12B1	1982	126	Refrigerant gas R-14
1975	124	Dinitrogen tetroxide and Nitric oxide mixture	1982	126	Refrigerant gas R-14, compressed
1975	124	Nitric oxide and Dinitrogen tetroxide mixture	1982	126	Tetrafluoromethane
1975	124	Nitric oxide and Nitrogen dioxide mixture	1982	126	Tetrafluoromethane, compressed
1975	124	Nitric oxide and Nitrogen tetroxide mixture	1983	126	1-Chloro-2,2,2-trifluoroethane
1975	124	Nitrogen dioxide and Nitric oxide mixture	1983	126	Chlorotrifluoroethane
1975	124	Nitrogen tetroxide and Nitric oxide mixture	1983	126	Refrigerant gas R-133a
			1984	126	Refrigerant gas R-23
			1984	126	Trifluoromethane
			1986	131	Alcohols, flammable, poisonous, n.o.s.
			1986	131	Alcohols, flammable, toxic, n.o.s.

ID No.	Guide No.	Name of Material
1986	131	Alcohols, poisonous, n.o.s.
1986	131	Alcohols, toxic, n.o.s.
1986	131	Denatured alcohol (toxic)
1986	131	Propargyl alcohol
1987	127	Alcohols, n.o.s.
1987	127	Denatured alcohol
1988	131	Aldehydes, flammable, poisonous, n.o.s.
1988	131	Aldehydes, flammable, toxic, n.o.s.
1988	131	Aldehydes, poisonous, n.o.s.
1988	131	Aldehydes, toxic, n.o.s.
1989	129	Aldehydes, n.o.s.
1990	129	Benzaldehyde
1991	131P	Chloroprene, stabilized
1992	131	Flammable liquid, poisonous, n.o.s.
1992	131	Flammable liquid, toxic, n.o.s.
1993	128	Combustible liquid, n.o.s.
1993	128	Compound, cleaning liquid (flammable)
1993	128	Compound, tree or weed killing, liquid (flammable)
1993	128	Diesel fuel
1993	128	Flammable liquid, n.o.s.
1993	128	Fuel oil
1993	128	Medicines, flammable, liquid, n.o.s.
1993	128	Refrigerating machine
1994	131	Iron pentacarbonyl
1999	130	Asphalt
1999	130	Tars, liquid
2000	133	Celluloid, in blocks, rods, rolls, sheets, tubes, etc., except scrap
2001	133	Cobalt naphthenates, powder
2002	135	Celluloid, scrap
2003	135	Metal alkyls, n.o.s.
2003	135	Metal alkyls, water-reactive, n.o.s.
2003	135	Metal aryls, n.o.s
2003	135	Metal aryls, water-reactive, n.o.s.
2004	135	Magnesium diamide
2005	135	Magnesium diphenyl
2006	135	Plastic, nitrocellulose-based, spontaneously combustible, n.o.s.
2006	135	Plastics, nitrocellulose-based, self-heating, n.o.s.
2008	135	Zirconium powder, dry
2009	135	Zirconium, dry, finished sheets, strips or coiled wire
2010	138	Magnesium hydride
2011	139	Magnesium phosphide
2012	139	Potassium phosphide
2013	139	Strontium phosphide
2014	140	Hydrogen peroxide, aqueous solution, with not less than 20% but not more than 60% Hydrogen peroxide (stabilized as necessary)
2015	143	Hydrogen peroxide, aqueous solution, stabilized, with more than 60% Hydrogen peroxide
2015	143	Hydrogen peroxide, stabilized
2016	151	Ammunition, poisonous, non-explosive
2016	151	Ammunition, toxic, non-explosive

ID No.	Guide No.	Name of Material
2017	159	Ammunition, tear-producing, non-explosive
2018	152	Chloroanilines, solid
2019	152	Chloroanilines, liquid
2020	153	Chlorophenols, solid
2021	153	Chlorophenols, liquid
2022	153	Cresylic acid
2023	131P	1-Chloro-2,3-epoxypropane
2023	131P	Epichlorohydrin
2024	151	Mercury compound, liquid, n.o.s.
2025	151	Mercury compound, solid, n.o.s.
2026	151	Phenylmercuric compound, n.o.s.
2027	151	Sodium arsenite, solid
2028	153	Bombs, smoke, non-explosive, with corrosive liquid, without initiating device
2029	132	Hydrazine, anhydrous
2029	132	Hydrazine, aqueous solutions, with more than 64% Hydrazine
2030	153	Hydrazine, aqueous solution, with more than 37% Hydrazine
2030	153	Hydrazine, aqueous solution, with not less than 37% but not more than 64% Hydrazine
2030	153	Hydrazine hydrate
2031	157	Nitric acid, other than red fuming
2032	157	Nitric acid, fuming
2032	157	Nitric acid, red fuming
2033	154	Potassium monoxide
2034	115	Hydrogen and Methane mixture, compressed
2034	115	Methane and Hydrogen mixture, compressed
2035	115	Refrigerant gas R-143a
2035	115	1,1,1-Trifluoroethane
2035	115	Trifluoroethane, compressed
2036	121	Xenon
2036	121	Xenon, compressed
2037	115	Gas cartridges
2037	115	Receptacles, small, containing gas
2038	152	Dinitrotoluenes
2038	152	Dinitrotoluenes, liquid
2038	152	Dinitrotoluenes, solid
2044	115	2,2-Dimethylpropane
2045	130	Isobutyl aldehyde
2045	130	Isobutyraldehyde
2046	130	Cymenes
2047	129	Dichloropropenes
2048	130	Dicyclopentadiene
2049	130	Diethylbenzene
2050	128	Diisobutylene, isomeric compounds
2051	132	2-Dimethylaminoethanol
2051	132	Dimethylethanolamine
2052	128	Dipentene
2053	129	Methylamyl alcohol
2053	129	Methyl isobutyl carbinol
2053	129	M.I.B.C.
2054	132	Morpholine
2055	128P	Styrene monomer, stabilized
2056	127	Tetrahydrofuran
2057	128	Tripropylene
2058	129	Valeraldehyde
2059	127	Nitrocellulose, solution, flammable
2059	127	Nitrocellulose, solution, in a flammable liquid

ID No.	Guide No.	Name of Material	ID No.	Guide No.	Name of Material
2067	140	Ammonium nitrate fertilizers	2189	119	Dichlorosilane
2068	140	Ammonium nitrate fertilizers, with Calcium carbonate	2190	124	Oxygen difluoride
			2190	124	Oxygen difluoride, compressed
2069	140	Ammonium nitrate fertilizers, with Ammonium sulfate	2191	123	Sulfuryl fluoride
			2191	123	Sulphuryl fluoride
2069	140	Ammonium nitrate fertilizers, with Ammonium sulphate	2192	119	Germane
2069	140	Ammonium nitrate mixed fertilizers	2193	126	Hexafluoroethane
			2193	126	Hexafluoroethane, compressed
2070	143	Ammonium nitrate fertilizers, with Phosphate or Potash	2193	126	Refrigerant gas R-116
			2193	126	Refrigerant gas R-116, compressed
2071	140	Ammonium nitrate fertilizer, with not more than 0.4% combustible material	2194	125	Selenium hexafluoride
			2195	125	Tellurium hexafluoride
2071	140	Ammonium nitrate fertilizers	2196	125	Tungsten hexafluoride
2072	140	Ammonium nitrate fertilizer, n.o.s.	2197	125	Hydrogen iodide, anhydrous
2072	140	Ammonium nitrate fertilizers	2198	125	Phosphorus pentafluoride
2073	125	Ammonia, solution, with more than 35% but not more than 50% Ammonia	2198	125	Phosphorus pentafluoride, compressed
2074	153P	Acrylamide	2199	119	Phosphine
2074	153P	Acrylamide, solid	2200	116P	Propadiene, stabilized
2075	153	Chloral, anhydrous, stabilized	2201	122	Nitrous oxide, refrigerated liquid
2076	153	Cresols	2202	117	Hydrogen selenide, anhydrous
2076	153	Cresols, liquid	2203	116	Silane
2076	153	Cresols, solid	2203	116	Silane, compressed
2077	153	alpha-Naphthylamine	2204	119	Carbonyl sulfide
2077	153	Naphthylamine (alpha)	2204	119	Carbonyl sulphide
2078	156	Toluene diisocyanate	2205	153	Adiponitrile
2079	154	Diethylenetriamine	2206	155	Isocyanate solution, poisonous, n.o.s.
2186	125	Hydrogen chloride, refrigerated liquid	2206	155	Isocyanate solution, toxic, n.o.s.
2187	120	Carbon dioxide, refrigerated liquid	2206	155	Isocyanate solutions, n.o.s.
			2206	155	Isocyanates, n.o.s.
2188	119	Arsine	2206	155	Isocyanates, poisonous, n.o.s.
2188	119	SA			

ID No.	Guide No.	Name of Material	ID No.	Guide No.	Name of Material
2206	155	Isocyanates, toxic, n.o.s.	2226	156	Benzotrichloride
2208	140	Bleaching powder	2227	130P	n-Butyl methacrylate, stabilized
2208	140	Calcium hypochlorite mixture, dry, with more than 10% but not more than 39% available Chlorine	2232	153	Chloroacetaldehyde
			2232	153	2-Chloroethanal
			2233	152	Chloroanisidines
2209	132	Formaldehyde, solutions (Formalin) (corrosive)	2234	130	Chlorobenzotrifluorides
			2235	153	Chlorobenzyl chlorides
2210	135	Maneb	2235	153	Chlorobenzyl chlorides, liquid
2210	135	Maneb preparation, with not less than 60% Maneb	2236	156	3-Chloro-4-methylphenyl isocyanate
2211	133	Polymeric beads, expandable	2236	156	3-Chloro-4-methylphenyl isocyanate, liquid
2211	133	Polystyrene beads, expandable	2237	153	Chloronitroanilines
2212	171	Asbestos	2238	129	Chlorotoluenes
2212	171	Asbestos, blue	2239	153	Chlorotoluidines
2212	171	Asbestos, brown	2239	153	Chlorotoluidines, liquid
2212	171	Blue asbestos	2239	153	Chlorotoluidines, solid
2212	171	Brown asbestos	2240	154	Chromosulfuric acid
2213	133	Paraformaldehyde	2240	154	Chromosulphuric acid
2214	156	Phthalic anhydride	2241	128	Cycloheptane
2215	156	Maleic acid	2242	128	Cycloheptene
2215	156	Maleic anhydride	2243	130	Cyclohexyl acetate
2215	156	Maleic anhydride, molten	2244	129	Cyclopentanol
2216	171	Fish meal, stabilized	2245	128	Cyclopentanone
2216	171	Fish scrap, stabilized	2246	128	Cyclopentene
2217	135	Seed cake, with not more than 1.5% oil and not more than 11% moisture	2247	128	n-Decane
			2248	132	Di-n-butylamine
2218	132P	Acrylic acid, stabilized	2249	131	Dichlorodimethyl ether, symmetrical
2219	129	Allyl glycidyl ether	2250	156	Dichlorophenyl isocyanates
2222	128	Anisole	2251	128P	Bicyclo[2.2.1]hepta-2,5-diene, stabilized
2224	152	Benzonitrile			
2225	156	Benzenesulfonyl chloride	2251	128P	2,5-Norbornadiene, stabilized
2225	156	Benzenesulphonyl chloride	2252	127	1,2-Dimethoxyethane

ID No.	Guide No.	Name of Material	ID No.	Guide No.	Name of Material
2253	153	N,N-Dimethylaniline	2281	156	Hexamethylene diisocyanate
2254	133	Matches, fusee	2282	129	Hexanols
2256	130	Cyclohexene	2283	130P	Isobutyl methacrylate, stabilized
2257	138	Potassium	2284	131	Isobutyronitrile
2257	138	Potassium, metal	2285	156	Isocyanatobenzotrifluorides
2258	132	1,2-Propylenediamine	2286	128	Pentamethylheptane
2258	132	1,3-Propylenediamine	2287	128	Isoheptenes
2259	153	Triethylenetetramine	2288	128	Isohexenes
2260	132	Tripropylamine	2289	153	Isophoronediamine
2261	153	Xylenols	2290	156	IPDI
2261	153	Xylenols, solid	2290	156	Isophorone diisocyanate
2262	156	Dimethylcarbamoyl chloride	2291	151	Lead compound, soluble, n.o.s.
2263	128	Dimethylcyclohexanes	2293	128	4-Methoxy-4-methylpentan-2-one
2264	132	N,N-Dimethylcyclohexylamine	2294	153	N-Methylaniline
2264	132	Dimethylcyclohexylamine	2295	155	Methyl chloroacetate
2265	129	N,N-Dimethylformamide	2296	128	Methylcyclohexane
2266	132	Dimethyl-N-propylamine	2297	128	Methylcyclohexanone
2267	156	Dimethyl thiophosphoryl chloride	2298	128	Methylcyclopentane
			2299	155	Methyl dichloroacetate
2269	153	3,3'-Iminodipropylamine	2300	153	2-Methyl-5-ethylpyridine
2270	132	Ethylamine, aqueous solution, with not less than 50% but not more than 70% Ethylamine	2301	128	2-Methylfuran
			2302	127	5-Methylhexan-2-one
2271	128	Ethyl amyl ketone	2303	128	Isopropenylbenzene
2272	153	N-Ethylaniline	2304	133	Naphthalene, molten
2273	153	2-Ethylaniline	2305	153	Nitrobenzenesulfonic acid
2274	153	N-Ethyl-N-benzylaniline	2305	153	Nitrobenzenesulphonic acid
2275	129	2-Ethylbutanol	2306	152	Nitrobenzotrifluorides
2276	132	2-Ethylhexylamine	2306	152	Nitrobenzotrifluorides, liquid
2277	130P	Ethyl methacrylate	2307	152	3-Nitro-4-chlorobenzotrifluoride
2277	130P	Ethyl methacrylate, stabilized	2308	157	Nitrosylsulfuric acid
2278	128	n-Heptene	2308	157	Nitrosylsulfuric acid, liquid
2279	151	Hexachlorobutadiene	2308	157	Nitrosylsulfuric acid, solid
2280	153	Hexamethylenediamine, solid	2308	157	Nitrosylsulphuric acid

ID No.	Guide No.	Name of Material	ID No.	Guide No.	Name of Material
2308	157	Nitrosylsulphuric acid, liquid	2325	129	1,3,5-Trimethylbenzene
2308	157	Nitrosylsulphuric acid, solid	2326	153	Trimethylcyclohexylamine
2309	128P	Octadiene	2327	153	Trimethylhexamethylenediamines
2310	131	Pentan-2,4-dione	2328	156	Trimethylhexamethylene diisocyanate
2310	131	2,4-Pentanedione	2329	130	Trimethyl phosphite
2310	131	Pentane-2,4-dione	2330	128	Undecane
2311	153	Phenetidines	2331	154	Zinc chloride, anhydrous
2312	153	Phenol, molten	2332	129	Acetaldehyde oxime
2313	129	Picolines	2333	131	Allyl acetate
2315	171	Articles containing Polychlorinated biphenyls (PCB)	2334	131	Allylamine
2315	171	PCB	2335	131	Allyl ethyl ether
2315	171	Polychlorinated biphenyls	2336	131	Allyl formate
2315	171	Polychlorinated biphenyls, liquid	2337	131	Phenyl mercaptan
2315	171	Polychlorinated biphenyls, solid	2338	127	Benzotrifluoride
2316	157	Sodium cuprocyanide, solid	2339	130	2-Bromobutane
2317	157	Sodium cuprocyanide, solution	2340	130	2-Bromoethyl ethyl ether
2318	135	Sodium hydrosulfide, solid, with less than 25% water of crystallization	2341	130	1-Bromo-3-methylbutane
			2342	130	Bromomethylpropanes
2318	135	Sodium hydrosulfide, with less than 25% water of crystallization	2343	130	2-Bromopentane
			2344	129	2-Bromopropane
2318	135	Sodium hydrosulphide, solid, with less than 25% water of crystallization	2344	129	Bromopropanes
			2345	130	3-Bromopropyne
2318	135	Sodium hydrosulphide, with less than 25% water of crystallization	2346	127	Butanedione
			2346	127	Diacetyl
2319	128	Terpene hydrocarbons, n.o.s.	2347	130	Butyl mercaptan
2320	153	Tetraethylenepentamine	2348	129P	Butyl acrylates, stabilized
2321	153	Trichlorobenzenes, liquid	2350	127	Butyl methyl ether
2322	152	Trichlorobutene	2351	129	Butyl nitrites
2323	130	Triethyl phosphite	2352	127P	Butyl vinyl ether, stabilized
2324	128	Triisobutylene	2353	132	Butyryl chloride
			2354	131	Chloromethyl ethyl ether
			2356	129	2-Chloropropane

ID No.	Guide No.	Name of Material	ID No.	Guide No.	Name of Material
2357	132	Cyclohexylamine	2385	129	Ethyl isobutyrate
2358	128P	Cyclooctatetraene	2386	132	1-Ethylpiperidine
2359	132	Diallylamine	2387	130	Fluorobenzene
2360	131P	Diallyl ether	2388	130	Fluorotoluenes
2361	132	Diisobutylamine	2389	128	Furan
2362	130	1,1-Dichloroethane	2390	129	2-Iodobutane
2363	129	Ethyl mercaptan	2391	129	Iodomethylpropanes
2364	128	n-Propyl benzene	2392	129	Iodopropanes
2366	128	Diethyl carbonate	2393	129	Isobutyl formate
2367	130	alpha-Methylvaleraldehyde	2394	129	Isobutyl propionate
2367	130	Methyl valeraldehyde (alpha)	2395	132	Isobutyryl chloride
2368	128	alpha-Pinene	2396	131P	Methacrylaldehyde, stabilized
2368	128	Pinene (alpha)	2397	127	3-Methylbutan-2-one
2369	152	Ethylene glycol monobutyl ether	2398	127	Methyl tert-butyl ether
2370	128	1-Hexene	2399	132	1-Methylpiperidine
2371	128	Isopentenes	2400	130	Methyl isovalerate
2372	129	1,2-Di-(dimethylamino)ethane	2401	132	Piperidine
2373	127	Diethoxymethane	2402	130	Propanethiols
2374	127	3,3-Diethoxypropene	2403	129P	Isopropenyl acetate
2375	129	Diethyl sulfide	2404	131	Propionitrile
2375	129	Diethyl sulphide	2405	129	Isopropyl butyrate
2376	127	2,3-Dihydropyran	2406	127	Isopropyl isobutyrate
2377	127	1,1-Dimethoxyethane	2407	155	Isopropyl chloroformate
2378	131	2-Dimethylaminoacetonitrile	2409	129	Isopropyl propionate
2379	132	1,3-Dimethylbutylamine	2410	129	1,2,3,6-Tetrahydropyridine
2380	127	Dimethyldiethoxysilane	2410	129	1,2,5,6-Tetrahydropyridine
2381	130	Dimethyl disulfide	2411	131	Butyronitrile
2381	130	Dimethyl disulphide	2412	130	Tetrahydrothiophene
2382	131	1,2-Dimethylhydrazine	2413	128	Tetrapropyl orthotitanate
2382	131	Dimethylhydrazine, symmetrical	2414	130	Thiophene
2383	132	Dipropylamine	2416	129	Trimethyl borate
2384	127	Di-n-propyl ether	2417	125	Carbonyl fluoride
2384	127	Dipropyl ether	2417	125	Carbonyl fluoride, compressed

ID No.	Guide No.	Name of Material
2418	125	Sulfur tetrafluoride
2418	125	Sulphur tetrafluoride
2419	116	Bromotrifluoroethylene
2420	125	Hexafluoroacetone
2421	124	Nitrogen trioxide
2422	126	Octafluorobut-2-ene
2422	126	Refrigerant gas R-1318
2424	126	Octafluoropropane
2424	126	Refrigerant gas R-218
2426	140	Ammonium nitrate, liquid (hot concentrated solution)
2427	140	Potassium chlorate, aqueous solution
2427	140	Potassium chlorate, solution
2428	140	Sodium chlorate, aqueous solution
2429	140	Calcium chlorate, aqueous solution
2429	140	Calcium chlorate, solution
2430	153	Alkyl phenols, solid, n.o.s. (including C2-C12 homologues)
2431	153	Anisidines
2431	153	Anisidines, liquid
2431	153	Anisidines, solid
2432	153	N,N-Diethylaniline
2433	152	Chloronitrotoluenes
2433	152	Chloronitrotoluenes, liquid
2433	152	Chloronitrotoluenes, solid
2434	156	Dibenzyldichlorosilane
2435	156	Ethylphenyldichlorosilane
2436	129	Thioacetic acid
2437	156	Methylphenyldichlorosilane
2438	132	Trimethylacetyl chloride
2439	154	Sodium hydrogendifluoride
2440	154	Stannic chloride, pentahydrate
2440	154	Tin tetrachloride, pentahydrate
2441	135	Titanium trichloride, pyrophoric
2441	135	Titanium trichloride mixture, pyrophoric
2442	156	Trichloroacetyl chloride
2443	137	Vanadium oxytrichloride
2444	137	Vanadium tetrachloride
2445	135	Lithium alkyls
2445	135	Lithium alkyls, liquid
2446	153	Nitrocresols
2446	153	Nitrocresols, solid
2447	136	Phosphorus, white, molten
2447	136	White phosphorus, molten
2447	136	Yellow phosphorus, molten
2448	133	Sulfur, molten
2448	133	Sulphur, molten
2451	122	Nitrogen trifluoride
2451	122	Nitrogen trifluoride, compressed
2452	116P	Ethylacetylene, stabilized
2453	115	Ethyl fluoride
2453	115	Refrigerant gas R-161
2454	115	Methyl fluoride
2454	115	Refrigerant gas R-41
2455	116	Methyl nitrite
2456	130P	2-Chloropropene
2457	128	2,3-Dimethylbutane
2458	130	Hexadiene
2459	128	2-Methyl-1-butene
2460	128	2-Methyl-2-butene
2461	128	Methylpentadiene
2463	138	Aluminum hydride

ID No.	Guide No.	Name of Material	ID No.	Guide No.	Name of Material
2464	141	Beryllium nitrate	2486	155	Isobutyl isocyanate
2465	140	Dichloroisocyanuric acid, dry	2487	155	Phenyl isocyanate
2465	140	Dichloroisocyanuric acid salts	2488	155	Cyclohexyl isocyanate
2465	140	Sodium dichloroisocyanurate	2490	153	Dichloroisopropyl ether
2465	140	Sodium dichloro-s-triazinetrione	2491	153	Ethanolamine
2466	143	Potassium superoxide	2491	153	Ethanolamine, solution
2467	140	Sodium percarbonates	2491	153	Monoethanolamine
2468	140	Trichloroisocyanuric acid, dry	2493	132	Hexamethyleneimine
2468	140	(mono)-(Trichloro)-tetra-(monopotassium dichloro)-penta-s-triazinetrione, dry	2495	144	Iodine pentafluoride
			2496	156	Propionic anhydride
2469	140	Zinc bromate	2498	129	1,2,3,6-Tetrahydrobenzaldehyde
2470	152	Phenylacetonitrile, liquid	2501	152	1-Aziridinyl phosphine oxide (Tris)
2471	154	Osmium tetroxide			
2473	154	Sodium arsanilate	2501	152	Tri-(1-aziridinyl)phosphine oxide, solution
2474	157	Thiophosgene			
2475	157	Vanadium trichloride	2501	152	Tris-(1-aziridinyl)phosphine oxide, solution
2477	131	Methyl isothiocyanate			
2478	155	Isocyanate solution, flammable, poisonous, n.o.s.	2502	132	Valeryl chloride
			2503	137	Zirconium tetrachloride
2478	155	Isocyanate solution, flammable, toxic, n.o.s.	2504	159	Acetylene tetrabromide
			2504	159	Tetrabromoethane
2478	155	Isocyanate solutions, n.o.s.	2505	154	Ammonium fluoride
2478	155	Isocyanates, flammable, poisonous, n.o.s.	2506	154	Ammonium hydrogen sulfate
			2506	154	Ammonium hydrogen sulphate
2478	155	Isocyanates, flammable, toxic, n.o.s.	2507	154	Chloroplatinic acid, solid
			2508	156	Molybdenum pentachloride
2478	155	Isocyanates, n.o.s.	2509	154	Potassium hydrogen sulfate
2480	155	Methyl isocyanate	2509	154	Potassium hydrogen sulphate
2481	155	Ethyl isocyanate	2511	153	2-Chloropropionic acid
2482	155	n-Propyl isocyanate	2511	153	2-Chloropropionic acid, solid
2483	155	Isopropyl isocyanate	2511	153	2-Chloropropionic acid, solution
2484	155	tert-Butyl isocyanate	2512	152	Aminophenols
2485	155	n-Butyl isocyanate	2513	156	Bromoacetyl bromide

ID No.	Guide No.	Name of Material
2514	130	Bromobenzene
2515	159	Bromoform
2516	151	Carbon tetrabromide
2517	115	1-Chloro-1,1-difluoroethane
2517	115	Chlorodifluoroethanes
2517	115	Difluorochloroethanes
2517	115	Refrigerant gas R-142b
2518	153	1,5,9-Cyclododecatriene
2520	130P	Cyclooctadienes
2521	131P	Diketene, stabilized
2522	153P	2-Dimethylaminoethyl methacrylate
2522	153P	Dimethylaminoethyl methacrylate
2524	129	Ethyl orthoformate
2525	156	Ethyl oxalate
2526	132	Furfurylamine
2527	129P	Isobutyl acrylate, stabilized
2528	130	Isobutyl isobutyrate
2529	132	Isobutyric acid
2530	132	Isobutyric anhydride
2531	153P	Methacrylic acid, stabilized
2533	156	Methyl trichloroacetate
2534	119	Methylchlorosilane
2535	132	4-Methylmorpholine
2535	132	N-Methylmorpholine
2535	132	Methylmorpholine
2536	127	Methyltetrahydrofuran
2538	133	Nitronaphthalene
2541	128	Terpinolene
2542	153	Tributylamine
2545	135	Hafnium powder, dry
2546	135	Titanium powder, dry

ID No.	Guide No.	Name of Material
2547	143	Sodium superoxide
2548	124	Chlorine pentafluoride
2552	151	Hexafluoroacetone hydrate
2552	151	Hexafluoroacetone hydrate, liquid
2554	130P	Methylallyl chloride
2555	113	Nitrocellulose with water, not less than 25% water
2556	113	Nitrocellulose with alcohol
2556	113	Nitrocellulose with not less than 25% alcohol
2557	133	Nitrocellulose
2557	133	Nitrocellulose mixture, without pigment
2557	133	Nitrocellulose mixture, without plasticizer
2557	133	Nitrocellulose mixture, with pigment
2557	133	Nitrocellulose mixture, with pigment and plasticizer
2557	133	Nitrocellulose mixture, with plasticizer
2558	131	Epibromohydrin
2560	129	2-Methylpentan-2-ol
2561	128	3-Methyl-1-butene
2564	153	Trichloroacetic acid, solution
2565	153	Dicyclohexylamine
2567	154	Sodium pentachlorophenate
2570	154	Cadmium compound
2571	156	Alkylsulfuric acids
2571	156	Alkylsulphuric acids
2571	156	Ethylsulfuric acid
2571	156	Ethylsulphuric acid
2572	153	Phenylhydrazine
2573	141	Thallium chlorate

ID No.	Guide No.	Name of Material	ID No.	Guide No.	Name of Material
2574	151	Tricresyl phosphate	2585	153	Alkyl sulphonic acids, solid, with not more than 5% free Sulphuric acid
2576	137	Phosphorus oxybromide, molten			
2577	156	Phenylacetyl chloride	2585	153	Aryl sulfonic acids, solid, with not more than 5% free Sulfuric acid
2578	157	Phosphorus trioxide			
2579	153	Piperazine	2585	153	Aryl sulphonic acids, solid, with not more than 5% free Sulphuric acid
2580	154	Aluminum bromide, solution			
2581	154	Aluminum chloride, solution	2586	153	Alkyl sulfonic acids, liquid, with not more than 5% free Sulfuric acid
2582	154	Ferric chloride, solution			
2583	153	Alkyl sulfonic acids, solid, with more than 5% free Sulfuric acid	2586	153	Alkyl sulphonic acids, liquid, with not more than 5% free Sulphuric acid
2583	153	Alkyl sulphonic acids, solid, with more than 5% free Sulphuric acid	2586	153	Aryl sulfonic acids, liquid, with not more than 5% free Sulfuric acid
2583	153	Aryl sulfonic acids, solid, with more than 5% free Sulfuric acid	2586	153	Aryl sulphonic acids, liquid, with not more than 5% free Sulphuric acid
2583	153	Aryl sulphonic acids, solid, with more than 5% free Sulphuric acid	2587	153	Benzoquinone
			2588	151	Pesticide, solid, poisonous
2584	153	Alkyl sulfonic acids, liquid, with more than 5% free Sulfuric acid	2588	151	Pesticide, solid, poisonous, n.o.s.
2584	153	Alkyl sulphonic acids, liquid, with more than 5% free Sulphuric acid	2588	151	Pesticide, solid, toxic, n.o.s.
			2589	155	Vinyl chloroacetate
2584	153	Aryl sulfonic acids, liquid, with more than 5% free Sulfuric acid	2590	171	Asbestos, white
			2590	171	White asbestos
2584	153	Aryl sulphonic acids, liquid, with more than 5% free Sulphuric acid	2591	120	Xenon, refrigerated liquid (cryogenic liquid)
2584	153	Dodecylbenzenesulfonic acid	2599	126	Chlorotrifluoromethane and Trifluoromethane azeotropic mixture with approximately 60% Chlorotrifluoromethane
2584	153	Dodecylbenzenesulphonic acid			
2585	153	Alkyl sulfonic acids, solid, with not more than 5% free Sulfuric acid	2599	126	Refrigerant gas R-13 and Refrigerant gas R-23 azeotropic mixture with 60% Refrigerant gas R-13

ID No.	Guide No.	Name of Material
2599	126	Refrigerant gas R-23 and Refrigerant gas R-13 azeotropic mixture with 60% Refrigerant gas R-13
2599	126	Refrigerant gas R-503 (azeotropic mixture of Refrigerant gas R-13 and Refrigerant gas R-23 with approximately 60% Refrigerant gas R-13)
2599	126	Trifluoromethane and Chlorotrifluoromethane azeotropic mixture with approximately 60% Chlorotrifluoromethane
2600	119	Carbon monoxide and Hydrogen mixture
2600	119	Carbon monoxide and Hydrogen mixture, compressed
2600	119	Hydrogen and Carbon monoxide mixture
2600	119	Hydrogen and Carbon monoxide mixture, compressed
2601	115	Cyclobutane
2602	126	Dichlorodifluoromethane and Difluoroethane azeotropic mixture with approximately 74% Dichlorodifluoromethane
2602	126	Difluoroethane and Dichlorodifluoromethane azeotropic mixture with approximately 74% Dichlorodifluoromethane
2602	126	Refrigerant gas R-12 and Refrigerant gas R-152a azeotropic mixture with 74% Refrigerant gas R-12
2602	126	Refrigerant gas R-152a and Refrigerant gas R-12 azeotropic mixture with 74% Refrigerant gas R-12
2602	126	Refrigerant gas R-500 (azeotropic mixture of Refrigerant gas R-12 and Refrigerant gas R-152a with approximately 74% Refrigerant gas R-12)
2603	131	Cycloheptatriene
2604	132	Boron trifluoride diethyl etherate
2605	155	Methoxymethyl isocyanate
2606	155	Methyl orthosilicate
2607	129P	Acrolein dimer, stabilized
2608	129	Nitropropanes
2609	156	Triallyl borate
2610	132	Triallylamine
2611	131	Propylene chlorohydrin
2612	127	Methyl propyl ether
2614	129	Methallyl alcohol
2615	127	Ethyl propyl ether
2616	129	Triisopropyl borate
2617	129	Methylcyclohexanols
2618	130P	Vinyltoluenes, stabilized
2619	132	Benzyldimethylamine
2620	130	Amyl butyrates
2621	127	Acetyl methyl carbinol
2622	131P	Glycidaldehyde
2623	133	Firelighters, solid, with flammable liquid
2624	138	Magnesium silicide
2626	140	Chloric acid, aqueous solution, with not more than 10% Chloric acid
2627	140	Nitrites, inorganic, n.o.s.
2628	151	Potassium fluoroacetate
2629	151	Sodium fluoroacetate
2630	151	Selenates

ID No.	Guide No.	Name of Material	ID No.	Guide No.	Name of Material
2630	151	Selenites	2670	157	Cyanuric chloride
2630	151	Sodium selenite	2671	153	Aminopyridines
2642	154	Fluoroacetic acid	2672	154	Ammonia, solution, with more than 10% but not more than 35% Ammonia
2643	155	Methyl bromoacetate			
2644	151	Methyl iodide	2672	154	Ammonium hydroxide
2645	153	Phenacyl bromide	2672	154	Ammonium hydroxide, with more than 10% but not more than 35% Ammonia
2646	151	Hexachlorocyclopentadiene			
2647	153	Malononitrile			
2648	154	1,2-Dibromobutan-3-one	2673	151	2-Amino-4-chlorophenol
2649	153	1,3-Dichloroacetone	2674	154	Sodium fluorosilicate
2650	153	1,1-Dichloro-1-nitroethane	2674	154	Sodium silicofluoride
2651	153	4,4'-Diaminodiphenylmethane	2676	119	Stibine
2653	156	Benzyl iodide	2677	154	Rubidium hydroxide, solution
2655	151	Potassium fluorosilicate	2678	154	Rubidium hydroxide
2655	151	Potassium silicofluoride	2678	154	Rubidium hydroxide, solid
2656	154	Quinoline	2679	154	Lithium hydroxide, solution
2657	153	Selenium disulfide	2680	154	Lithium hydroxide
2657	153	Selenium disulphide	2680	154	Lithium hydroxide, monohydrate
2658	152	Selenium powder	2680	154	Lithium hydroxide, solid
2659	151	Sodium chloroacetate	2681	154	Caesium hydroxide, solution
2660	153	Mononitrotoluidines	2681	154	Cesium hydroxide, solution
2660	153	Nitrotoluidines (mono)	2682	157	Caesium hydroxide
2661	153	Hexachloroacetone	2682	157	Cesium hydroxide
2662	153	Hydroquinone	2683	132	Ammonium sulfide, solution
2662	153	Hydroquinone, solid	2683	132	Ammonium sulphide, solution
2664	160	Dibromomethane	2684	132	3-Diethylaminopropylamine
2666	156	Ethyl cyanoacetate	2684	132	Diethylaminopropylamine
2667	152	Butyltoluenes	2685	132	N,N-Diethylethylenediamine
2668	131	Chloroacetonitrile	2686	132	2-Diethylaminoethanol
2669	152	Chlorocresols	2686	132	Diethylaminoethanol
2669	152	Chlorocresols, liquid	2687	133	Dicyclohexylammonium nitrite
2669	152	Chlorocresols, solid	2688	159	1-Bromo-3-chloropropane
2669	152	Chlorocresols, solution	2688	159	1-Chloro-3-bromopropane

ID No.	Guide No.	Name of Material	ID No.	Guide No.	Name of Material
2689	153	Glycerol alpha-monochlorohydrin	2726	140	Nickel nitrite
2690	152	N,n-Butylimidazole	2727	141	Thallium nitrate
2691	137	Phosphorus pentabromide	2728	140	Zirconium nitrate
2692	157	Boron tribromide	2729	152	Hexachlorobenzene
2693	154	Bisulfites, aqueous solution, n.o.s.	2730	152	Nitroanisoles
			2730	152	Nitroanisoles, liquid
2693	154	Bisulfites, inorganic, aqueous solution, n.o.s.	2730	152	Nitroanisoles, solid
			2732	152	Nitrobromobenzenes
2693	154	Bisulphites, aqueous solution, n.o.s.	2732	152	Nitrobromobenzenes, liquid
			2732	152	Nitrobromobenzenes, solid
2693	154	Bisulphites, inorganic, aqueous solution, n.o.s.	2733	132	Alkylamines, n.o.s.
			2733	132	Amines, flammable, corrosive, n.o.s.
2698	156	Tetrahydrophthalic anhydrides	2733	132	Polyalkylamines, n.o.s.
2699	154	Trifluoroacetic acid	2733	132	Polyamines, flammable, corrosive, n.o.s.
2705	153P	1-Pentol			
2707	127	Dimethyldioxanes	2734	132	Alkylamines, n.o.s.
2708	127	Butoxyl	2734	132	Amines, liquid, corrosive, flammable, n.o.s.
2709	128	Butylbenzenes			
2710	128	Dipropyl ketone	2734	132	Polyalkylamines, n.o.s.
2711	129	Dibromobenzene	2734	132	Polyamines, liquid, corrosive, flammable, n.o.s.
2713	153	Acridine			
2714	133	Zinc resinate	2735	153	Alkylamines, n.o.s.
2715	133	Aluminum resinate	2735	153	Amines, liquid, corrosive, n.o.s.
2716	153	1,4-Butynediol	2735	153	Polyalkylamines, n.o.s.
2717	133	Camphor	2735	153	Polyamines, liquid, corrosive, n.o.s.
2717	133	Camphor, synthetic			
2719	141	Barium bromate	2738	153	N-Butylaniline
2720	141	Chromium nitrate	2739	156	Butyric anhydride
2721	141	Copper chlorate	2740	155	n-Propyl chloroformate
2722	140	Lithium nitrate	2741	141	Barium hypochlorite, with more than 22% available Chlorine
2723	140	Magnesium chlorate			
2724	140	Manganese nitrate	2742	155	sec-Butyl chloroformate
2725	140	Nickel nitrate	2742	155	Chloroformates, n.o.s.

ID No.	Guide No.	Name of Material
2742	155	Chloroformates, poisonous, corrosive, flammable, n.o.s.
2742	155	Chloroformates, toxic, corrosive, flammable, n.o.s.
2742	155	Isobutyl chloroformate
2743	155	n-Butyl chloroformate
2744	155	Cyclobutyl chloroformate
2745	157	Chloromethyl chloroformate
2746	156	Phenyl chloroformate
2747	156	tert-Butylcyclohexyl chloroformate
2748	156	2-Ethylhexyl chloroformate
2749	130	Tetramethylsilane
2750	153	1,3-Dichloropropanol-2
2751	155	Diethylthiophosphoryl chloride
2752	127	1,2-Epoxy-3-ethoxypropane
2753	153	N-Ethylbenzyltoluidines
2753	153	N-Ethylbenzyltoluidines, liquid
2753	153	N-Ethylbenzyltoluidines, solid
2754	153	N-Ethyltoluidines
2757	151	Carbamate pesticide, solid, poisonous
2757	151	Carbamate pesticide, solid, toxic
2758	131	Carbamate pesticide, liquid, flammable, poisonous
2758	131	Carbamate pesticide, liquid, flammable, toxic
2759	151	Arsenical pesticide, solid, poisonous
2759	151	Arsenical pesticide, solid, toxic
2760	131	Arsenical pesticide, liquid, flammable, poisonous
2760	131	Arsenical pesticide, liquid, flammable, toxic

ID No.	Guide No.	Name of Material
2761	151	Aldrin, solid
2761	151	Dieldrin
2761	151	Organochlorine pesticide, solid, poisonous
2761	151	Organochlorine pesticide, solid, toxic
2762	131	Aldrin, liquid
2762	131	Organochlorine pesticide, liquid, flammable, poisonous
2762	131	Organochlorine pesticide, liquid, flammable, toxic
2763	151	Triazine pesticide, solid, poisonous
2763	151	Triazine pesticide, solid, toxic
2764	131	Triazine pesticide, liquid, flammable, poisonous
2764	131	Triazine pesticide, liquid, flammable, toxic
2765	152	Phenoxy pesticide, solid, poisonous
2765	152	Phenoxy pesticide, solid, toxic
2766	131	Phenoxy pesticide, liquid, flammable, poisonous
2766	131	Phenoxy pesticide, liquid, flammable, toxic
2767	151	Phenyl urea pesticide, solid, poisonous
2767	151	Phenyl urea pesticide, solid, toxic
2768	131	Phenyl urea pesticide, liquid, flammable, poisonous
2768	131	Phenyl urea pesticide, liquid, flammable, toxic
2769	151	Benzoic derivative pesticide, solid, poisonous
2769	151	Benzoic derivative pesticide, solid, toxic

ID No.	Guide No.	Name of Material
2770	131	Benzoic derivative pesticide, liquid, flammable, poisonous
2770	131	Benzoic derivative pesticide, liquid, flammable, toxic
2771	151	Dithiocarbamate pesticide, solid, poisonous
2771	151	Dithiocarbamate pesticide, solid, toxic
2771	151	Thiocarbamate pesticide, solid, poisonous
2771	151	Thiocarbamate pesticide, solid, toxic
2772	131	Dithiocarbamate pesticide, liquid, flammable, poisonous
2772	131	Dithiocarbamate pesticide, liquid, flammable, toxic
2772	131	Thiocarbamate pesticide, liquid, flammable, poisonous
2772	131	Thiocarbamate pesticide, liquid, flammable, toxic
2773	151	Phthalimide derivative pesticide, solid, poisonous
2773	151	Phthalimide derivative pesticide, solid, toxic
2774	131	Phthalimide derivative pesticide, liquid, flammable, poisonous
2774	131	Phthalimide derivative pesticide, liquid, flammable, toxic
2775	151	Copper based pesticide, solid, poisonous
2775	151	Copper based pesticide, solid, toxic
2776	131	Copper based pesticide, liquid, flammable, poisonous
2776	131	Copper based pesticide, liquid, flammable, toxic
2777	151	Mercury based pesticide, solid, poisonous

ID No.	Guide No.	Name of Material
2777	151	Mercury based pesticide, solid, toxic
2778	131	Mercury based pesticide, liquid, flammable, poisonous
2778	131	Mercury based pesticide, liquid, flammable, toxic
2779	153	Substituted nitrophenol pesticide, solid, poisonous
2779	153	Substituted nitrophenol pesticide, solid, toxic
2780	131	Substituted nitrophenol pesticide, liquid, flammable, poisonous
2780	131	Substituted nitrophenol pesticide, liquid, flammable, toxic
2781	151	Bipyridilium pesticide, solid, poisonous
2781	151	Bipyridilium pesticide, solid, toxic
2782	131	Bipyridilium pesticide, liquid, flammable, poisonous
2782	131	Bipyridilium pesticide, liquid, flammable, toxic
2783	152	Methyl parathion, solid
2783	152	Organophosphorus pesticide, solid, poisonous
2783	152	Organophosphorus pesticide, solid, toxic
2783	152	Parathion
2783	152	Tetraethyl pyrophosphate, solid
2784	131	Organophosphorus pesticide, liquid, flammable, poisonous
2784	131	Organophosphorus pesticide, liquid, flammable, toxic
2785	152	4-Thiapentanal
2785	152	Thia-4-pentanal

ID No.	Guide No.	Name of Material
2786	153	Organotin pesticide, solid, poisonous
2786	153	Organotin pesticide, solid, toxic
2787	131	Organotin pesticide, liquid, flammable, poisonous
2787	131	Organotin pesticide, liquid, flammable, toxic
2788	153	Organotin compound, liquid, n.o.s.
2789	132	Acetic acid, glacial
2789	132	Acetic acid, solution, more than 80% acid
2790	153	Acetic acid, solution, more than 10% but not more than 80% acid
2793	170	Ferrous metal borings, shavings, turnings or cuttings
2794	154	Batteries, wet, filled with acid
2795	154	Batteries, wet, filled with alkali
2796	157	Battery fluid, acid
2796	157	Sulfuric acid, with not more than 51% acid
2796	157	Sulphuric acid, with not more than 51% acid
2797	154	Battery fluid, alkali
2797	154	Battery fluid, alkali, with battery
2797	154	Battery fluid, alkali, with electronic equipment or actuating device
2798	137	Benzene phosphorus dichloride
2798	137	Phenylphosphorus dichloride
2799	137	Benzene phosphorus thiodichloride
2799	137	Phenylphosphorus thiodichloride
2800	154	Batteries, wet, non-spillable
2801	154	Dye, liquid, corrosive, n.o.s.
2801	154	Dye intermediate, liquid, corrosive, n.o.s.
2802	154	Copper chloride
2803	172	Gallium
2805	138	Lithium hydride, fused solid
2806	138	Lithium nitride
2807	171	Magnetized material
2809	172	Mercury
2809	172	Mercury metal
2810	153	Buzz
2810	153	BZ
2810	153	Compound, tree or weed killing, liquid (toxic)
2810	153	CS
2810	153	DC
2810	153	GA
2810	153	GB
2810	153	GD
2810	153	GF
2810	153	H
2810	153	HD
2810	153	HL
2810	153	HN-1
2810	153	HN-2
2810	153	HN-3
2810	153	L (Lewisite)
2810	153	Lewisite
2810	153	Mustard
2810	153	Mustard Lewisite
2810	153	Poison B, liquid, n.o.s.
2810	153	Poisonous liquid, n.o.s.
2810	153	Poisonous liquid, n.o.s. (Inhalation Hazard Zone A)

ID No.	Guide No.	Name of Material
2810	153	Poisonous liquid, n.o.s. (Inhalation Hazard Zone B)
2810	153	Poisonous liquid, organic, n.o.s.
2810	153	Poisonous liquid, organic, n.o.s. (Inhalation Hazard Zone A)
2810	153	Poisonous liquid, organic, n.o.s. (Inhalation Hazard Zone B)
2810	153	Sarin
2810	153	Soman
2810	153	Tabun
2810	153	Thickened GD
2810	153	Toxic liquid, n.o.s.
2810	153	Toxic liquid, n.o.s. (Inhalation Hazard Zone A)
2810	153	Toxic liquid, n.o.s. (Inhalation Hazard Zone B)
2810	153	Toxic liquid, organic, n.o.s.
2810	153	Toxic liquid, organic, n.o.s. (Inhalation Hazard Zone A)
2810	153	Toxic liquid, organic, n.o.s. (Inhalation Hazard Zone B)
2810	153	VX
2811	154	CX
2811	154	Poisonous solid, organic, n.o.s.
2811	154	Selenium oxide
2811	154	Toxic solid, organic, n.o.s.
2812	154	Sodium aluminate, solid
2813	138	Water-reactive solid, n.o.s.
2814	158	Infectious substance, affecting humans
2815	153	N-Aminoethylpiperazine
2817	154	Ammonium bifluoride, solution
2817	154	Ammonium hydrogendifluoride, solution
2817	154	Ammonium hydrogen fluoride, solution
2818	154	Ammonium polysulfide, solution
2818	154	Ammonium polysulphide, solution
2819	153	Amyl acid phosphate
2820	153	Butyric acid
2821	153	Phenol solution
2822	153	2-Chloropyridine
2823	153	Crotonic acid
2823	153	Crotonic acid, liquid
2823	153	Crotonic acid, solid
2826	155	Ethyl chlorothioformate
2829	153	Caproic acid
2829	153	Hexanoic acid
2830	139	Lithium ferrosilicon
2831	160	1,1,1-Trichloroethane
2834	154	Phosphorous acid
2834	154	Phosphorous acid, ortho
2835	138	Sodium aluminum hydride
2837	154	Bisulfates, aqueous solution
2837	154	Bisulphates, aqueous solution
2837	154	Sodium bisulfate, solution
2837	154	Sodium bisulphate, solution
2837	154	Sodium hydrogen sulfate, solution
2837	154	Sodium hydrogen sulphate, solution
2838	129P	Vinyl butyrate, stabilized
2839	153	Aldol
2840	129	Butyraldoxime
2841	131	Di-n-amylamine
2842	129	Nitroethane
2844	138	Calcium manganese silicon
2845	135	Ethyl phosphonous dichloride, anhydrous

ID No.	Guide No.	Name of Material
2845	135	Methyl phosphonous dichloride
2845	135	Pyrophoric liquid, n.o.s.
2845	135	Pyrophoric liquid, organic, n.o.s.
2846	135	Pyrophoric solid, n.o.s.
2846	135	Pyrophoric solid, organic, n.o.s.
2849	153	3-Chloropropanol-1
2850	128	Propylene tetramer
2851	157	Boron trifluoride, dihydrate
2852	113	Dipicryl sulfide, wetted with not less than 10% water
2852	113	Dipicryl sulphide, wetted with not less than 10% water
2853	151	Magnesium fluorosilicate
2853	151	Magnesium silicofluoride
2854	151	Ammonium fluorosilicate
2854	151	Ammonium silicofluoride
2855	151	Zinc fluorosilicate
2855	151	Zinc silicofluoride
2856	151	Fluorosilicates, n.o.s.
2856	151	Silicofluorides, n.o.s.
2857	126	Refrigerating machines, containing Ammonia solutions (UN2672)
2857	126	Refrigerating machines, containing non-flammable, non-poisonous gases
2857	126	Refrigerating machines, containing non-flammable, non-toxic gases
2858	170	Zirconium, dry, coiled wire, finished metal sheets or strips
2859	154	Ammonium metavanadate
2861	151	Ammonium polyvanadate
2862	151	Vanadium pentoxide
2863	154	Sodium ammonium vanadate
2864	151	Potassium metavanadate
2865	154	Hydroxylamine sulfate
2865	154	Hydroxylamine sulphate
2869	157	Titanium trichloride mixture
2870	135	Aluminum borohydride
2870	135	Aluminum borohydride in devices
2871	170	Antimony powder
2872	159	Dibromochloropropanes
2873	153	Dibutylaminoethanol
2874	153	Furfuryl alcohol
2875	151	Hexachlorophene
2876	153	Resorcinol
2878	170	Titanium sponge granules
2878	170	Titanium sponge powders
2879	157	Selenium oxychloride
2880	140	Calcium hypochlorite, hydrated, with not less than 5.5% but not more than 16% water
2880	140	Calcium hypochlorite, hydrated mixture, with not less than 5.5% but not more than 16% water
2881	135	Metal catalyst, dry
2881	135	Nickel catalyst, dry
2900	158	Infectious substance, affecting animals only
2901	124	Bromine chloride
2902	151	Pesticide, liquid, poisonous, n.o.s.
2902	151	Pesticide, liquid, toxic, n.o.s.
2903	131	Pesticide, liquid, poisonous, flammable, n.o.s.
2903	131	Pesticide, liquid, toxic, flammable, n.o.s.

ID No.	Guide No.	Name of Material	ID No.	Guide No.	Name of Material
2904	154	Chlorophenates, liquid	2910	161	Radioactive material, excepted package, limited quantity of material
2904	154	Chlorophenolates, liquid			
2904	154	Phenolates, liquid	2911	161	Radioactive material, excepted package, instruments or articles
2905	154	Chlorophenates, solid			
2905	154	Chlorophenolates, solid	2912	162	Radioactive material, low specific activity (LSA), n.o.s.
2905	154	Phenolates, solid			
2907	133	Isosorbide dinitrate mixture	2912	162	Radioactive material, low specific activity (LSA-I) non fissile or fissile-excepted
2908	161	Radioactive material, excepted package, empty packaging			
2909	161	Radioactive material, excepted package, articles manufactured from depleted Uranium	2913	162	Radioactive material, surface contaminated objects (SCO)
			2913	162	Radioactive material, surface contaminated objects (SCO-I) non fissile or fissile-excepted
2909	161	Radioactive material, excepted package, articles manufactured from natural Thorium	2913	162	Radioactive material, surface contaminated objects (SCO-II) non fissile or fissile-excepted
2909	161	Radioactive material, excepted package, articles manufactured from natural Uranium	2915	163	Radioactive material, Type A package non-special form, non fissile or fissile-excepted
2910	161	Radioactive material, excepted package, articles manufactured from depleted Uranium	2916	163	Radioactive material, Type B(U) package non fissile or fissile-excepted
2910	161	Radioactive material, excepted package, articles manufactured from natural Thorium	2917	163	Radioactive material, Type B(M) package non fissile or fissile-excepted
2910	161	Radioactive material, excepted package, articles manufactured from natural Uranium	2918	165	Radioactive material, fissile, n.o.s.
			2919	163	Radioactive material, transported under special arrangement non fissile or fissile-excepted
2910	161	Radioactive material, excepted package, empty packaging			
			2920	132	Corrosive liquid, flammable, n.o.s.
2910	161	Radioactive material, excepted package, instruments or articles	2920	132	Dichlorobutene
			2921	134	Corrosive solid, flammable, n.o.s.

ID No.	Guide No.	Name of Material
2922	154	Corrosive liquid, poisonous, n.o.s.
2922	154	Corrosive liquid, toxic, n.o.s.
2922	154	Sodium hydrosulfide, solution
2922	154	Sodium hydrosulphide, solution
2923	154	Corrosive solid, poisonous, n.o.s.
2923	154	Corrosive solid, toxic, n.o.s.
2924	132	Flammable liquid, corrosive, n.o.s
2925	134	Flammable solid, corrosive, n.o.s.
2925	134	Flammable solid, corrosive, organic, n.o.s.
2926	134	Flammable solid, poisonous, n.o.s.
2926	134	Flammable solid, poisonous, organic, n.o.s.
2926	134	Flammable solid, toxic, organic, n.o.s.
2927	154	Ethyl phosphonothioic dichloride, anhydrous
2927	154	Ethyl phosphorodichloridate
2927	154	Poisonous liquid, corrosive, n.o.s.
2927	154	Poisonous liquid, corrosive, n.o.s. (Inhalation Hazard Zone A)
2927	154	Poisonous liquid, corrosive, n.o.s. (Inhalation Hazard Zone B)
2927	154	Poisonous liquid, corrosive, organic, n.o.s.
2927	154	Poisonous liquid, corrosive, organic, n.o.s. (Inhalation Hazard Zone A)
2927	154	Poisonous liquid, corrosive, organic, n.o.s. (Inhalation Hazard Zone B)
2927	154	Toxic liquid, corrosive, n.o.s.
2927	154	Toxic liquid, corrosive, n.o.s. (Inhalation Hazard Zone A)
2927	154	Toxic liquid, corrosive, n.o.s. (Inhalation Hazard Zone B)
2927	154	Toxic liquid, corrosive, organic, n.o.s.
2927	154	Toxic liquid, corrosive, organic, n.o.s. (Inhalation Hazard Zone A)
2927	154	Toxic liquid, corrosive, organic, n.o.s. (Inhalation Hazard Zone B)
2928	154	Poisonous solid, corrosive, n.o.s.
2928	154	Toxic solid, corrosive, organic, n.o.s.
2929	131	Poisonous liquid, flammable, n.o.s.
2929	131	Poisonous liquid, flammable, n.o.s. (Inhalation Hazard Zone A)
2929	131	Poisonous liquid, flammable, n.o.s. (Inhalation Hazard Zone B)
2929	131	Poisonous liquid, flammable, organic, n.o.s.
2929	131	Poisonous liquid, flammable, organic, n.o.s. (Inhalation Hazard Zone A)
2929	131	Poisonous liquid, flammable, organic, n.o.s. (Inhalation Hazard Zone B)
2929	131	Toxic liquid, flammable, n.o.s.
2929	131	Toxic liquid, flammable, n.o.s. (Inhalation Hazard Zone A)
2929	131	Toxic liquid, flammable, n.o.s. (Inhalation Hazard Zone B)
2929	131	Toxic liquid, flammable, organic, n.o.s.

ID No.	Guide No.	Name of Material
2929	**131**	Toxic liquid, flammable, organic, n.o.s. (Inhalation Hazard Zone A)
2929	**131**	Toxic liquid, flammable, organic, n.o.s. (Inhalation Hazard Zone B)
2930	**134**	Poisonous solid, flammable, n.o.s.
2930	**134**	Poisonous solid, flammable, organic, n.o.s.
2930	**134**	Toxic solid, flammable, n.o.s.
2930	**134**	Toxic solid, flammable, organic, n.o.s.
2931	**151**	Vanadyl sulfate
2931	**151**	Vanadyl sulphate
2933	**129**	Methyl 2-chloropropionate
2934	**129**	Isopropyl 2-chloropropionate
2935	**129**	Ethyl 2-chloropropionate
2936	**153**	Thiolactic acid
2937	**153**	alpha-Methylbenzyl alcohol
2937	**153**	alpha-Methylbenzyl alcohol, liquid
2937	**153**	Methylbenzyl alcohol (alpha)
2938	**152**	Methyl benzoate
2940	**135**	Cyclooctadiene phosphines
2940	**135**	9-Phosphabicyclononanes
2941	**153**	Fluoroanilines
2942	**153**	2-Trifluoromethylaniline
2943	**129**	Tetrahydrofurfurylamine
2945	**132**	N-Methylbutylamine
2946	**153**	2-Amino-5-diethylaminopentane
2947	**155**	Isopropyl chloroacetate
2948	**153**	3-Trifluoromethylaniline
2949	**154**	Sodium hydrosulfide, with not less than 25% water of crystallization
2949	**154**	Sodium hydrosulphide, with not less than 25% water of crystallization
2950	**138**	Magnesium granules, coated
2956	**149**	5-tert-Butyl-2,4,6-trinitro-m-xylene
2956	**149**	Musk xylene
2965	**139**	Boron trifluoride dimethyl etherate
2966	**153**	Thioglycol
2967	**154**	Sulfamic acid
2967	**154**	Sulphamic acid
2968	**135**	Maneb, stabilized
2968	**135**	Maneb preparation, stabilized
2969	**171**	Castor beans, meal, pomace or flake
2974	**164**	Radioactive material, special form, n.o.s.
2975	**162**	Thorium metal, pyrophoric
2976	**162**	Thorium nitrate, solid
2977	**166**	Radioactive material, Uranium hexafluoride, fissile
2977	**166**	Uranium hexafluoride, fissile containing more than 1% Uranium-235
2978	**166**	Radioactive material, Uranium hexafluoride
2978	**166**	Uranium hexafluoride
2978	**166**	Uranium hexafluoride non fissile or fissile-excepted
2979	**162**	Uranium metal, pyrophoric
2980	**162**	Uranyl nitrate, hexahydrate, solution
2981	**162**	Uranyl nitrate, solid
2982	**163**	Radioactive material, n.o.s.

ID No.	Guide No.	Name of Material
2983	129P	Ethylene oxide and Propylene oxide mixture, with not more than 30% Ethylene oxide
2983	129P	Propylene oxide and Ethylene oxide mixture, with not more than 30% Ethylene oxide
2984	140	Hydrogen peroxide, aqueous solution, with not less than 8% but less than 20% Hydrogen peroxide
2985	155	Chlorosilanes, flammable, corrosive, n.o.s.
2985	155	Chlorosilanes, n.o.s.
2986	155	Chlorosilanes, corrosive, flammable, n.o.s.
2986	155	Chlorosilanes, n.o.s.
2987	156	Chlorosilanes, corrosive, n.o.s.
2987	156	Chlorosilanes, n.o.s.
2988	139	Chlorosilanes, n.o.s.
2988	139	Chlorosilanes, water-reactive, flammable, corrosive, n.o.s.
2989	133	Lead phosphite, dibasic
2990	171	Life-saving appliances, self-inflating
2991	131	Carbamate pesticide, liquid, poisonous, flammable
2991	131	Carbamate pesticide, liquid, toxic, flammable
2992	151	Carbamate pesticide, liquid, poisonous
2992	151	Carbamate pesticide, liquid, toxic
2993	131	Arsenical pesticide, liquid, poisonous, flammable
2993	131	Arsenical pesticide, liquid, toxic, flammable
2994	151	Arsenical pesticide, liquid, poisonous
2994	151	Arsenical pesticide, liquid, toxic
2995	131	Organochlorine pesticide, liquid, poisonous, flammable
2995	131	Organochlorine pesticide, liquid, toxic, flammable
2996	151	Organochlorine pesticide, liquid, poisonous
2996	151	Organochlorine pesticide, liquid, toxic
2997	131	Triazine pesticide, liquid, poisonous, flammable
2997	131	Triazine pesticide, liquid, toxic, flammable
2998	151	Triazine pesticide, liquid, poisonous
2998	151	Triazine pesticide, liquid, toxic
2999	131	Phenoxy pesticide, liquid, poisonous, flammable
2999	131	Phenoxy pesticide, liquid, toxic, flammable
3000	152	Phenoxy pesticide, liquid, poisonous
3000	152	Phenoxy pesticide, liquid, toxic
3001	131	Phenyl urea pesticide, liquid, poisonous, flammable
3001	131	Phenyl urea pesticide, liquid, toxic, flammable
3002	151	Phenyl urea pesticide, liquid, poisonous
3002	151	Phenyl urea pesticide, liquid, toxic
3003	131	Benzoic derivative pesticide, liquid, poisonous, flammable
3003	131	Benzoic derivative pesticide, liquid, toxic, flammable
3004	151	Benzoic derivative pesticide, liquid, poisonous

ID No.	Guide No.	Name of Material
3004	151	Benzoic derivative pesticide, liquid, toxic
3005	131	Dithiocarbamate pesticide, liquid, poisonous, flammable
3005	131	Dithiocarbamate pesticide, liquid, toxic, flammable
3005	131	Thiocarbamate pesticide, liquid, poisonous, flammable
3005	131	Thiocarbamate pesticide, liquid, toxic, flammable
3006	151	Dithiocarbamate pesticide, liquid, poisonous
3006	151	Dithiocarbamate pesticide, liquid, toxic
3006	151	Thiocarbamate pesticide, liquid, poisonous
3006	151	Thiocarbamate pesticide, liquid, toxic
3007	131	Phthalimide derivative pesticide, liquid, poisonous, flammable
3007	131	Phthalimide derivative pesticide, liquid, toxic, flammable
3008	151	Phthalimide derivative pesticide, liquid, poisonous
3008	151	Phthalimide derivative pesticide, liquid, toxic
3009	131	Copper based pesticide, liquid, poisonous, flammable
3009	131	Copper based pesticide, liquid, toxic, flammable
3010	151	Copper based pesticide, liquid, poisonous
3010	151	Copper based pesticide, liquid, toxic
3011	131	Mercury based pesticide, liquid, poisonous, flammable
3011	131	Mercury based pesticide, liquid, toxic, flammable
3012	151	Mercury based pesticide, liquid, poisonous
3012	151	Mercury based pesticide, liquid, toxic
3013	131	Substituted nitrophenol pesticide, liquid, poisonous, flammable
3013	131	Substituted nitrophenol pesticide, liquid, toxic, flammable
3014	153	Substituted nitrophenol pesticide, liquid, poisonous
3014	153	Substituted nitrophenol pesticide, liquid, toxic
3015	131	Bipyridilium pesticide, liquid, poisonous, flammable
3015	131	Bipyridilium pesticide, liquid, toxic, flammable
3016	151	Bipyridilium pesticide, liquid, poisonous
3016	151	Bipyridilium pesticide, liquid, toxic
3017	131	Organophosphorus pesticide, liquid, poisonous, flammable
3017	131	Organophosphorus pesticide, liquid, toxic, flammable
3018	152	Methyl parathion, liquid
3018	152	Organophosphorus pesticide, liquid, poisonous
3018	152	Organophosphorus pesticide, liquid, toxic
3018	152	Tetraethyl pyrophosphate, liquid
3019	131	Organotin pesticide, liquid, poisonous, flammable
3019	131	Organotin pesticide, liquid, toxic, flammable
3020	153	Organotin pesticide, liquid, poisonous

ID No.	Guide No.	Name of Material
3020	153	Organotin pesticide, liquid, toxic
3021	131	Pesticide, liquid, flammable, poisonous, n.o.s.
3021	131	Pesticide, liquid, flammable, toxic, n.o.s.
3022	127P	1,2-Butylene oxide, stabilized
3023	131	2-Methyl-2-heptanethiol
3023	131	tert-Octyl mercaptan
3024	131	Coumarin derivative pesticide, liquid, flammable, poisonous
3024	131	Coumarin derivative pesticide, liquid, flammable, toxic
3025	131	Coumarin derivative pesticide, liquid, poisonous, flammable
3025	131	Coumarin derivative pesticide, liquid, toxic, flammable
3026	151	Coumarin derivative pesticide, liquid, poisonous
3026	151	Coumarin derivative pesticide, liquid, toxic
3027	151	Coumarin derivative pesticide, solid, poisonous
3027	151	Coumarin derivative pesticide, solid, toxic
3028	154	Batteries, dry, containing Potassium hydroxide solid
3048	157	Aluminum phosphide pesticide
3049	138	Metal alkyl halides, n.o.s.
3049	138	Metal alkyl halides, water-reactive, n.o.s.
3049	138	Metal aryl halides, n.o.s.
3049	138	Metal aryl halides, water-reactive, n.o.s.
3050	138	Metal alkyl hydrides, n.o.s.
3050	138	Metal alkyl hydrides, water-reactive, n.o.s.
3050	138	Metal aryl hydrides, n.o.s.
3050	138	Metal aryl hydrides, water-reactive, n.o.s.
3051	135	Aluminum alkyls
3052	135	Aluminum alkyl halides
3052	135	Aluminum alkyl halides, liquid
3052	135	Aluminum alkyl halides, solid
3053	135	Magnesium alkyls
3054	129	Cyclohexanethiol
3054	129	Cyclohexyl mercaptan
3055	154	2-(2-Aminoethoxy)ethanol
3056	129	n-Heptaldehyde
3057	125	Trifluoroacetyl chloride
3064	127	Nitroglycerin, solution in alcohol, with more than 1% but not more than 5% Nitroglycerin
3065	127	Alcoholic beverages
3066	153	Paint (corrosive)
3066	153	Paint related material (corrosive)
3070	126	Dichlorodifluoromethane and Ethylene oxide mixture, with not more than 12.5% Ethylene oxide
3070	126	Dichlorodifluoromethane and Ethylene oxide mixtures, with not more than 12% Ethylene oxide
3070	126	Ethylene oxide and Dichlorodifluoromethane mixture, with not more than 12.5% Ethylene oxide
3070	126	Ethylene oxide and Dichlorodifluoromethane mixtures, with not more than 12% Ethylene oxide

ID No.	Guide No.	Name of Material
3071	131	Mercaptan mixture, liquid, poisonous, flammable, n.o.s.
3071	131	Mercaptan mixture, liquid, toxic, flammable, n.o.s.
3071	131	Mercaptans, liquid, poisonous, flammable, n.o.s.
3071	131	Mercaptans, liquid, toxic, flammable, n.o.s.
3072	171	Life-saving appliances, not self-inflating
3073	131P	Vinylpyridines, stabilized
3076	138	Aluminum alkyl hydrides
3077	171	Environmentally hazardous substances, solid, n.o.s.
3077	171	Hazardous waste, solid, n.o.s.
3077	171	Other regulated substances, solid, n.o.s.
3078	138	Cerium, turnings or gritty powder
3079	131P	Methacrylonitrile, stabilized
3080	155	Isocyanate solution, poisonous, flammable, n.o.s.
3080	155	Isocyanate solution, toxic, flammable, n.o.s.
3080	155	Isocyanate solutions, n.o.s.
3080	155	Isocyanates, n.o.s.
3080	155	Isocyanates, poisonous, flammable, n.o.s.
3080	155	Isocyanates, toxic, flammable, n.o.s.
3082	171	Environmentally hazardous substances, liquid, n.o.s.
3082	171	Hazardous waste, liquid, n.o.s.
3082	171	Other regulated substances, liquid, n.o.s.
3083	124	Perchloryl fluoride
3084	140	Corrosive solid, oxidizing, n.o.s.
3085	140	Oxidizing solid, corrosive, n.o.s.
3086	141	Poisonous solid, oxidizing, n.o.s.
3086	141	Toxic solid, oxidizing, n.o.s.
3087	141	Oxidizing solid, poisonous, n.o.s.
3087	141	Oxidizing solid, toxic, n.o.s.
3088	135	Self-heating solid, organic, n.o.s.
3089	170	Metal powder, flammable, n.o.s.
3090	138	Lithium batteries
3090	138	Lithium batteries, liquid or solid cathode
3090	138	Lithium metal batteries (including lithium alloy batteries)
3091	138	Lithium batteries contained in equipment
3091	138	Lithium batteries packed with equipment
3091	138	Lithium metal batteries contained in equipment (including lithium alloy batteries)
3091	138	Lithium metal batteries packed with equipment (including lithium alloy batteries)
3092	129	1-Methoxy-2-propanol
3093	140	Corrosive liquid, oxidizing, n.o.s.
3094	138	Corrosive liquid, water-reactive, n.o.s.
3094	138	Corrosive liquid, which in contact with water emits flammable gases, n.o.s.
3095	136	Corrosive solid, self-heating, n.o.s.
3096	138	Corrosive solid, water-reactive, n.o.s.

ID No.	Guide No.	Name of Material
3096	138	Corrosive solid, which in contact with water emits flammable gases, n.o.s.
3097	140	Flammable solid, oxidizing, n.o.s.
3098	140	Oxidizing liquid, corrosive, n.o.s.
3099	142	Oxidizing liquid, poisonous, n.o.s.
3099	142	Oxidizing liquid, toxic, n.o.s.
3100	135	Oxidizing solid, self-heating, n.o.s.
3101	146	Organic peroxide type B, liquid
3102	146	Organic peroxide type B, solid
3103	146	Organic peroxide type C, liquid
3104	146	Organic peroxide type C, solid
3105	145	Organic peroxide type D, liquid
3106	145	Organic peroxide type D, solid
3107	145	Organic peroxide type E, liquid
3108	145	Organic peroxide type E, solid
3109	145	Organic peroxide type F, liquid
3110	145	Organic peroxide type F, solid
3111	148	Organic peroxide type B, liquid, temperature controlled
3112	148	Organic peroxide type B, solid, temperature controlled
3113	148	Organic peroxide type C, liquid, temperature controlled
3114	148	Organic peroxide type C, solid, temperature controlled
3115	148	Organic peroxide type D, liquid, temperature controlled
3116	148	Organic peroxide type D, solid, temperature controlled
3117	148	Organic peroxide type E, liquid, temperature controlled
3118	148	Organic peroxide type E, solid, temperature controlled
3119	148	Organic peroxide type F, liquid, temperature controlled
3120	148	Organic peroxide type F, solid, temperature controlled
3121	144	Oxidizing solid, water-reactive, n.o.s.
3122	142	Poisonous liquid, oxidizing, n.o.s.
3122	142	Poisonous liquid, oxidizing, n.o.s. (Inhalation Hazard Zone A)
3122	142	Poisonous liquid, oxidizing, n.o.s. (Inhalation Hazard Zone B)
3122	142	Toxic liquid, oxidizing, n.o.s.
3122	142	Toxic liquid, oxidizing, n.o.s. (Inhalation Hazard Zone A)
3122	142	Toxic liquid, oxidizing, n.o.s. (Inhalation Hazard Zone B)
3123	139	Poisonous liquid, water-reactive, n.o.s.
3123	139	Poisonous liquid, water-reactive, n.o.s. (Inhalation Hazard Zone A)
3123	139	Poisonous liquid, water-reactive, n.o.s. (Inhalation Hazard Zone B)
3123	139	Poisonous liquid, which in contact with water emits flammable gases, n.o.s.
3123	139	Poisonous liquid, which in contact with water emits flammable gases, n.o.s. (Inhalation Hazard Zone A)
3123	139	Poisonous liquid, which in contact with water emits flammable gases, n.o.s. (Inhalation Hazard Zone B)

ID No.	Guide No.	Name of Material
3123	139	Toxic liquid, water-reactive, n.o.s.
3123	139	Toxic liquid, water-reactive, n.o.s. (Inhalation Hazard Zone A)
3123	139	Toxic liquid, water-reactive, n.o.s. (Inhalation Hazard Zone B)
3123	139	Toxic liquid, which in contact with water emits flammable gases, n.o.s.
3123	139	Toxic liquid, which in contact with water emits flammable gases, n.o.s. (Inhalation Hazard Zone A)
3123	139	Toxic liquid, which in contact with water emits flammable gases, n.o.s. (Inhalation Hazard Zone B)
3124	136	Poisonous solid, self-heating, n.o.s.
3124	136	Toxic solid, self-heating, n.o.s.
3125	139	Poisonous solid, water-reactive, n.o.s.
3125	139	Poisonous solid, which in contact with water emits flammable gases, n.o.s.
3125	139	Toxic solid, water-reactive, n.o.s.
3125	139	Toxic solid, which in contact with water emits flammable gases, n.o.s.
3126	136	Self-heating solid, corrosive, organic, n.o.s.
3127	135	Self-heating solid, oxidizing, n.o.s.
3128	136	Self-heating solid, poisonous, organic, n.o.s.
3128	136	Self-heating solid, toxic, organic, n.o.s.
3129	138	Water-reactive liquid, corrosive, n.o.s.
3130	139	Water-reactive liquid, poisonous, n.o.s.
3130	139	Water-reactive liquid, toxic, n.o.s.
3131	138	Water-reactive solid, corrosive, n.o.s.
3132	138	Water-reactive solid, flammable, n.o.s.
3133	138	Water-reactive solid, oxidizing, n.o.s.
3134	139	Water-reactive solid, poisonous, n.o.s.
3134	139	Water-reactive solid, toxic, n.o.s.
3135	138	Water-reactive solid, self-heating, n.o.s.
3136	120	Trifluoromethane, refrigerated liquid
3137	140	Oxidizing solid, flammable, n.o.s.
3138	115	Acetylene, Ethylene and Propylene in mixture, refrigerated liquid containing at least 71.5% Ethylene with not more than 22.5% Acetylene and not more than 6% Propylene
3138	115	Ethylene, Acetylene and Propylene in mixture, refrigerated liquid containing at least 71.5% Ethylene with not more than 22.5% Acetylene and not more than 6% Propylene

ID No.	Guide No.	Name of Material
3138	115	Propylene, Ethylene and Acetylene in mixture, refrigerated liquid containing at least 71.5% Ethylene with not more than 22.5% Acetylene and not more than 6% Propylene
3139	140	Oxidizing liquid, n.o.s.
3140	151	Alkaloids, liquid, n.o.s. (poisonous)
3140	151	Alkaloid salts, liquid, n.o.s. (poisonous)
3141	157	Antimony compound, inorganic, liquid, n.o.s.
3142	151	Disinfectant, liquid, poisonous, n.o.s.
3142	151	Disinfectant, liquid, toxic, n.o.s.
3142	151	Disinfectants, liquid, n.o.s. (poisonous)
3143	151	Dye, solid, poisonous, n.o.s.
3143	151	Dye, solid, toxic, n.o.s.
3143	151	Dye intermediate, solid, poisonous, n.o.s.
3143	151	Dye intermediate, solid, toxic, n.o.s.
3144	151	Nicotine compound, liquid, n.o.s.
3144	151	Nicotine preparation, liquid, n.o.s.
3145	153	Alkyl phenols, liquid, n.o.s. (including C2-C12 homologues)
3146	153	Organotin compound, solid, n.o.s.
3147	154	Dye, solid, corrosive, n.o.s.
3147	154	Dye intermediate, solid, corrosive, n.o.s.
3148	138	Water-reactive liquid, n.o.s.
3149	140	Hydrogen peroxide and Peroxyacetic acid mixture, with acid(s), water and not more than 5% Peroxyacetic acid, stabilized
3150	115	Devices, small, hydrocarbon gas powered, with release device
3150	115	Hydrocarbon gas refills for small devices, with release device
3151	171	Polyhalogenated biphenyls, liquid
3151	171	Polyhalogenated terphenyls, liquid
3152	171	Polyhalogenated biphenyls, solid
3152	171	Polyhalogenated terphenyls, solid
3153	115	Perfluoromethyl vinyl ether
3153	115	Perfluoro(methyl vinyl ether)
3154	115	Perfluoroethyl vinyl ether
3154	115	Perfluoro(ethyl vinyl ether)
3155	154	Pentachlorophenol
3156	122	Compressed gas, oxidizing, n.o.s.
3157	122	Liquefied gas, oxidizing, n.o.s.
3158	120	Gas, refrigerated liquid, n.o.s.
3159	126	Refrigerant gas R-134a
3159	126	1,1,1,2-Tetrafluoroethane
3160	119	Liquefied gas, poisonous, flammable, n.o.s.
3160	119	Liquefied gas, poisonous, flammable, n.o.s. (Inhalation Hazard Zone A)
3160	119	Liquefied gas, poisonous, flammable, n.o.s. (Inhalation Hazard Zone B)

ID No.	Guide No.	Name of Material	ID No.	Guide No.	Name of Material
3160	119	Liquefied gas, poisonous, flammable, n.o.s. (Inhalation Hazard Zone C)	3163	126	Liquefied gas, n.o.s.
3160	119	Liquefied gas, poisonous, flammable, n.o.s. (Inhalation Hazard Zone D)	3164	126	Articles, pressurized, hydraulic (containing non-flammable gas)
3160	119	Liquefied gas, toxic, flammable, n.o.s.	3164	126	Articles, pressurized, pneumatic (containing non-flammable gas)
3160	119	Liquefied gas, toxic, flammable, n.o.s. (Inhalation Hazard Zone A)	3165	131	Aircraft hydraulic power unit fuel tank
3160	119	Liquefied gas, toxic, flammable, n.o.s. (Inhalation Hazard Zone B)	3166	128	Engines, internal combustion, flammable gas powered
3160	119	Liquefied gas, toxic, flammable, n.o.s. (Inhalation Hazard Zone C)	3166	128	Engines, internal combustion, flammable liquid powered
3160	119	Liquefied gas, toxic, flammable, n.o.s. (Inhalation Hazard Zone D)	3166	128	Engines, internal combustion, including when fitted in machinery or vehicles
3161	115	Liquefied gas, flammable, n.o.s.	3166	128	Vehicle, flammable gas powered
3162	123	Liquefied gas, poisonous, n.o.s.	3166	128	Vehicle, flammable liquid powered
3162	123	Liquefied gas, poisonous, n.o.s. (Inhalation Hazard Zone A)	3167	115	Gas sample, non-pressurized, flammable, n.o.s., not refrigerated liquid
3162	123	Liquefied gas, poisonous, n.o.s. (Inhalation Hazard Zone B)	3168	119	Gas sample, non-pressurized, poisonous, flammable, n.o.s., not refrigerated liquid
3162	123	Liquefied gas, poisonous, n.o.s. (Inhalation Hazard Zone C)	3168	119	Gas sample, non-pressurized, toxic, flammable, n.o.s., not refrigerated liquid
3162	123	Liquefied gas, poisonous, n.o.s. (Inhalation Hazard Zone D)	3169	123	Gas sample, non-pressurized, poisonous, n.o.s., not refrigerated liquid
3162	123	Liquefied gas, toxic, n.o.s.	3169	123	Gas sample, non-pressurized, toxic, n.o.s., not refrigerated liquid
3162	123	Liquefied gas, toxic, n.o.s. (Inhalation Hazard Zone A)	3170	138	Aluminum dross
3162	123	Liquefied gas, toxic, n.o.s. (Inhalation Hazard Zone B)	3170	138	Aluminum processing by-products
3162	123	Liquefied gas, toxic, n.o.s. (Inhalation Hazard Zone C)	3170	138	Aluminum remelting by-products
3162	123	Liquefied gas, toxic, n.o.s. (Inhalation Hazard Zone D)			

ID No.	Guide No.	Name of Material	ID No.	Guide No.	Name of Material
3170	138	Aluminum smelting by-products	3184	136	Self-heating liquid, toxic, organic, n.o.s.
3171	154	Battery-powered equipment (wet battery)	3185	136	Self-heating liquid, corrosive, organic, n.o.s.
3171	154	Battery-powered vehicle (wet battery)	3186	135	Self-heating liquid, inorganic, n.o.s.
3171	154	Wheelchair, electric, with batteries	3187	136	Self-heating liquid, poisonous, inorganic, n.o.s.
3172	153	Toxins, extracted from living sources, liquid, n.o.s.	3187	136	Self-heating liquid, toxic, inorganic, n.o.s.
3172	153	Toxins, extracted from living sources, n.o.s.	3188	136	Self-heating liquid, corrosive, inorganic, n.o.s.
3172	153	Toxins, extracted from living sources, solid, n.o.s.	3189	135	Metal powder, self-heating, n.o.s.
3174	135	Titanium disulfide	3189	135	Self-heating metal powders, n.o.s.
3174	135	Titanium disulphide	3190	135	Self-heating solid, inorganic, n.o.s.
3175	133	Solids containing flammable liquid, n.o.s.	3191	136	Self-heating solid, inorganic, poisonous, n.o.s.
3176	133	Flammable solid, organic, molten, n.o.s.	3191	136	Self-heating solid, inorganic, toxic, n.o.s.
3178	133	Flammable solid, inorganic, n.o.s.	3191	136	Self-heating solid, poisonous, inorganic, n.o.s.
3178	133	Smokeless powder for small arms	3191	136	Self-heating solid, toxic, inorganic, n.o.s.
3179	134	Flammable solid, poisonous, inorganic, n.o.s.	3192	136	Self-heating solid, corrosive, inorganic, n.o.s.
3179	134	Flammable solid, toxic, inorganic, n.o.s.	3194	135	Pyrophoric liquid, inorganic, n.o.s.
3180	134	Flammable solid, corrosive, inorganic, n.o.s.	3200	135	Pyrophoric solid, inorganic, n.o.s.
3180	134	Flammable solid, inorganic, corrosive, n.o.s.	3203	135	Pyrophoric organometallic compound, n.o.s.
3181	133	Metal salts of organic compounds, flammable, n.o.s.	3203	135	Pyrophoric organometallic compound, water-reactive, n.o.s.
3182	170	Metal hydrides, flammable, n.o.s.	3205	135	Alkaline earth metal alcoholates, n.o.s.
3183	135	Self-heating liquid, organic, n.o.s.	3206	136	Alkali metal alcoholates, self-heating, corrosive, n.o.s.
3184	136	Self-heating liquid, poisonous, organic, n.o.s.			

ID No.	Guide No.	Name of Material	ID No.	Guide No.	Name of Material
3207	138	Organometallic compound, water-reactive, flammable, n.o.s.	3223	149	Self-reactive liquid type C
3207	138	Organometallic compound dispersion, water-reactive, flammable, n.o.s.	3224	149	Self-reactive solid type C
			3225	149	Self-reactive liquid type D
			3226	149	Self-reactive solid type D
3207	138	Organometallic compound solution, water-reactive, flammable, n.o.s.	3227	149	Self-reactive liquid type E
			3228	149	Self-reactive solid type E
3208	138	Metallic substance, water-reactive, n.o.s.	3229	149	Self-reactive liquid type F
			3230	149	Self-reactive solid type F
3209	138	Metallic substance, water-reactive, self-heating, n.o.s.	3231	150	Self-reactive liquid type B, temperature controlled
3210	140	Chlorates, inorganic, aqueous solution, n.o.s.	3232	150	Self-reactive solid type B, temperature controlled
3211	140	Perchlorates, inorganic, aqueous solution, n.o.s.	3233	150	Self-reactive liquid type C, temperature controlled
3212	140	Hypochlorites, inorganic, n.o.s.	3234	150	Self-reactive solid type C, temperature controlled
3213	140	Bromates, inorganic, aqueous solution, n.o.s.	3235	150	Self-reactive liquid type D, temperature controlled
3214	140	Permanganates, inorganic, aqueous solution, n.o.s.	3236	150	Self-reactive solid type D, temperature controlled
3215	140	Persulfates, inorganic, n.o.s.	3237	150	Self-reactive liquid type E, temperature controlled
3215	140	Persulphates, inorganic, n.o.s.	3238	150	Self-reactive solid type E, temperature controlled
3216	140	Persulfates, inorganic, aqueous solution, n.o.s.	3239	150	Self-reactive liquid type F, temperature controlled
3216	140	Persulphates, inorganic, aqueous solution, n.o.s.	3240	150	Self-reactive solid type F, temperature controlled
3217	140	Percarbonates, inorganic, n.o.s.			
3218	140	Nitrates, inorganic, aqueous solution, n.o.s.	3241	133	2-Bromo-2-nitropropane-1, 3-diol
3219	140	Nitrites, inorganic, aqueous solution, n.o.s.	3242	149	Azodicarbonamide
3220	126	Pentafluoroethane	3243	151	Solids containing poisonous liquid, n.o.s.
3220	126	Refrigerant gas R-125	3243	151	Solids containing toxic liquid, n.o.s.
3221	149	Self-reactive liquid type B			
3222	149	Self-reactive solid type B	3244	154	Solids containing corrosive liquid, n.o.s.

ID No.	Guide No.	Name of Material	ID No.	Guide No.	Name of Material
3245	171	Genetically modified micro-organisms	3258	171	Elevated temperature solid, n.o.s., at or above 240°C (464°F)
3245	171	Genetically modified organisms	3259	154	Amines, solid, corrosive, n.o.s.
3246	156	Methanesulfonyl chloride	3259	154	Polyamines, solid, corrosive, n.o.s.
3246	156	Methanesulphonyl chloride	3260	154	Corrosive solid, acidic, inorganic, n.o.s.
3247	140	Sodium peroxoborate, anhydrous	3261	154	Corrosive solid, acidic, organic, n.o.s.
3248	131	Medicine, liquid, flammable, poisonous, n.o.s.	3262	154	Corrosive solid, basic, inorganic, n.o.s.
3248	131	Medicine, liquid, flammable, toxic, n.o.s.	3263	154	Corrosive solid, basic, organic, n.o.s.
3249	151	Medicine, solid, poisonous, n.o.s.	3264	154	Corrosive liquid, acidic, inorganic, n.o.s.
3249	151	Medicine, solid, toxic, n.o.s.	3265	153	Corrosive liquid, acidic, organic, n.o.s.
3250	153	Chloroacetic acid, molten	3266	154	Corrosive liquid, basic, inorganic, n.o.s.
3251	133	Isosorbide-5-mononitrate	3267	153	Corrosive liquid, basic, organic, n.o.s.
3252	115	Difluoromethane			
3252	115	Refrigerant gas R-32	3268	171	Air bag inflators
3253	154	Disodium trioxosilicate	3268	171	Air bag inflators, pyrotechnic
3253	154	Disodium trioxosilicate, pentahydrate	3268	171	Air bag modules
3254	135	Tributylphosphane	3268	171	Air bag modules, pyrotechnic
3254	135	Tributylphosphine	3268	171	Seat-belt modules
3255	135	tert-Butyl hypochlorite	3268	171	Seat-belt pre-tensioners
3256	128	Elevated temperature liquid, flammable, n.o.s., with flash point above 37.8°C (100°F), at or above its flash point	3268	171	Seat-belt pre-tensioners, pyrotechnic
3256	128	Elevated temperature liquid, flammable, n.o.s., with flash point above 60.5°C (141°F), at or above its flash point	3269	128	Polyester resin kit
			3270	133	Nitrocellulose membrane filters
			3271	127	Ethers, n.o.s.
3257	128	Elevated temperature liquid, n.o.s., at or above 100°C (212°F), and below its flash point	3272	127	Esters, n.o.s.
			3273	131	Nitriles, flammable, poisonous, n.o.s.

ID No.	Guide No.	Name of Material	ID No.	Guide No.	Name of Material
3273	131	Nitriles, flammable, toxic, n.o.s.	3282	151	Organometallic compound, toxic, liquid, n.o.s.
3274	132	Alcoholates solution, n.o.s., in alcohol	3282	151	Organometallic compound, toxic, n.o.s.
3275	131	Nitriles, poisonous, flammable, n.o.s.	3283	151	Selenium compound, n.o.s.
3275	131	Nitriles, toxic, flammable, n.o.s.	3283	151	Selenium compound, solid, n.o.s.
3276	151	Nitriles, poisonous, liquid, n.o.s.	3284	151	Tellurium compound, n.o.s.
3276	151	Nitriles, poisonous, n.o.s.	3285	151	Vanadium compound, n.o.s.
3276	151	Nitriles, toxic, liquid, n.o.s.	3286	131	Flammable liquid, poisonous, corrosive, n.o.s.
3276	151	Nitriles, toxic, n.o.s.	3286	131	Flammable liquid, toxic, corrosive, n.o.s.
3277	154	Chloroformates, poisonous, corrosive, n.o.s.	3287	151	Poisonous liquid, inorganic, n.o.s.
3277	154	Chloroformates, toxic, corrosive, n.o.s.	3287	151	Poisonous liquid, inorganic, n.o.s. (Inhalation Hazard Zone A)
3278	151	Organophosphorus compound, poisonous, liquid, n.o.s.	3287	151	Poisonous liquid, inorganic, n.o.s. (Inhalation Hazard Zone B)
3278	151	Organophosphorus compound, poisonous, n.o.s.	3287	151	Toxic liquid, inorganic, n.o.s.
3278	151	Organophosphorus compound, toxic, liquid, n.o.s.	3287	151	Toxic liquid, inorganic, n.o.s. (Inhalation Hazard Zone A)
3278	151	Organophosphorus compound, toxic, n.o.s.	3287	151	Toxic liquid, inorganic, n.o.s. (Inhalation Hazard Zone B)
3279	131	Organophosphorus compound, poisonous, flammable, n.o.s.	3288	151	Poisonous solid, inorganic, n.o.s.
3279	131	Organophosphorus compound, toxic, flammable, n.o.s.	3288	151	Toxic solid, inorganic, n.o.s.
3280	151	Organoarsenic compound, liquid, n.o.s.	3289	154	Poisonous liquid, corrosive, inorganic, n.o.s.
3280	151	Organoarsenic compound, n.o.s.	3289	154	Poisonous liquid, corrosive, inorganic, n.o.s. (Inhalation Hazard Zone A)
3281	151	Metal carbonyls, liquid, n.o.s.	3289	154	Poisonous liquid, corrosive, inorganic, n.o.s. (Inhalation Hazard Zone B)
3281	151	Metal carbonyls, n.o.s.			
3282	151	Organometallic compound, poisonous, liquid, n.o.s.			
3282	151	Organometallic compound, poisonous, n.o.s.			

ID No.	Guide No.	Name of Material
3289	154	Toxic liquid, corrosive, inorganic, n.o.s.
3289	154	Toxic liquid, corrosive, inorganic, n.o.s. (Inhalation Hazard Zone A)
3289	154	Toxic liquid, corrosive, inorganic, n.o.s. (Inhalation Hazard Zone B)
3290	154	Poisonous solid, corrosive, inorganic, n.o.s.
3290	154	Toxic solid, corrosive, inorganic, n.o.s.
3291	158	(Bio)Medical waste, n.o.s.
3291	158	Clinical waste, unspecified, n.o.s.
3291	158	Medical waste, n.o.s.
3291	158	Regulated medical waste, n.o.s.
3292	138	Batteries, containing Sodium
3292	138	Cells, containing Sodium
3293	152	Hydrazine, aqueous solution, with not more than 37% Hydrazine
3294	131	Hydrogen cyanide, solution in alcohol, with not more than 45% Hydrogen cyanide
3295	128	Hydrocarbons, liquid, n.o.s.
3296	126	Heptafluoropropane
3296	126	Refrigerant gas R-227
3297	126	Chlorotetrafluoroethane and Ethylene oxide mixture, with not more than 8.8% Ethylene oxide
3297	126	Ethylene oxide and Chlorotetrafluoroethane mixture, with not more than 8.8% Ethylene oxide
3298	126	Ethylene oxide and Pentafluoroethane mixture, with not more than 7.9% Ethylene oxide
3298	126	Pentafluoroethane and Ethylene oxide mixture, with not more than 7.9% Ethylene oxide
3299	126	Ethylene oxide and Tetrafluoroethane mixture, with not more than 5.6% Ethylene oxide
3299	126	Tetrafluoroethane and Ethylene oxide mixture, with not more than 5.6% Ethylene oxide
3300	119P	Carbon dioxide and Ethylene oxide mixture, with more than 87% Ethylene oxide
3300	119P	Ethylene oxide and Carbon dioxide mixture, with more than 87% Ethylene oxide
3301	136	Corrosive liquid, self-heating, n.o.s.
3302	152	2-Dimethylaminoethyl acrylate
3303	124	Compressed gas, poisonous, oxidizing, n.o.s.
3303	124	Compressed gas, poisonous, oxidizing, n.o.s. (Inhalation Hazard Zone A)
3303	124	Compressed gas, poisonous, oxidizing, n.o.s. (Inhalation Hazard Zone B)
3303	124	Compressed gas, poisonous, oxidizing, n.o.s. (Inhalation Hazard Zone C)
3303	124	Compressed gas, poisonous, oxidizing, n.o.s. (Inhalation Hazard Zone D)
3303	124	Compressed gas, toxic, oxidizing, n.o.s.

ID No.	Guide No.	Name of Material	ID No.	Guide No.	Name of Material
3303	124	Compressed gas, toxic, oxidizing, n.o.s. (Inhalation Hazard Zone A)	3305	119	Compressed gas, poisonous, flammable, corrosive, n.o.s.
3303	124	Compressed gas, toxic, oxidizing, n.o.s. (Inhalation Hazard Zone B)	3305	119	Compressed gas, poisonous, flammable, corrosive, n.o.s. (Inhalation Hazard Zone A)
3303	124	Compressed gas, toxic, oxidizing, n.o.s. (Inhalation Hazard Zone C)	3305	119	Compressed gas, poisonous, flammable, corrosive, n.o.s. (Inhalation Hazard Zone B)
3303	124	Compressed gas, toxic, oxidizing, n.o.s. (Inhalation Hazard Zone D)	3305	119	Compressed gas, poisonous, flammable, corrosive, n.o.s. (Inhalation Hazard Zone C)
3304	123	Compressed gas, poisonous, corrosive, n.o.s.	3305	119	Compressed gas, poisonous, flammable, corrosive, n.o.s. (Inhalation Hazard Zone D)
3304	123	Compressed gas, poisonous, corrosive, n.o.s. (Inhalation Hazard Zone A)	3305	119	Compressed gas, toxic, flammable, corrosive, n.o.s.
3304	123	Compressed gas, poisonous, corrosive, n.o.s. (Inhalation Hazard Zone B)	3305	119	Compressed gas, toxic, flammable, corrosive, n.o.s. (Inhalation Hazard Zone A)
3304	123	Compressed gas, poisonous, corrosive, n.o.s. (Inhalation Hazard Zone C)	3305	119	Compressed gas, toxic, flammable, corrosive, n.o.s. (Inhalation Hazard Zone B)
3304	123	Compressed gas, poisonous, corrosive, n.o.s. (Inhalation Hazard Zone D)	3305	119	Compressed gas, toxic, flammable, corrosive, n.o.s. (Inhalation Hazard Zone C)
3304	123	Compressed gas, toxic, corrosive, n.o.s.	3305	119	Compressed gas, toxic, flammable, corrosive, n.o.s. (Inhalation Hazard Zone D)
3304	123	Compressed gas, toxic, corrosive, n.o.s. (Inhalation Hazard Zone A)	3306	124	Compressed gas, poisonous, oxidizing, corrosive, n.o.s.
3304	123	Compressed gas, toxic, corrosive, n.o.s. (Inhalation Hazard Zone B)	3306	124	Compressed gas, poisonous, oxidizing, corrosive, n.o.s. (Inhalation Hazard Zone A)
3304	123	Compressed gas, toxic, corrosive, n.o.s. (Inhalation Hazard Zone C)	3306	124	Compressed gas, poisonous, oxidizing, corrosive, n.o.s. (Inhalation Hazard Zone B)
3304	123	Compressed gas, toxic, corrosive, n.o.s. (Inhalation Hazard Zone D)	3306	124	Compressed gas, poisonous, oxidizing, corrosive, n.o.s. (Inhalation Hazard Zone C)

ID No.	Guide No.	Name of Material
3306	124	Compressed gas, poisonous, oxidizing, corrosive, n.o.s. (Inhalation Hazard Zone D)
3306	124	Compressed gas, toxic, oxidizing, corrosive, n.o.s.
3306	124	Compressed gas, toxic, oxidizing, corrosive, n.o.s. (Inhalation Hazard Zone A)
3306	124	Compressed gas, toxic, oxidizing, corrosive, n.o.s. (Inhalation Hazard Zone B)
3306	124	Compressed gas, toxic, oxidizing, corrosive, n.o.s. (Inhalation Hazard Zone C)
3306	124	Compressed gas, toxic, oxidizing, corrosive, n.o.s. (Inhalation Hazard Zone D)
3307	124	Liquefied gas, poisonous, oxidizing, n.o.s.
3307	124	Liquefied gas, poisonous, oxidizing, n.o.s. (Inhalation Hazard Zone A)
3307	124	Liquefied gas, poisonous, oxidizing, n.o.s. (Inhalation Hazard Zone B)
3307	124	Liquefied gas, poisonous, oxidizing, n.o.s. (Inhalation Hazard Zone C)
3307	124	Liquefied gas, poisonous, oxidizing, n.o.s. (Inhalation Hazard Zone D)
3307	124	Liquefied gas, toxic, oxidizing, n.o.s.
3307	124	Liquefied gas, toxic, oxidizing, n.o.s. (Inhalation Hazard Zone A)
3307	124	Liquefied gas, toxic, oxidizing, n.o.s. (Inhalation Hazard Zone B)
3307	124	Liquefied gas, toxic, oxidizing, n.o.s. (Inhalation Hazard Zone C)
3307	124	Liquefied gas, toxic, oxidizing, n.o.s. (Inhalation Hazard Zone D)
3308	123	Liquefied gas, poisonous, corrosive, n.o.s.
3308	123	Liquefied gas, poisonous, corrosive, n.o.s. (Inhalation Hazard Zone A)
3308	123	Liquefied gas, poisonous, corrosive, n.o.s. (Inhalation Hazard Zone B)
3308	123	Liquefied gas, poisonous, corrosive, n.o.s. (Inhalation Hazard Zone C)
3308	123	Liquefied gas, poisonous, corrosive, n.o.s. (Inhalation Hazard Zone D)
3308	123	Liquefied gas, toxic, corrosive, n.o.s.
3308	123	Liquefied gas, toxic, corrosive, n.o.s. (Inhalation Hazard Zone A)
3308	123	Liquefied gas, toxic, corrosive, n.o.s. (Inhalation Hazard Zone B)
3308	123	Liquefied gas, toxic, corrosive, n.o.s. (Inhalation Hazard Zone C)
3308	123	Liquefied gas, toxic, corrosive, n.o.s. (Inhalation Hazard Zone D)
3309	119	Liquefied gas, poisonous, flammable, corrosive, n.o.s.
3309	119	Liquefied gas, poisonous, flammable, corrosive, n.o.s. (Inhalation Hazard Zone A)

ID No.	Guide No.	Name of Material
3309	119	Liquefied gas, poisonous, flammable, corrosive, n.o.s. (Inhalation Hazard Zone B)
3309	119	Liquefied gas, poisonous, flammable, corrosive, n.o.s. (Inhalation Hazard Zone C)
3309	119	Liquefied gas, poisonous, flammable, corrosive, n.o.s. (Inhalation Hazard Zone D)
3309	119	Liquefied gas, toxic, flammable, corrosive, n.o.s.
3309	119	Liquefied gas, toxic, flammable, corrosive, n.o.s. (Inhalation Hazard Zone A)
3309	119	Liquefied gas, toxic, flammable, corrosive, n.o.s. (Inhalation Hazard Zone B)
3309	119	Liquefied gas, toxic, flammable, corrosive, n.o.s. (Inhalation Hazard Zone C)
3309	119	Liquefied gas, toxic, flammable, corrosive, n.o.s. (Inhalation Hazard Zone D)
3310	124	Liquefied gas, poisonous, oxidizing, corrosive, n.o.s.
3310	124	Liquefied gas, poisonous, oxidizing, corrosive, n.o.s. (Inhalation Hazard Zone A)
3310	124	Liquefied gas, poisonous, oxidizing, corrosive, n.o.s. (Inhalation Hazard Zone B)
3310	124	Liquefied gas, poisonous, oxidizing, corrosive, n.o.s. (Inhalation Hazard Zone C)
3310	124	Liquefied gas, poisonous, oxidizing, corrosive, n.o.s. (Inhalation Hazard Zone D)
3310	124	Liquefied gas, toxic, oxidizing, corrosive, n.o.s.
3310	124	Liquefied gas, toxic, oxidizing, corrosive, n.o.s. (Inhalation Hazard Zone A)
3310	124	Liquefied gas, toxic, oxidizing, corrosive, n.o.s. (Inhalation Hazard Zone B)
3310	124	Liquefied gas, toxic, oxidizing, corrosive, n.o.s. (Inhalation Hazard Zone C)
3310	124	Liquefied gas, toxic, oxidizing, corrosive, n.o.s. (Inhalation Hazard Zone D)
3311	122	Gas, refrigerated liquid, oxidizing, n.o.s.
3312	115	Gas, refrigerated liquid, flammable, n.o.s.
3313	135	Organic pigments, self-heating
3314	171	Plastic molding compound
3314	171	Plastics moulding compound
3315	151	Chemical sample, poisonous
3315	151	Chemical sample, poisonous liquid
3315	151	Chemical sample, poisonous solid
3315	151	Chemical sample, toxic
3315	151	Chemical sample, toxic liquid
3315	151	Chemical sample, toxic solid
3316	171	Chemical kit
3316	171	First aid kit
3317	113	2-Amino-4,6-dinitrophenol, wetted with not less than 20% water
3318	125	Ammonia solution, with more than 50% Ammonia
3319	113	Nitroglycerin mixture, desensitized, solid, n.o.s., with more than 2% but not more than 10% Nitroglycerin

ID No.	Guide No.	Name of Material
3319	113	Nitroglycerin mixture with more than 2% but not more than 10% Nitroglycerin, desensitized
3320	157	Sodium borohydride and Sodium hydroxide solution, with not more than 12% Sodium borohydride and not more than 40% Sodium hydroxide
3321	162	Radioactive material, low specific activity (LSA-II) non fissile or fissile-excepted
3322	162	Radioactive material, low specific activity (LSA-III) non fissile or fissile-excepted
3323	163	Radioactive material, Type C package
3324	165	Radioactive material, low specific activity (LSA-II), fissile
3325	165	Radioactive material, low specific activity (LSA-III), fissile
3326	165	Radioactive material, surface contaminated objects (SCO-I), fissile
3326	165	Radioactive material, surface contaminated objects (SCO-II), fissile
3327	165	Radioactive material, Type A package, fissile, non-special form
3328	165	Radioactive material, Type B(U) package, fissile
3329	165	Radioactive material, Type B(M) package, fissile
3330	165	Radioactive material, Type C package, fissile
3331	165	Radioactive material, transported under special arrangement, fissile
3332	164	Radioactive material, Type A package, special form, non fissile or fissile-excepted
3333	165	Radioactive material, Type A package, special form, fissile
3334	171	Aviation regulated liquid, n.o.s.
3334	171	Self-defense spray, non-pressurized
3335	171	Aviation regulated solid, n.o.s.
3336	130	Mercaptan mixture, liquid, flammable, n.o.s.
3336	130	Mercaptans, liquid, flammable, n.o.s.
3337	126	Refrigerant gas R-404A
3338	126	Refrigerant gas R-407A
3339	126	Refrigerant gas R-407B
3340	126	Refrigerant gas R-407C
3341	135	Thiourea dioxide
3342	135	Xanthates
3343	113	Nitroglycerin mixture, desensitized, liquid, flammable, n.o.s., with not more than 30% Nitroglycerin
3344	113	Pentaerythrite tetranitrate mixture, desensitized, solid, n.o.s., with more than 10% but not more than 20% PETN
3344	113	Pentaerythritol tetranitrate mixture, desensitized, solid, n.o.s., with more than 10% but not more than 20% PETN
3344	113	PETN mixture, desensitized, solid, n.o.s., with more than 10% but not more than 20% PETN
3345	153	Phenoxyacetic acid derivative pesticide, solid, poisonous

ID No.	Guide No.	Name of Material	ID No.	Guide No.	Name of Material
3345	153	Phenoxyacetic acid derivative pesticide, solid, toxic	3355	119	Insecticide gas, poisonous, flammable, n.o.s.
3346	131	Phenoxyacetic acid derivative pesticide, liquid, flammable, poisonous	3355	119	Insecticide gas, poisonous, flammable, n.o.s. (Inhalation Hazard Zone A)
3346	131	Phenoxyacetic acid derivative pesticide, liquid, flammable, toxic	3355	119	Insecticide gas, poisonous, flammable, n.o.s. (Inhalation Hazard Zone B)
3347	131	Phenoxyacetic acid derivative pesticide, liquid, poisonous, flammable	3355	119	Insecticide gas, poisonous, flammable, n.o.s. (Inhalation Hazard Zone C)
3347	131	Phenoxyacetic acid derivative pesticide, liquid, toxic, flammable	3355	119	Insecticide gas, poisonous, flammable, n.o.s. (Inhalation Hazard Zone D)
3348	153	Phenoxyacetic acid derivative pesticide, liquid, poisonous	3355	119	Insecticide gas, toxic, flammable, n.o.s.
3348	153	Phenoxyacetic acid derivative pesticide, liquid, toxic	3355	119	Insecticide gas, toxic, flammable, n.o.s. (Inhalation Hazard Zone A)
3349	151	Pyrethroid pesticide, solid, poisonous	3355	119	Insecticide gas, toxic, flammable, n.o.s. (Inhalation Hazard Zone B)
3349	151	Pyrethroid pesticide, solid, toxic	3355	119	Insecticide gas, toxic, flammable, n.o.s. (Inhalation Hazard Zone C)
3350	131	Pyrethroid pesticide, liquid, flammable, poisonous	3355	119	Insecticide gas, toxic, flammable, n.o.s. (Inhalation Hazard Zone D)
3350	131	Pyrethroid pesticide, liquid, flammable, toxic	3356	140	Oxygen generator, chemical
3351	131	Pyrethroid pesticide, liquid, poisonous, flammable	3356	140	Oxygen generator, chemical, spent
3351	131	Pyrethroid pesticide, liquid, toxic, flammable	3357	113	Nitroglycerin mixture, desensitized, liquid, n.o.s., with not more than 30% Nitroglycerin
3352	151	Pyrethroid pesticide, liquid, poisonous			
3352	151	Pyrethroid pesticide, liquid, toxic	3358	115	Refrigerating machines, containing flammable, non-poisonous, liquefied gases
3353	126	Air bag inflators, compressed gas			
3353	126	Air bag modules, compressed gas			
3353	126	Seat-belt pre-tensioners, compressed gas			
3354	115	Insecticide gas, flammable, n.o.s.			

ID No.	Guide No.	Name of Material
3358	115	Refrigerating machines, containing flammable, non-toxic, liquefied gases
3359	171	Fumigated unit
3360	133	Fibers, vegetable, dry
3360	133	Fibres, vegetable, dry
3361	156	Chlorosilanes, poisonous, corrosive, n.o.s.
3361	156	Chlorosilanes, toxic, corrosive, n.o.s.
3362	155	Chlorosilanes, poisonous, corrosive, flammable, n.o.s.
3362	155	Chlorosilanes, toxic, corrosive, flammable, n.o.s.
3363	171	Dangerous goods in apparatus
3363	171	Dangerous goods in machinery
3364	113	Picric acid, wetted with not less than 10% water
3364	113	Trinitrophenol, wetted with not less than 10% water
3365	113	Picryl chloride, wetted with not less than 10% water
3365	113	Trinitrochlorobenzene, wetted with not less than 10% water
3366	113	TNT, wetted with not less than 10% water
3366	113	Trinitrotoluene, wetted with not less than 10% water
3367	113	Trinitrobenzene, wetted with not less than 10% water
3368	113	Trinitrobenzoic acid, wetted with not less than 10% water
3369	113	Sodium dinitro-o-cresolate, wetted with not less than 10% water
3370	113	Urea nitrate, wetted with not less than 10% water
3371	129	2-Methylbutanal
3372	138	Organometallic compound, solid, water-reactive, flammable, n.o.s.
3373	158	Biological substance, category B
3373	158	Clinical specimens
3373	158	Diagnostic specimens
3374	116	Acetylene, solvent free
3375	140	Ammonium nitrate emulsion
3375	140	Ammonium nitrate gel
3375	140	Ammonium nitrate suspension
3376	113	4-Nitrophenylhydrazine, with not less than 30% water
3377	140	Sodium perborate monohydrate
3378	140	Sodium carbonate peroxyhydrate
3379	128	Desensitized explosive, liquid, n.o.s.
3380	133	Desensitized explosive, solid, n.o.s.
3381	151	Poisonous by inhalation liquid, n.o.s. (Inhalation Hazard Zone A)
3381	151	Toxic by inhalation liquid, n.o.s. (Inhalation Hazard Zone A)
3382	151	Poisonous by inhalation liquid, n.o.s. (Inhalation Hazard Zone B)
3382	151	Toxic by inhalation liquid, n.o.s. (Inhalation Hazard Zone B)
3383	131	Poisonous by inhalation liquid, flammable, n.o.s. (Inhalation Hazard Zone A)
3383	131	Toxic by inhalation liquid, flammable, n.o.s. (Inhalation Hazard Zone A)

ID No.	Guide No.	Name of Material
3384	131	Poisonous by inhalation liquid, flammable, n.o.s. (Inhalation Hazard Zone B)
3384	131	Toxic by inhalation liquid, flammable, n.o.s. (Inhalation Hazard Zone B)
3385	139	Poisonous by inhalation liquid, water-reactive, n.o.s. (Inhalation Hazard Zone A)
3385	139	Toxic by inhalation liquid, water-reactive, n.o.s. (Inhalation Hazard Zone A)
3386	139	Poisonous by inhalation liquid, water-reactive, n.o.s. (Inhalation Hazard Zone B)
3386	139	Toxic by inhalation liquid, water-reactive, n.o.s. (Inhalation Hazard Zone B)
3387	142	Poisonous by inhalation liquid, oxidizing, n.o.s. (Inhalation Hazard Zone A)
3387	142	Toxic by inhalation liquid, oxidizing, n.o.s. (Inhalation Hazard Zone A)
3388	142	Poisonous by inhalation liquid, oxidizing, n.o.s. (Inhalation Hazard Zone B)
3388	142	Toxic by inhalation liquid, oxidizing, n.o.s. (Inhalation Hazard Zone B)
3389	154	Poisonous by inhalation liquid, corrosive, n.o.s. (Inhalation Hazard Zone A)
3389	154	Toxic by inhalation liquid, corrosive, n.o.s. (Inhalation Hazard Zone A)
3390	154	Poisonous by inhalation liquid, corrosive, n.o.s. (Inhalation Hazard Zone B)
3390	154	Toxic by inhalation liquid, corrosive, n.o.s. (Inhalation Hazard Zone B)
3391	135	Organometallic substance, solid, pyrophoric
3392	135	Organometallic substance, liquid, pyrophoric
3393	135	Organometallic substance, solid, pyrophoric, water-reactive
3394	135	Organometallic substance, liquid, pyrophoric, water-reactive
3395	135	Organometallic substance, solid, water-reactive
3396	138	Organometallic substance, solid, water-reactive, flammable
3397	138	Organometallic substance, solid, water-reactive, self-heating
3398	135	Organometallic substance, liquid, water-reactive
3399	138	Organometallic substance, liquid, water-reactive, flammable
3400	138	Organometallic substance, solid, self-heating
3401	138	Alkali metal amalgam, solid
3402	138	Alkaline earth metal amalgam, solid
3403	138	Potassium, metal alloys, solid
3404	138	Potassium sodium alloys, solid
3404	138	Sodium potassium alloys, solid
3405	141	Barium chlorate, solution
3406	141	Barium perchlorate, solution
3407	140	Chlorate and Magnesium chloride mixture, solution

ID No.	Guide No.	Name of Material
3407	140	Magnesium chloride and Chlorate mixture, solution
3408	141	Lead perchlorate, solution
3409	152	Chloronitrobenzenes, liquid
3410	153	4-Chloro-o-toluidine hydrochloride, solution
3411	153	beta-Naphthylamine, solution
3411	153	Naphthylamine (beta), solution
3412	153	Formic acid, with not less than 5% but less than 10% acid
3412	153	Formic acid, with not less than 10% but not more than 85% acid
3413	157	Potassium cyanide, solution
3414	157	Sodium cyanide, solution
3415	154	Sodium fluoride, solution
3416	153	Chloroacetophenone, liquid
3417	152	Xylyl bromide, solid
3418	151	2,4-Toluylenediamine, solution
3419	157	Boron trifluoride acetic acid complex, solid
3420	157	Boron trifluoride propionic acid complex, solid
3421	154	Potassium hydrogen difluoride, solution
3422	154	Potassium fluoride, solution
3423	153	Tetramethylammonium hydroxide, solid
3424	141	Ammonium dinitro-o-cresolate, solution
3425	156	Bromoacetic acid, solid
3426	153P	Acrylamide, solution
3427	153	Chlorobenzyl chlorides, solid
3428	156	3-Chloro-4-methylphenyl isocyanate, solid
3429	153	Chlorotoluidines, liquid
3430	153	Xylenols, liquid
3431	152	Nitrobenzotrifluorides, solid
3432	171	Polychlorinated biphenyls, solid
3433	135	Lithium alkyls, solid
3434	153	Nitrocresols, liquid
3435	153	Hydroquinone, solution
3436	151	Hexafluoroacetone hydrate, solid
3437	152	Chlorocresols, solid
3438	153	alpha-Methylbenzyl alcohol, solid
3439	151	Nitriles, poisonous, solid, n.o.s.
3439	151	Nitriles, toxic, solid, n.o.s.
3440	151	Selenium compound, liquid, n.o.s.
3441	153	Chlorodinitrobenzenes, solid
3442	153	Dichloroanilines, solid
3443	152	Dinitrobenzenes, solid
3444	151	Nicotine hydrochloride, solid
3445	151	Nicotine sulfate, solid
3445	151	Nicotine sulphate, solid
3446	152	Nitrotoluenes, solid
3447	152	Nitroxylenes, solid
3448	159	Tear gas substance, solid, n.o.s.
3449	159	Bromobenzyl cyanides, solid
3450	151	Diphenylchloroarsine, solid
3451	153	Toluidines, solid
3452	153	Xylidines, solid
3453	154	Phosphoric acid, solid
3454	152	Dinitrotoluenes, solid
3455	153	Cresols, solid
3456	157	Nitrosylsulfuric acid, solid
3456	157	Nitrosylsulphuric acid, solid

ID No.	Guide No.	Name of Material
3457	**152**	Chloronitrotoluenes, solid
3458	**152**	Nitroanisoles, solid
3459	**152**	Nitrobromobenzenes, solid
3460	**153**	N-Ethylbenzyltoluidines, solid
3461	**135**	Aluminum alkyl halides, solid
3462	**153**	Toxins, extracted from living sources, solid, n.o.s.
3463	**132**	Propionic acid, with not less than 90% acid
3464	**151**	Organophosphorus compound, poisonous, solid, n.o.s.
3464	**151**	Organophosphorus compound, toxic, solid, n.o.s.
3465	**151**	Organoarsenic compound, solid, n.o.s.
3466	**151**	Metal carbonyls, solid, n.o.s.
3467	**151**	Organometallic compound, poisonous, solid, n.o.s.
3467	**151**	Organometallic compound, toxic, solid, n.o.s.
3468	**115**	Hydrogen in a metal hydride storage system
3468	**115**	Hydrogen in a metal hydride storage system contained in equipment
3468	**115**	Hydrogen in a metal hydride storage system packed with equipment
3469	**132**	Paint, flammable, corrosive
3469	**132**	Paint related material, flammable, corrosive
3470	**132**	Paint, corrosive, flammable
3470	**132**	Paint related material, corrosive, flammable
3471	**154**	Hydrogendifluorides, solution, n.o.s.
3472	**153**	Crotonic acid, liquid
3473	**128**	Fuel cell cartridges contained in equipment, containing flammable liquids
3473	**128**	Fuel cell cartridges containing flammable liquids
3473	**128**	Fuel cell cartridges packed with equipment, containing flammable liquids
3474	**113**	1-Hydroxybenzotriazole, anhydrous, wetted with not less than 20% water
3475	**127**	Ethanol and gasoline mixture, with more than 10% ethanol
3475	**127**	Ethanol and motor spirit mixture, with more than 10% ethanol
3475	**127**	Ethanol and petrol mixture, with more than 10% ethanol
3475	**127**	Gasoline and ethanol mixture, with more than 10% ethanol
3475	**127**	Motor spirit and ethanol mixture, with more than 10% ethanol
3475	**127**	Petrol and ethanol mixture, with more than 10% ethanol
3476	**138**	Fuel cell cartridges contained in equipment, containing water-reactive substances
3476	**138**	Fuel cell cartridges, containing water-reactive substances
3476	**138**	Fuel cell cartridges packed with equipment, containing water-reactive substances
3477	**153**	Fuel cell cartridges contained in equipment, containing corrosive substances
3477	**153**	Fuel cell cartridges, containing corrosive substances

ID No.	Guide No.	Name of Material
3477	153	Fuel cell cartridges packed with equipment, containing corrosive substances
3478	115	Fuel cell cartridges contained in equipment, containing liquefied flammable gas
3478	115	Fuel cell cartridges, containing liquefied flammable gas
3478	115	Fuel cell cartridges packed with equipment, containing liquefied flammable gas
3479	115	Fuel cell cartridges contained in equipment, containing hydrogen in metal hydride
3479	115	Fuel cell cartridges, containing hydrogen in metal hydride
3479	115	Fuel cell cartridges packed with equipment, containing hydrogen in metal hydride
3480	147	Lithium ion batteries (including lithium ion polymer batteries)
3481	147	Lithium ion batteries contained in equipment (including lithium ion polymer batteries)
3481	147	Lithium ion batteries packed with equipment (including lithium ion polymer batteries)
8000	171	Consumer commodity
8013	171	Gas generator assemblies
8038	171	Heat producing article
9035	123	Gas identification set
9163	171	Zirconium sulfate
9163	171	Zirconium sulphate
9191	143	Chlorine dioxide, hydrate, frozen
9192	167	Fluorine, refrigerated liquid (cryogenic liquid)
9195	135	Metal alkyl, solution, n.o.s.
9202	168	Carbon monoxide, refrigerated liquid (cryogenic liquid)
9206	137	Methyl phosphonic dichloride
9260	169	Aluminum, molten
9263	156	Chloropivaloyl chloride
9264	151	3,5-Dichloro-2,4,6-trifluoropyridine
9269	132	Trimethoxysilane
9279	115	Hydrogen absorbed in metal hydride

Note: If an entry is highlighted in green in either the yellow-bordered or blue-bordered pages AND THERE IS NO FIRE, go directly to Table 1 - Initial Isolation and Protective Action Distances (green bordered pages) and look up the ID number and name of material to obtain initial isolation and protective action distances. IF THERE IS A FIRE, or IF A FIRE IS INVOLVED, ALSO CONSULT the assigned guide (orange-bordered pages) and apply as appropriate the evacuation information shown under PUBLIC SAFETY. Please remember that, if the name in Table 1 is shown with (when spilled in water), and the material has not been spilled in water, Table 1 does not apply and safety distances can be found within the appropriate guide.

Name of Material	Guide No.	ID No.	Name of Material	Guide No.	ID No.
AC	117	1051	Acrylamide	153P	2074
Accumulators, pressurized, pneumatic or hydraulic	126	1956	Acrylamide, solid	153P	2074
			Acrylamide, solution	153P	3426
Acetal	127	1088	Acrylic acid, stabilized	132P	2218
Acetaldehyde	129	1089	Acrylonitrile, stabilized	131P	1093
Acetaldehyde ammonia	171	1841	Adamsite	154	1698
Acetaldehyde oxime	129	2332	Adhesives (flammable)	128	1133
Acetic acid, glacial	132	2789	Adiponitrile	153	2205
Acetic acid, solution, more than 10% but not more than 80% acid	153	2790	Aerosol dispensers	126	1950
			Aerosols	126	1950
			Air, compressed	122	1002
Acetic acid, solution, more than 80% acid	132	2789	Air, refrigerated liquid (cryogenic liquid)	122	1003
Acetic anhydride	137	1715	Air, refrigerated liquid (cryogenic liquid), non-pressurized	122	1003
Acetone	127	1090			
Acetone cyanohydrin, stabilized	155	1541			
Acetone oils	127	1091	Air bag inflators	171	3268
Acetonitrile	127	1648	Air bag inflators, compressed gas	126	3353
Acetyl bromide	156	1716	Air bag inflators, pyrotechnic	171	3268
Acetyl chloride	155	1717	Air bag modules	171	3268
Acetylene	116	1001	Air bag modules, compressed gas	126	3353
Acetylene, dissolved	116	1001	Air bag modules, pyrotechnic	171	3268
Acetylene, solvent free	116	3374	Aircraft hydraulic power unit fuel tank	131	3165
Acetylene, Ethylene and Propylene in mixture, refrigerated liquid containing at least 71.5% Ethylene with not more than 22.5% Acetylene and not more than 6% Propylene	115	3138	Alcoholates solution, n.o.s., in alcohol	132	3274
			Alcoholic beverages	127	3065
			Alcohols, flammable, poisonous, n.o.s.	131	1986
Acetylene tetrabromide	159	2504	Alcohols, flammable, toxic, n.o.s.	131	1986
Acetyl iodide	156	1898			
Acetyl methyl carbinol	127	2621	Alcohols, n.o.s.	127	1987
Acid, sludge	153	1906	Alcohols, poisonous, n.o.s.	131	1986
Acid butyl phosphate	153	1718	Alcohols, toxic, n.o.s.	131	1986
Acridine	153	2713	Aldehydes, flammable, poisonous, n.o.s.	131	1988
Acrolein, stabilized	131P	1092			
Acrolein dimer, stabilized	129P	2607			

Name of Material	Guide No.	ID No.	Name of Material	Guide No.	ID No.
Aldehydes, flammable, toxic, n.o.s.	131	1988	Alkylamines, n.o.s.	132	2734
Aldehydes, n.o.s.	129	1989	Alkylamines, n.o.s.	153	2735
Aldehydes, poisonous, n.o.s.	131	1988	Alkyl phenols, liquid, n.o.s. (including C2-C12 homologues)	153	3145
Aldehydes, toxic, n.o.s.	131	1988			
Aldol	153	2839	Alkyl phenols, solid, n.o.s. (including C2-C12 homologues)	153	2430
Aldrin, liquid	131	2762			
Aldrin, solid	151	2761			
Alkali metal alcoholates, self-heating, corrosive, n.o.s.	136	3206	Alkyl sulfonic acids, liquid, with more than 5% free Sulfuric acid	153	2584
Alkali metal alloy, liquid, n.o.s.	138	1421	Alkyl sulfonic acids, liquid, with not more than 5% free Sulfuric acid	153	2586
Alkali metal amalgam	138	1389			
Alkali metal amalgam, liquid	138	1389			
Alkali metal amalgam, solid	138	1389	Alkyl sulfonic acids, solid, with more than 5% free Sulfuric acid	153	2583
Alkali metal amalgam, solid	138	3401			
Alkali metal amides	139	1390	Alkyl sulfonic acids, solid, with not more than 5% free Sulfuric acid	153	2585
Alkali metal dispersion	138	1391			
Alkaline earth metal alcoholates, n.o.s.	135	3205	Alkylsulfuric acids	156	2571
Alkaline earth metal alloy, n.o.s.	138	1393	Alkyl sulphonic acids, liquid, with more than 5% free Sulphuric acid	153	2584
Alkaline earth metal amalgam	138	1392			
Alkaline earth metal amalgam, liquid	138	1392	Alkyl sulphonic acids, liquid, with not more than 5% free Sulphuric acid	153	2586
Alkaline earth metal amalgam, solid	138	3402	Alkyl sulphonic acids, solid, with more than 5% free Sulphuric acid	153	2583
Alkaline earth metal dispersion	138	1391			
Alkaloids, liquid, n.o.s. (poisonous)	151	3140	Alkyl sulphonic acids, solid, with not more than 5% free Sulphuric acid	153	2585
Alkaloids, solid, n.o.s. (poisonous)	151	1544			
Alkaloid salts, liquid, n.o.s. (poisonous)	151	3140	Alkylsulphuric acids	156	2571
			Allyl acetate	131	2333
Alkaloid salts, solid, n.o.s. (poisonous)	151	1544	Allyl alcohol	131	1098
			Allylamine	131	2334
Alkylamines, n.o.s.	132	2733	Allyl bromide	131	1099

Name of Material	Guide No.	ID No.	Name of Material	Guide No.	ID No.
Allyl chloride	131	1100	Aluminum processing by-products	138	3170
Allyl chlorocarbonate	155	1722	Aluminum remelting by-products	138	3170
Allyl chloroformate	155	1722	Aluminum resinate	133	2715
Allyl ethyl ether	131	2335	Aluminum silicon powder, uncoated	138	1398
Allyl formate	131	2336			
Allyl glycidyl ether	129	2219	Aluminum smelting by-products	138	3170
Allyl iodide	132	1723	Amines, flammable, corrosive, n.o.s.	132	2733
Allyl isothiocyanate, stabilized	155	1545			
Allyltrichlorosilane, stabilized	155	1724	Amines, liquid, corrosive, flammable, n.o.s.	132	2734
Aluminum, molten	169	9260			
Aluminum alkyl halides	135	3052	Amines, liquid, corrosive, n.o.s.	153	2735
Aluminum alkyl halides, liquid	135	3052	Amines, solid, corrosive, n.o.s.	154	3259
Aluminum alkyl halides, solid	135	3052	2-Amino-4-chlorophenol	151	2673
Aluminum alkyl halides, solid	135	3461	2-Amino-5-diethylaminopentane	153	2946
Aluminum alkyl hydrides	138	3076	2-Amino-4,6-dinitrophenol, wetted with not less than 20% water	113	3317
Aluminum alkyls	135	3051			
Aluminum borohydride	135	2870			
Aluminum borohydride in devices	135	2870	2-(2-Aminoethoxy)ethanol	154	3055
			N-Aminoethylpiperazine	153	2815
Aluminum bromide, anhydrous	137	1725	Aminophenols	152	2512
Aluminum bromide, solution	154	2580	Aminopyridines	153	2671
Aluminum carbide	138	1394	Ammonia, anhydrous	125	1005
Aluminum chloride, anhydrous	137	1726	Ammonia, solution, with more than 10% but not more than 35% Ammonia	154	2672
Aluminum chloride, solution	154	2581			
Aluminum dross	138	3170	Ammonia, solution, with more than 35% but not more than 50% Ammonia	125	2073
Aluminum ferrosilicon powder	139	1395			
Aluminum hydride	138	2463			
Aluminum nitrate	140	1438	Ammonia solution, with more than 50% Ammonia	125	3318
Aluminum phosphide	139	1397			
Aluminum phosphide pesticide	157	3048	Ammonium arsenate	151	1546
Aluminum powder, coated	170	1309	Ammonium bifluoride, solid	154	1727
Aluminum powder, pyrophoric	135	1383	Ammonium bifluoride, solution	154	2817
Aluminum powder, uncoated	138	1396	Ammonium dichromate	141	1439
			Ammonium dinitro-o-cresolate	141	1843

Name of Material	Guide No.	ID No.	Name of Material	Guide No.	ID No.
Ammonium dinitro-o-cresolate, solid	141	1843	Ammonium nitrate fertilizers, with Ammonium sulphate	140	2069
Ammonium dinitro-o-cresolate, solution	141	3424	Ammonium nitrate fertilizers, with Calcium carbonate	140	2068
Ammonium fluoride	154	2505	Ammonium nitrate fertilizers, with Phosphate or Potash	143	2070
Ammonium fluorosilicate	151	2854			
Ammonium hydrogendifluoride, solid	154	1727	Ammonium nitrate-fuel oil mixtures	112	——
Ammonium hydrogendifluoride, solution	154	2817	Ammonium nitrate gel	140	3375
			Ammonium nitrate mixed fertilizers	140	2069
Ammonium hydrogen fluoride, solid	154	1727	Ammonium nitrate suspension	140	3375
Ammonium hydrogen fluoride, solution	154	2817	Ammonium perchlorate	143	1442
			Ammonium persulfate	140	1444
Ammonium hydrogen sulfate	154	2506	Ammonium persulphate	140	1444
Ammonium hydrogen sulphate	154	2506	Ammonium picrate, wetted with not less than 10% water	113	1310
Ammonium hydroxide	154	2672			
Ammonium hydroxide, with more than 10% but not more than 35% Ammonia	154	2672	Ammonium polysulfide, solution	154	2818
			Ammonium polysulphide, solution	154	2818
Ammonium metavanadate	154	2859	Ammonium polyvanadate	151	2861
Ammonium nitrate, liquid (hot concentrated solution)	140	2426	Ammonium silicofluoride	151	2854
			Ammonium sulfide, solution	132	2683
Ammonium nitrate, with not more than 0.2% combustible substances	140	1942	Ammonium sulphide, solution	132	2683
			Ammunition, poisonous, non-explosive	151	2016
Ammonium nitrate emulsion	140	3375	Ammunition, tear-producing, non-explosive	159	2017
Ammonium nitrate fertilizer, n.o.s.	140	2072	Ammunition, toxic, non-explosive	151	2016
Ammonium nitrate fertilizer, with not more than 0.4% combustible material	140	2071			
			Amyl acetates	129	1104
Ammonium nitrate fertilizers	140	2067	Amyl acid phosphate	153	2819
Ammonium nitrate fertilizers	140	2071	Amyl alcohols	129	1105
Ammonium nitrate fertilizers	140	2072	Amylamines	132	1106
Ammonium nitrate fertilizers, with Ammonium sulfate	140	2069	Amyl butyrates	130	2620
			Amyl chloride	129	1107

Name of Material	Guide No.	ID No.	Name of Material	Guide No.	ID No.
n-Amylene	128	1108	Antimony trichloride, solution	157	1733
Amyl formates	129	1109	Antimony trifluoride, solid	157	1549
Amyl mercaptan	130	1111	Antimony trifluoride, solution	157	1549
n-Amyl methyl ketone	127	1110	Aqua regia	157	1798
Amyl methyl ketone	127	1110	Argon	121	1006
Amyl nitrate	140	1112	Argon, compressed	121	1006
Amyl nitrite	129	1113	Argon, refrigerated liquid (cryogenic liquid)	120	1951
Amyltrichlorosilane	155	1728	Arsenic	152	1558
Anhydrous ammonia	125	1005	Arsenic acid, liquid	154	1553
Aniline	153	1547	Arsenic acid, solid	154	1554
Aniline hydrochloride	153	1548	Arsenical dust	152	1562
Anisidines	153	2431	Arsenical pesticide, liquid, flammable, poisonous	131	2760
Anisidines, liquid	153	2431	Arsenical pesticide, liquid, flammable, toxic	131	2760
Anisidines, solid	153	2431	Arsenical pesticide, liquid, poisonous	151	2994
Anisole	128	2222	Arsenical pesticide, liquid, poisonous, flammable	131	2993
Anisoyl chloride	156	1729	Arsenical pesticide, liquid, toxic	151	2994
Antimony compound, inorganic, liquid, n.o.s.	157	3141	Arsenical pesticide, liquid, toxic, flammable	131	2993
Antimony compound, inorganic, n.o.s.	157	1549	Arsenical pesticide, solid, poisonous	151	2759
Antimony compound, inorganic, solid, n.o.s.	157	1549	Arsenical pesticide, solid, toxic	151	2759
Antimony lactate	151	1550	Arsenic bromide	151	1555
Antimony pentachloride, liquid	157	1730	Arsenic chloride	157	1560
Antimony pentachloride, solution	157	1731	Arsenic compound, liquid, n.o.s.	152	1556
Antimony pentafluoride	157	1732	Arsenic compound, liquid, n.o.s., inorganic	152	1556
Antimony potassium tartrate	151	1551	Arsenic compound, solid, n.o.s.	152	1557
Antimony powder	170	2871	Arsenic compound, solid, n.o.s., inorganic	152	1557
Antimony tribromide, solid	157	1549	Arsenic pentoxide	151	1559
Antimony tribromide, solution	157	1549	Arsenic sulfide	152	1557
Antimony trichloride	157	1733			
Antimony trichloride, liquid	157	1733			
Antimony trichloride, solid	157	1733			

Name of Material	Guide No.	ID No.	Name of Material	Guide No.	ID No.
Arsenic sulphide	152	1557	Asbestos	171	2212
Arsenic trichloride	157	1560	Asbestos, blue	171	2212
Arsenic trioxide	151	1561	Asbestos, brown	171	2212
Arsenic trisulfide	152	1557	Asbestos, white	171	2590
Arsenic trisulphide	152	1557	Asphalt	130	1999
Arsine	119	2188	Aviation regulated liquid, n.o.s.	171	3334
Articles containing Polychlorinated biphenyls (PCB)	171	2315	Aviation regulated solid, n.o.s.	171	3335
			1-Aziridinyl phosphine oxide (Tris)	152	2501
Articles, pressurized, hydraulic (containing non-flammable gas)	126	3164	Azodicarbonamide	149	3242
			Barium	138	1400
Articles, pressurized, pneumatic (containing non-flammable gas)	126	3164	Barium alloys, pyrophoric	135	1854
			Barium azide, wetted with not less than 50% water	113	1571
Aryl sulfonic acids, liquid, with more than 5% free Sulfuric acid	153	2584	Barium bromate	141	2719
			Barium chlorate	141	1445
Aryl sulfonic acids, liquid, with not more than 5% free Sulfuric acid	153	2586	Barium chlorate, solid	141	1445
			Barium chlorate, solution	141	3405
			Barium compound, n.o.s.	154	1564
Aryl sulfonic acids, solid, with more than 5% free Sulfuric acid	153	2583	Barium cyanide	157	1565
Aryl sulfonic acids, solid, with not more than 5% free Sulfuric acid	153	2585	Barium hypochlorite, with more than 22% available Chlorine	141	2741
			Barium nitrate	141	1446
			Barium oxide	157	1884
Aryl sulphonic acids, liquid, with more than 5% free Sulphuric acid	153	2584	Barium perchlorate	141	1447
			Barium perchlorate, solid	141	1447
Aryl sulphonic acids, liquid, with not more than 5% free Sulphuric acid	153	2586	Barium perchlorate, solution	141	3406
			Barium permanganate	141	1448
			Barium peroxide	141	1449
Aryl sulphonic acids, solid, with more than 5% free Sulphuric acid	153	2583	Batteries, containing Sodium	138	3292
			Batteries, dry, containing Potassium hydroxide solid	154	3028
Aryl sulphonic acids, solid, with not more than 5% free Sulphuric acid	153	2585	Batteries, wet, filled with acid	154	2794
			Batteries, wet, filled with alkali	154	2795

Name of Material	Guide No.	ID No.	Name of Material	Guide No.	ID No.
Batteries, wet, non-spillable	154	2800	Benzoquinone	153	2587
Battery fluid, acid	157	2796	Benzotrichloride	156	2226
Battery fluid, alkali	154	2797	Benzotrifluoride	127	2338
Battery fluid, alkali, with battery	154	2797	Benzoyl chloride	137	1736
Battery fluid, alkali, with electronic equipment or actuating device	154	2797	Benzyl bromide	156	1737
			Benzyl chloride	156	1738
			Benzyl chloroformate	137	1739
Battery-powered equipment (wet battery)	154	3171	Benzyldimethylamine	132	2619
Battery-powered vehicle (wet battery)	154	3171	Benzylidene chloride	156	1886
			Benzyl iodide	156	2653
Benzaldehyde	129	1990	Beryllium compound, n.o.s.	154	1566
Benzene	130	1114	Beryllium nitrate	141	2464
Benzene phosphorus dichloride	137	2798	Beryllium powder	134	1567
Benzene phosphorus thiodichloride	137	2799	Bhusa, wet, damp or contaminated with oil	133	1327
Benzenesulfonyl chloride	156	2225	Bicyclo[2.2.1]hepta-2,5-diene, stabilized	128P	2251
Benzenesulphonyl chloride	156	2225			
Benzidine	153	1885	Biological agents	158	——
Benzoic derivative pesticide, liquid, flammable, poisonous	131	2770	Biological substance, category B	158	3373
			(Bio)Medical waste, n.o.s.	158	3291
Benzoic derivative pesticide, liquid, flammable, toxic	131	2770	Bipyridilium pesticide, liquid, flammable, poisonous	131	2782
Benzoic derivative pesticide, liquid, poisonous	151	3004	Bipyridilium pesticide, liquid, flammable, toxic	131	2782
Benzoic derivative pesticide, liquid, poisonous, flammable	131	3003	Bipyridilium pesticide, liquid, poisonous	151	3016
Benzoic derivative pesticide, liquid, toxic	151	3004	Bipyridilium pesticide, liquid, poisonous, flammable	131	3015
Benzoic derivative pesticide, liquid, toxic, flammable	131	3003	Bipyridilium pesticide, liquid, toxic	151	3016
Benzoic derivative pesticide, solid, poisonous	151	2769	Bipyridilium pesticide, liquid, toxic, flammable	131	3015
Benzoic derivative pesticide, solid, toxic	151	2769	Bipyridilium pesticide, solid, poisonous	151	2781
Benzonitrile	152	2224	Bipyridilium pesticide, solid, toxic	151	2781

Name of Material	Guide No.	ID No.
Bisulfates, aqueous solution	154	2837
Bisulfites, aqueous solution, n.o.s.	154	2693
Bisulfites, inorganic, aqueous solution, n.o.s.	154	2693
Bisulphates, aqueous solution	154	2837
Bisulphites, aqueous solution, n.o.s.	154	2693
Bisulphites, inorganic, aqueous solution, n.o.s.	154	2693
Blasting agent, n.o.s.	112	——
Bleaching powder	140	2208
Blue asbestos	171	2212
Bombs, smoke, non-explosive, with corrosive liquid, without initiating device	153	2028
Borate and Chlorate mixtures	140	1458
Borneol	133	1312
Boron tribromide	157	2692
Boron trichloride	125	1741
Boron trifluoride	125	1008
Boron trifluoride, compressed	125	1008
Boron trifluoride, dihydrate	157	2851
Boron trifluoride acetic acid complex	157	1742
Boron trifluoride acetic acid complex, liquid	157	1742
Boron trifluoride acetic acid complex, solid	157	3419
Boron trifluoride diethyl etherate	132	2604
Boron trifluoride dimethyl etherate	139	2965
Boron trifluoride propionic acid complex	157	1743
Boron trifluoride propionic acid complex, liquid	157	1743
Boron trifluoride propionic acid complex, solid	157	3420
Bromates, inorganic, aqueous solution, n.o.s.	140	3213
Bromates, inorganic, n.o.s.	141	1450
Bromine	154	1744
Bromine, solution	154	1744
Bromine, solution (Inhalation Hazard Zone A)	154	1744
Bromine, solution (Inhalation Hazard Zone B)	154	1744
Bromine chloride	124	2901
Bromine pentafluoride	144	1745
Bromine trifluoride	144	1746
Bromoacetic acid	156	1938
Bromoacetic acid, solid	156	3425
Bromoacetic acid, solution	156	1938
Bromoacetone	131	1569
Bromoacetyl bromide	156	2513
Bromobenzene	130	2514
Bromobenzyl cyanides	159	1694
Bromobenzyl cyanides, liquid	159	1694
Bromobenzyl cyanides, solid	159	1694
Bromobenzyl cyanides, solid	159	3449
1-Bromobutane	130	1126
2-Bromobutane	130	2339
Bromochlorodifluoromethane	126	1974
Bromochloromethane	160	1887
1-Bromo-3-chloropropane	159	2688
2-Bromoethyl ethyl ether	130	2340
Bromoform	159	2515
1-Bromo-3-methylbutane	130	2341
Bromomethylpropanes	130	2342
2-Bromo-2-nitropropane-1,3-diol	133	3241

Name of Material	Guide No.	ID No.	Name of Material	Guide No.	ID No.
2-Bromopentane	130	2343	Butyl ethers	128	1149
2-Bromopropane	129	2344	n-Butyl formate	129	1128
Bromopropanes	129	2344	tert-Butyl hypochlorite	135	3255
3-Bromopropyne	130	2345	N,n-Butylimidazole	152	2690
Bromotrifluoroethylene	116	2419	n-Butyl isocyanate	155	2485
Bromotrifluoromethane	126	1009	tert-Butyl isocyanate	155	2484
Brown asbestos	171	2212	Butyl mercaptan	130	2347
Brucine	152	1570	n-Butyl methacrylate, stabilized	130P	2227
Butadienes, stabilized	116P	1010	Butyl methyl ether	127	2350
Butadienes and hydrocarbon mixture, stabilized	116P	1010	Butyl nitrites	129	2351
			Butyl propionates	130	1914
Butane	115	1011	Butyltoluenes	152	2667
Butane	115	1075	Butyltrichlorosilane	155	1747
Butanedione	127	2346	5-tert-Butyl-2,4,6-trinitro-m-xylene	149	2956
Butane mixture	115	1011			
Butane mixture	115	1075	Butyl vinyl ether, stabilized	127P	2352
Butanols	129	1120	1,4-Butynediol	153	2716
Butoxyl	127	2708	Butyraldehyde	129	1129
Butyl acetates	129	1123	Butyraldoxime	129	2840
Butyl acid phosphate	153	1718	Butyric acid	153	2820
Butyl acrylates, stabilized	129P	2348	Butyric anhydride	156	2739
n-Butylamine	132	1125	Butyronitrile	131	2411
N-Butylaniline	153	2738	Butyryl chloride	132	2353
Butylbenzenes	128	2709	Buzz	153	2810
n-Butyl bromide	130	1126	BZ	153	2810
Butyl chloride	130	1127	CA	159	1694
n-Butyl chloroformate	155	2743	Cacodylic acid	151	1572
sec-Butyl chloroformate	155	2742	Cadmium compound	154	2570
tert-Butylcyclohexyl chloroformate	156	2747	Caesium	138	1407
			Caesium hydroxide	157	2682
Butylene	115	1012	Caesium hydroxide, solution	154	2681
Butylene	115	1075	Caesium nitrate	140	1451
1,2-Butylene oxide, stabilized	127P	3022	Calcium	138	1401

Name of Material	Guide No.	ID No.	Name of Material	Guide No.	ID No.
Calcium, metal and alloys, pyrophoric	135	1855	Calcium hypochlorite mixture, dry, with more than 39% available Chlorine (8.8% available Oxygen)	140	1748
Calcium, pyrophoric	135	1855			
Calcium alloys, pyrophoric	135	1855			
Calcium arsenate	151	1573	Calcium manganese silicon	138	2844
Calcium arsenate and Calcium arsenite mixture, solid	151	1574	Calcium nitrate	140	1454
			Calcium oxide	157	1910
Calcium arsenite, solid	151	1574	Calcium perchlorate	140	1455
Calcium arsenite and Calcium arsenate mixture, solid	151	1574	Calcium permanganate	140	1456
			Calcium peroxide	140	1457
Calcium carbide	138	1402	Calcium phosphide	139	1360
Calcium chlorate	140	1452	Calcium resinate	133	1313
Calcium chlorate, aqueous solution	140	2429	Calcium resinate, fused	133	1314
			Calcium silicide	138	1405
Calcium chlorate, solution	140	2429	Calcium silicon	138	1406
Calcium chlorite	140	1453	Camphor	133	2717
Calcium cyanamide, with more than 0.1% Calcium carbide	138	1403	Camphor, synthetic	133	2717
			Camphor oil	128	1130
Calcium cyanide	157	1575	Caproic acid	153	2829
Calcium dithionite	135	1923	Carbamate pesticide, liquid, flammable, poisonous	131	2758
Calcium hydride	138	1404			
Calcium hydrosulfite	135	1923	Carbamate pesticide, liquid, flammable, toxic	131	2758
Calcium hydrosulphite	135	1923			
Calcium hypochlorite, dry	140	1748	Carbamate pesticide, liquid, poisonous	151	2992
Calcium hypochlorite, hydrated, with not less than 5.5% but not more than 16% water	140	2880			
			Carbamate pesticide, liquid, poisonous, flammable	131	2991
Calcium hypochlorite, hydrated mixture, with not less than 5.5% but not more than 16% water	140	2880	Carbamate pesticide, liquid, toxic	151	2992
			Carbamate pesticide, liquid, toxic, flammable	131	2991
Calcium hypochlorite mixture, dry, with more than 10% but not more than 39% available Chlorine	140	2208	Carbamate pesticide, solid, poisonous	151	2757
			Carbamate pesticide, solid, toxic	151	2757
			Carbon, activated	133	1362

Name of Material	Guide No.	ID No.	Name of Material	Guide No.	ID No.
Carbon, animal or vegetable origin	133	1361	Carbon monoxide and Hydrogen mixture	119	2600
Carbon bisulfide	131	1131	Carbon monoxide and Hydrogen mixture, compressed	119	2600
Carbon bisulphide	131	1131	Carbon tetrabromide	151	2516
Carbon dioxide	120	1013	Carbon tetrachloride	151	1846
Carbon dioxide, compressed	120	1013	Carbonyl fluoride	125	2417
Carbon dioxide, refrigerated liquid	120	2187	Carbonyl fluoride, compressed	125	2417
Carbon dioxide, solid	120	1845	Carbonyl sulfide	119	2204
Carbon dioxide and Ethylene oxide mixture, with more than 9% but not more than 87% Ethylene oxide	115	1041	Carbonyl sulphide	119	2204
			Castor beans, meal, pomace or flake	171	2969
Carbon dioxide and Ethylene oxide mixture, with more than 87% Ethylene oxide	119P	3300	Caustic alkali liquid, n.o.s.	154	1719
			Caustic potash, dry, solid	154	1813
			Caustic potash, liquid	154	1814
Carbon dioxide and Ethylene oxide mixtures, with more than 6% Ethylene oxide	115	1041	Caustic potash, solution	154	1814
			Caustic soda, bead	154	1823
			Caustic soda, flake	154	1823
Carbon dioxide and Ethylene oxide mixtures, with not more than 6% Ethylene oxide	126	1952	Caustic soda, granular	154	1823
			Caustic soda, solid	154	1823
Carbon dioxide and Ethylene oxide mixtures, with not more than 9% Ethylene oxide	126	1952	Caustic soda, solution	154	1824
			Cells, containing Sodium	138	3292
Carbon dioxide and Nitrous oxide mixture	126	1015	Celluloid, in blocks, rods, rolls, sheets, tubes, etc., except scrap	133	2000
Carbon dioxide and Oxygen mixture	122	1014	Celluloid, scrap	135	2002
Carbon dioxide and Oxygen mixture, compressed	122	1014	Cerium, slabs, ingots or rods	170	1333
			Cerium, turnings or gritty powder	138	3078
Carbon disulfide	131	1131	Cesium	138	1407
Carbon disulphide	131	1131	Cesium hydroxide	157	2682
Carbon monoxide	119	1016	Cesium hydroxide, solution	154	2681
Carbon monoxide, compressed	119	1016	Cesium nitrate	140	1451
Carbon monoxide, refrigerated liquid (cryogenic liquid)	168	9202	CG	125	1076
			Charcoal	133	1361

Name of Material	Guide No.	ID No.	Name of Material	Guide No.	ID No.
Chemical kit	154	1760	Chloroacetic acid, solid	153	1751
Chemical kit	171	3316	Chloroacetic acid, solution	153	1750
Chemical sample, poisonous	151	3315	Chloroacetone, stabilized	131	1695
Chemical sample, poisonous liquid	151	3315	Chloroacetonitrile	131	2668
Chemical sample, poisonous solid	151	3315	Chloroacetophenone	153	1697
			Chloroacetophenone, liquid	153	1697
Chemical sample, toxic	151	3315	Chloroacetophenone, liquid	153	3416
Chemical sample, toxic liquid	151	3315	Chloroacetophenone, solid	153	1697
Chemical sample, toxic solid	151	3315	Chloroacetyl chloride	156	1752
Chloral, anhydrous, stabilized	153	2075	Chloroanilines, liquid	152	2019
Chlorate and Borate mixtures	140	1458	Chloroanilines, solid	152	2018
Chlorate and Magnesium chloride mixture	140	1459	Chloroanisidines	152	2233
			Chlorobenzene	130	1134
Chlorate and Magnesium chloride mixture, solid	140	1459	Chlorobenzotrifluorides	130	2234
			Chlorobenzyl chlorides	153	2235
Chlorate and Magnesium chloride mixture, solution	140	3407	Chlorobenzyl chlorides, liquid	153	2235
			Chlorobenzyl chlorides, solid	153	3427
Chlorates, inorganic, aqueous solution, n.o.s.	140	3210	1-Chloro-3-bromopropane	159	2688
Chlorates, inorganic, n.o.s.	140	1461	Chlorobutanes	130	1127
Chloric acid, aqueous solution, with not more than 10% Chloric acid	140	2626	Chlorocresols	152	2669
			Chlorocresols, liquid	152	2669
			Chlorocresols, solid	152	2669
Chlorine	124	1017	Chlorocresols, solid	152	3437
Chlorine dioxide, hydrate, frozen	143	9191	Chlorocresols, solution	152	2669
Chlorine pentafluoride	124	2548	Chlorodifluorobromomethane	126	1974
Chlorine trifluoride	124	1749	1-Chloro-1,1-difluoroethane	115	2517
Chlorite solution	154	1908	Chlorodifluoroethanes	115	2517
Chlorite solution, with more than 5% available Chlorine	154	1908	Chlorodifluoromethane	126	1018
			Chlorodifluoromethane and Chloropentafluoroethane mixture	126	1973
Chlorites, inorganic, n.o.s.	143	1462			
Chloroacetaldehyde	153	2232	Chlorodinitrobenzenes	153	1577
Chloroacetic acid, liquid	153	1750	Chlorodinitrobenzenes, liquid	153	1577
Chloroacetic acid, molten	153	3250	Chlorodinitrobenzenes, solid	153	1577

Name of Material	Guide No.	ID No.	Name of Material	Guide No.	ID No.
Chlorodinitrobenzenes, solid	153	3441	Chlorophenates, solid	154	2905
1-Chloro-2,3-epoxypropane	131P	2023	Chlorophenolates, liquid	154	2904
2-Chloroethanal	153	2232	Chlorophenolates, solid	154	2905
Chloroform	151	1888	Chlorophenols, liquid	153	2021
Chloroformates, n.o.s.	155	2742	Chlorophenols, solid	153	2020
Chloroformates, poisonous, corrosive, flammable, n.o.s.	155	2742	Chlorophenyltrichlorosilane	156	1753
			Chloropicrin	154	1580
Chloroformates, poisonous, corrosive, n.o.s.	154	3277	Chloropicrin and Methyl bromide mixture	123	1581
Chloroformates, toxic, corrosive, flammable, n.o.s.	155	2742	Chloropicrin and Methyl chloride mixture	119	1582
Chloroformates, toxic, corrosive, n.o.s.	154	3277	Chloropicrin mixture, n.o.s.	154	1583
			Chloropivaloyl chloride	156	9263
Chloromethyl chloroformate	157	2745	Chloroplatinic acid, solid	154	2507
Chloromethyl ethyl ether	131	2354	Chloroprene, stabilized	131P	1991
3-Chloro-4-methylphenyl isocyanate	156	2236	1-Chloropropane	129	1278
			2-Chloropropane	129	2356
3-Chloro-4-methylphenyl isocyanate, liquid	156	2236	3-Chloropropanol-1	153	2849
3-Chloro-4-methylphenyl isocyanate, solid	156	3428	2-Chloropropene	130P	2456
			2-Chloropropionic acid	153	2511
Chloronitroanilines	153	2237	2-Chloropropionic acid, solid	153	2511
Chloronitrobenzenes	152	1578	2-Chloropropionic acid, solution	153	2511
Chloronitrobenzenes, liquid	152	1578	2-Chloropyridine	153	2822
Chloronitrobenzenes, liquid	152	3409	Chlorosilanes, corrosive, flammable, n.o.s.	155	2986
Chloronitrobenzenes, solid	152	1578	Chlorosilanes, corrosive, n.o.s.	156	2987
Chloronitrotoluenes	152	2433	Chlorosilanes, flammable, corrosive, n.o.s.	155	2985
Chloronitrotoluenes, liquid	152	2433			
Chloronitrotoluenes, solid	152	2433	Chlorosilanes, n.o.s.	155	2985
Chloronitrotoluenes, solid	152	3457	Chlorosilanes, n.o.s.	155	2986
Chloropentafluoroethane	126	1020	Chlorosilanes, n.o.s.	156	2987
Chloropentafluoroethane and Chlorodifluoromethane mixture	126	1973	Chlorosilanes, n.o.s.	139	2988
			Chlorosilanes, poisonous, corrosive, flammable, n.o.s.	155	3362
Chlorophenates, liquid	154	2904			

Name of Material	Guide No.	ID No.
Chlorosilanes, poisonous, corrosive, n.o.s.	156	3361
Chlorosilanes, toxic, corrosive flammable, n.o.s.	155	3362
Chlorosilanes, toxic, corrosive, n.o.s.	156	3361
Chlorosilanes, water-reactive, flammable, corrosive, n.o.s.	139	2988
Chlorosulfonic acid	137	1754
Chlorosulfonic acid and Sulfur trioxide mixture	137	1754
Chlorosulphonic acid	137	1754
Chlorosulphonic acid and Sulphur trioxide mixture	137	1754
1-Chloro-1,2,2,2-tetrafluoroethane	126	1021
Chlorotetrafluoroethane	126	1021
Chlorotetrafluoroethane and Ethylene oxide mixture, with not more than 8.8% Ethylene oxide	126	3297
Chlorotoluenes	129	2238
4-Chloro-o-toluidine hydrochloride	153	1579
4-Chloro-o-toluidine hydrochloride, solid	153	1579
4-Chloro-o-toluidine hydrochloride, solution	153	3410
Chlorotoluidines	153	2239
Chlorotoluidines, liquid	153	2239
Chlorotoluidines, liquid	153	3429
Chlorotoluidines, solid	153	2239
1-Chloro-2,2,2-trifluoroethane	126	1983
Chlorotrifluoroethane	126	1983
Chlorotrifluoromethane	126	1022
Chlorotrifluoromethane and Trifluoromethane azeotropic mixture with approximately 60% Chlorotrifluoromethane	126	2599
Chromic acid, solid	141	1463
Chromic acid, solution	154	1755
Chromic fluoride, solid	154	1756
Chromic fluoride, solution	154	1757
Chromium nitrate	141	2720
Chromium oxychloride	137	1758
Chromium trioxide, anhydrous	141	1463
Chromosulfuric acid	154	2240
Chromosulphuric acid	154	2240
CK	125	1589
Clinical specimens	158	3373
Clinical waste, unspecified, n.o.s.	158	3291
CN	153	1697
Coal gas	119	1023
Coal gas, compressed	119	1023
Coal tar distillates, flammable	128	1136
Coating solution	127	1139
Cobalt naphthenates, powder	133	2001
Cobalt resinate, precipitated	133	1318
Combustible liquid, n.o.s.	128	1993
Compound, cleaning liquid (corrosive)	154	1760
Compound, cleaning liquid (flammable)	128	1993
Compound, tree or weed killing, liquid (corrosive)	154	1760
Compound, tree or weed killing, liquid (flammable)	128	1993
Compound, tree or weed killing, liquid (toxic)	153	2810

Name of Material	Guide No.	ID No.	Name of Material	Guide No.	ID No.
Compressed gas, flammable, n.o.s.	115	1954	Compressed gas, poisonous, corrosive, n.o.s. (Inhalation Hazard Zone D)	123	3304
Compressed gas, flammable, poisonous, n.o.s. (Inhalation Hazard Zone A)	119	1953	Compressed gas, poisonous, flammable, corrosive, n.o.s.	119	3305
Compressed gas, flammable, poisonous, n.o.s. (Inhalation Hazard Zone B)	119	1953	Compressed gas, poisonous, flammable, corrosive, n.o.s. (Inhalation Hazard Zone A)	119	3305
Compressed gas, flammable, poisonous, n.o.s. (Inhalation Hazard Zone C)	119	1953	Compressed gas, poisonous, flammable, corrosive, n.o.s. (Inhalation Hazard Zone B)	119	3305
Compressed gas, flammable, poisonous, n.o.s. (Inhalation Hazard Zone D)	119	1953	Compressed gas, poisonous, flammable, corrosive, n.o.s. (Inhalation Hazard Zone C)	119	3305
Compressed gas, flammable, toxic, n.o.s. (Inhalation Hazard Zone A)	119	1953	Compressed gas, poisonous, flammable, corrosive, n.o.s. (Inhalation Hazard Zone D)	119	3305
Compressed gas, flammable, toxic, n.o.s. (Inhalation Hazard Zone B)	119	1953	Compressed gas, poisonous, flammable, n.o.s.	119	1953
Compressed gas, flammable, toxic, n.o.s. (Inhalation Hazard Zone C)	119	1953	Compressed gas, poisonous, flammable, n.o.s. (Inhalation Hazard Zone A)	119	1953
Compressed gas, flammable, toxic, n.o.s. (Inhalation Hazard Zone D)	119	1953	Compressed gas, poisonous, flammable, n.o.s. (Inhalation Hazard Zone B)	119	1953
Compressed gas, n.o.s.	126	1956	Compressed gas, poisonous, flammable, n.o.s. (Inhalation Hazard Zone C)	119	1953
Compressed gas, oxidizing, n.o.s.	122	3156	Compressed gas, poisonous, flammable, n.o.s. (Inhalation Hazard Zone D)	119	1953
Compressed gas, poisonous, corrosive, n.o.s.	123	3304	Compressed gas, poisonous, n.o.s.	123	1955
Compressed gas, poisonous, corrosive, n.o.s. (Inhalation Hazard Zone A)	123	3304	Compressed gas, poisonous, n.o.s. (Inhalation Hazard Zone A)	123	1955
Compressed gas, poisonous, corrosive, n.o.s. (Inhalation Hazard Zone B)	123	3304	Compressed gas, poisonous, n.o.s. (Inhalation Hazard Zone B)	123	1955
Compressed gas, poisonous, corrosive, n.o.s. (Inhalation Hazard Zone C)	123	3304			

Name of Material	Guide No.	ID No.	Name of Material	Guide No.	ID No.
Compressed gas, poisonous, n.o.s. (Inhalation Hazard Zone C)	123	1955	Compressed gas, toxic, corrosive, n.o.s. (Inhalation Hazard Zone B)	123	3304
Compressed gas, poisonous, n.o.s. (Inhalation Hazard Zone D)	123	1955	Compressed gas, toxic, corrosive, n.o.s. (Inhalation Hazard Zone C)	123	3304
Compressed gas, poisonous, oxidizing, corrosive, n.o.s.	124	3306	Compressed gas, toxic, corrosive, n.o.s. (Inhalation Hazard Zone D)	123	3304
Compressed gas, poisonous, oxidizing, corrosive, n.o.s. (Inhalation Hazard Zone A)	124	3306	Compressed gas, toxic, flammable, corrosive, n.o.s.	119	3305
Compressed gas, poisonous, oxidizing, corrosive, n.o.s. (Inhalation Hazard Zone B)	124	3306	Compressed gas, toxic, flammable, corrosive, n.o.s. (Inhalation Hazard Zone A)	119	3305
Compressed gas, poisonous, oxidizing, corrosive, n.o.s. (Inhalation Hazard Zone C)	124	3306	Compressed gas, toxic, flammable, corrosive, n.o.s. (Inhalation Hazard Zone B)	119	3305
Compressed gas, poisonous, oxidizing, corrosive, n.o.s. (Inhalation Hazard Zone D)	124	3306	Compressed gas, toxic, flammable, corrosive, n.o.s. (Inhalation Hazard Zone C)	119	3305
Compressed gas, poisonous, oxidizing, n.o.s.	124	3303	Compressed gas, toxic, flammable, corrosive, n.o.s. (Inhalation Hazard Zone D)	119	3305
Compressed gas, poisonous, oxidizing, n.o.s. (Inhalation Hazard Zone A)	124	3303	Compressed gas, toxic, flammable, n.o.s.	119	1953
Compressed gas, poisonous, oxidizing, n.o.s. (Inhalation Hazard Zone B)	124	3303	Compressed gas, toxic, flammable, n.o.s. (Inhalation Hazard Zone A)	119	1953
Compressed gas, poisonous, oxidizing, n.o.s. (Inhalation Hazard Zone C)	124	3303	Compressed gas, toxic, flammable, n.o.s. (Inhalation Hazard Zone B)	119	1953
Compressed gas, poisonous, oxidizing, n.o.s. (Inhalation Hazard Zone D)	124	3303	Compressed gas, toxic, flammable, n.o.s. (Inhalation Hazard Zone C)	119	1953
Compressed gas, toxic, corrosive, n.o.s.	123	3304	Compressed gas, toxic, flammable, n.o.s. (Inhalation Hazard Zone D)	119	1953
Compressed gas, toxic, corrosive, n.o.s. (Inhalation Hazard Zone A)	123	3304	Compressed gas, toxic, n.o.s.	123	1955

Name of Material	Guide No.	ID No.
Compressed gas, toxic, n.o.s. (Inhalation Hazard Zone A)	123	1955
Compressed gas, toxic, n.o.s. (Inhalation Hazard Zone B)	123	1955
Compressed gas, toxic, n.o.s. (Inhalation Hazard Zone C)	123	1955
Compressed gas, toxic, n.o.s. (Inhalation Hazard Zone D)	123	1955
Compressed gas, toxic, oxidizing, corrosive, n.o.s.	124	3306
Compressed gas, toxic, oxidizing, corrosive, n.o.s. (Inhalation Hazard Zone A)	124	3306
Compressed gas, toxic, oxidizing, corrosive, n.o.s. (Inhalation Hazard Zone B)	124	3306
Compressed gas, toxic, oxidizing, corrosive, n.o.s. (Inhalation Hazard Zone C)	124	3306
Compressed gas, toxic, oxidizing, corrosive, n.o.s. (Inhalation Hazard Zone D)	124	3306
Compressed gas, toxic, oxidizing, n.o.s.	124	3303
Compressed gas, toxic, oxidizing, n.o.s. (Inhalation Hazard Zone A)	124	3303
Compressed gas, toxic, oxidizing, n.o.s. (Inhalation Hazard Zone B)	124	3303
Compressed gas, toxic, oxidizing, n.o.s. (Inhalation Hazard Zone C)	124	3303
Compressed gas, toxic, oxidizing, n.o.s. (Inhalation Hazard Zone D)	124	3303
Consumer commodity	171	8000
Copper acetoarsenite	151	1585

Name of Material	Guide No.	ID No.
Copper arsenite	151	1586
Copper based pesticide, liquid, flammable, poisonous	131	2776
Copper based pesticide, liquid, flammable, toxic	131	2776
Copper based pesticide, liquid, poisonous	151	3010
Copper based pesticide, liquid, poisonous, flammable	131	3009
Copper based pesticide, liquid, toxic	151	3010
Copper based pesticide, liquid, toxic, flammable	131	3009
Copper based pesticide, solid, poisonous	151	2775
Copper based pesticide, solid, toxic	151	2775
Copper chlorate	141	2721
Copper chloride	154	2802
Copper cyanide	151	1587
Copra	135	1363
Corrosive liquid, acidic, inorganic, n.o.s.	154	3264
Corrosive liquid, acidic, organic, n.o.s.	153	3265
Corrosive liquid, basic, inorganic, n.o.s.	154	3266
Corrosive liquid, basic, organic, n.o.s.	153	3267
Corrosive liquid, flammable, n.o.s.	132	2920
Corrosive liquid, n.o.s.	154	1760
Corrosive liquid, oxidizing, n.o.s.	140	3093
Corrosive liquid, poisonous, n.o.s.	154	2922

Name of Material	Guide No.	ID No.	Name of Material	Guide No.	ID No.
Corrosive liquid, self-heating, n.o.s.	136	3301	Coumarin derivative pesticide, liquid, poisonous	151	3026
Corrosive liquid, toxic, n.o.s.	154	2922	Coumarin derivative pesticide, liquid, poisonous, flammable	131	3025
Corrosive liquid, water-reactive, n.o.s.	138	3094	Coumarin derivative pesticide, liquid, toxic	151	3026
Corrosive liquid, which in contact with water emits flammable gases, n.o.s.	138	3094	Coumarin derivative pesticide, liquid, toxic, flammable	131	3025
Corrosive solid, acidic, inorganic, n.o.s.	154	3260	Coumarin derivative pesticide, solid, poisonous	151	3027
Corrosive solid, acidic, organic, n.o.s.	154	3261	Coumarin derivative pesticide, solid, toxic	151	3027
Corrosive solid, basic, inorganic, n.o.s.	154	3262	Cresols	153	2076
Corrosive solid, basic, organic, n.o.s.	154	3263	Cresols, liquid	153	2076
			Cresols, solid	153	2076
Corrosive solid, flammable, n.o.s.	134	2921	Cresols, solid	153	3455
Corrosive solid, n.o.s.	154	1759	Cresylic acid	153	2022
Corrosive solid, oxidizing, n.o.s.	140	3084	Crotonaldehyde	131P	1143
Corrosive solid, poisonous, n.o.s.	154	2923	Crotonaldehyde, stabilized	131P	1143
			Crotonic acid	153	2823
Corrosive solid, self-heating, n.o.s.	136	3095	Crotonic acid, liquid	153	2823
			Crotonic acid, liquid	153	3472
Corrosive solid, toxic, n.o.s.	154	2923	Crotonic acid, solid	153	2823
Corrosive solid, water-reactive, n.o.s.	138	3096	Crotonylene	128	1144
			CS	153	2810
Corrosive solid, which in contact with water emits flammable gases, n.o.s.	138	3096	Cumene	130	1918
			Cupriethylenediamine, solution	154	1761
Cotton	133	1365	CX	154	2811
Cotton, wet	133	1365	Cyanide solution, n.o.s.	157	1935
Cotton waste, oily	133	1364	Cyanides, inorganic, n.o.s.	157	1588
Coumarin derivative pesticide, liquid, flammable, poisonous	131	3024	Cyanides, inorganic, solid, n.o.s.	157	1588
Coumarin derivative pesticide, liquid, flammable, toxic	131	3024	Cyanogen	119	1026
			Cyanogen bromide	157	1889

Name of Material	Guide No.	ID No.
Cyanogen chloride, stabilized	125	1589
Cyanogen gas	119	1026
Cyanuric chloride	157	2670
Cyclobutane	115	2601
Cyclobutyl chloroformate	155	2744
1,5,9-Cyclododecatriene	153	2518
Cycloheptane	128	2241
Cycloheptatriene	131	2603
Cycloheptene	128	2242
Cyclohexane	128	1145
Cyclohexanethiol	129	3054
Cyclohexanone	127	1915
Cyclohexene	130	2256
Cyclohexenyltrichlorosilane	156	1762
Cyclohexyl acetate	130	2243
Cyclohexylamine	132	2357
Cyclohexyl isocyanate	155	2488
Cyclohexyl mercaptan	129	3054
Cyclohexyltrichlorosilane	156	1763
Cyclooctadiene phosphines	135	2940
Cyclooctadienes	130P	2520
Cyclooctatetraene	128P	2358
Cyclopentane	128	1146
Cyclopentanol	129	2244
Cyclopentanone	128	2245
Cyclopentene	128	2246
Cyclopropane	115	1027
Cymenes	130	2046
DA	151	1699
Dangerous goods in apparatus	171	3363
Dangerous goods in machinery	171	3363
DC	153	2810

Name of Material	Guide No.	ID No.
Decaborane	134	1868
Decahydronaphthalene	130	1147
n-Decane	128	2247
Denatured alcohol	127	1987
Denatured alcohol (toxic)	131	1986
Desensitized explosive, liquid, n.o.s.	128	3379
Desensitized explosive, solid, n.o.s.	133	3380
Deuterium	115	1957
Deuterium, compressed	115	1957
Devices, small, hydrocarbon gas powered, with release device	115	3150
Diacetone alcohol	129	1148
Diacetyl	127	2346
Diagnostic specimens	158	3373
Diallylamine	132	2359
Diallyl ether	131P	2360
4,4'-Diaminodiphenylmethane	153	2651
Di-n-amylamine	131	2841
Dibenzyldichlorosilane	156	2434
Diborane	119	1911
Diborane, compressed	119	1911
Diborane mixtures	119	1911
Dibromobenzene	129	2711
1,2-Dibromobutan-3-one	154	2648
Dibromochloropropanes	159	2872
Dibromodifluoromethane	171	1941
Dibromomethane	160	2664
Di-n-butylamine	132	2248
Dibutylaminoethanol	153	2873
Dibutyl ethers	128	1149
Dichloroacetic acid	153	1764
1,3-Dichloroacetone	153	2649

Name of Material	Guide No.	ID No.	Name of Material	Guide No.	ID No.
Dichloroacetyl chloride	156	1765	Dichlorophenyltrichlorosilane	156	1766
Dichloroanilines	153	1590	1,2-Dichloropropane	130	1279
Dichloroanilines, liquid	153	1590	Dichloropropane	130	1279
Dichloroanilines, solid	153	1590	1,3-Dichloropropanol-2	153	2750
Dichloroanilines, solid	153	3442	Dichloropropenes	129	2047
o-Dichlorobenzene	152	1591	Dichlorosilane	119	2189
Dichlorobutene	132	2920	1,2-Dichloro-1,1,2,2-tetrafluoroethane	126	1958
2,2'-Dichlorodiethyl ether	152	1916	Dichlorotetrafluoroethane	126	1958
Dichlorodifluoromethane	126	1028	3,5-Dichloro-2,4,6-trifluoropyridine	151	9264
Dichlorodifluoromethane and Difluoroethane azeotropic mixture with approximately 74% Dichlorodifluoromethane	126	2602	Dicyclohexylamine	153	2565
			Dicyclohexylammonium nitrite	133	2687
Dichlorodifluoromethane and Ethylene oxide mixture, with not more than 12.5% Ethylene oxide	126	3070	Dicyclopentadiene	130	2048
			1,2-Di-(dimethylamino)ethane	129	2372
			Didymium nitrate	140	1465
Dichlorodifluoromethane and Ethylene oxide mixture, with not more than 12% Ethylene oxide	126	3070	Dieldrin	151	2761
			Diesel fuel	128	1202
			Diesel fuel	128	1993
Dichlorodimethyl ether, symmetrical	131	2249	Diethoxymethane	127	2373
			3,3-Diethoxypropene	127	2374
1,1-Dichloroethane	130	2362	Diethylamine	132	1154
1,2-Dichloroethylene	130P	1150	2-Diethylaminoethanol	132	2686
Dichloroethylene	130P	1150	Diethylaminoethanol	132	2686
Dichloroethyl ether	152	1916	3-Diethylaminopropylamine	132	2684
Dichlorofluoromethane	126	1029	Diethylaminopropylamine	132	2684
Dichloroisocyanuric acid, dry	140	2465	N,N-Diethylaniline	153	2432
Dichloroisocyanuric acid salts	140	2465	Diethylbenzene	130	2049
Dichloroisopropyl ether	153	2490	Diethyl carbonate	128	2366
Dichloromethane	160	1593	Diethyldichlorosilane	155	1767
1,1-Dichloro-1-nitroethane	153	2650	Diethylenetriamine	154	2079
Dichloropentanes	130	1152	Diethyl ether	127	1155
Dichlorophenyl isocyanates	156	2250	N,N-Diethylethylenediamine	132	2685

Name of Material	Guide No.	ID No.	Name of Material	Guide No.	ID No.
Diethyl ketone	127	1156	2-Dimethylaminoethanol	132	2051
Diethyl sulfate	152	1594	2-Dimethylaminoethyl acrylate	152	3302
Diethyl sulfide	129	2375	2-Dimethylaminoethyl methacrylate	153P	2522
Diethyl sulphate	152	1594	Dimethylaminoethyl methacrylate	153P	2522
Diethyl sulphide	129	2375	N,N-Dimethylaniline	153	2253
Diethylthiophosphoryl chloride	155	2751	2,3-Dimethylbutane	128	2457
Diethylzinc	135	1366	1,3-Dimethylbutylamine	132	2379
Difluorochloroethanes	115	2517	Dimethylcarbamoyl chloride	156	2262
1,1-Difluoroethane	115	1030	Dimethyl carbonate	129	1161
Difluoroethane	115	1030	Dimethylcyclohexanes	128	2263
Difluoroethane and Dichlorodifluoromethane azeotropic mixture with approximately 74% Dichlorodifluoromethane	126	2602	N,N-Dimethylcyclohexylamine	132	2264
			Dimethylcyclohexylamine	132	2264
			Dimethyldichlorosilane	155	1162
1,1-Difluoroethylene	116P	1959	Dimethyldiethoxysilane	127	2380
Difluoromethane	115	3252	Dimethyldioxanes	127	2707
Difluorophosphoric acid, anhydrous	154	1768	Dimethyl disulfide	130	2381
			Dimethyl disulphide	130	2381
2,3-Dihydropyran	127	2376	Dimethylethanolamine	132	2051
Diisobutylamine	132	2361	Dimethyl ether	115	1033
Diisobutylene, isomeric compounds	128	2050	N,N-Dimethylformamide	129	2265
Diisobutyl ketone	128	1157	1,1-Dimethylhydrazine	131	1163
Diisooctyl acid phosphate	153	1902	1,2-Dimethylhydrazine	131	2382
Diisopropylamine	132	1158	Dimethylhydrazine, symmetrical	131	2382
Diisopropyl ether	127	1159	Dimethylhydrazine, unsymmetrical	131	1163
Diketene, stabilized	131P	2521	2,2-Dimethylpropane	115	2044
1,1-Dimethoxyethane	127	2377	Dimethyl-N-propylamine	132	2266
1,2-Dimethoxyethane	127	2252	Dimethyl sulfate	156	1595
Dimethylamine, anhydrous	118	1032	Dimethyl sulfide	130	1164
Dimethylamine, aqueous solution	132	1160	Dimethyl sulphate	156	1595
Dimethylamine, solution	132	1160	Dimethyl sulphide	130	1164
2-Dimethylaminoacetonitrile	131	2378	Dimethyl thiophosphoryl chloride	156	2267

Name of Material	Guide No.	ID No.
Dimethylzinc	135	1370
Dinitroanilines	153	1596
Dinitrobenzenes	152	1597
Dinitrobenzenes, liquid	152	1597
Dinitrobenzenes, solid	152	1597
Dinitrobenzenes, solid	152	3443
Dinitrochlorobenzenes	153	1577
Dinitro-o-cresol	153	1598
Dinitrogen tetroxide	124	1067
Dinitrogen tetroxide and Nitric oxide mixture	124	1975
Dinitrophenol, solution	153	1599
Dinitrophenol, wetted with not less than 15% water	113	1320
Dinitrophenolates, wetted with not less than 15% water	113	1321
Dinitroresorcinol, wetted with not less than 15% water	113	1322
Dinitrotoluenes	152	2038
Dinitrotoluenes, liquid	152	2038
Dinitrotoluenes, molten	152	1600
Dinitrotoluenes, solid	152	2038
Dinitrotoluenes, solid	152	3454
Dioxane	127	1165
Dioxolane	127	1166
Dipentene	128	2052
Diphenylamine chloroarsine	154	1698
Diphenylchloroarsine	151	1699
Diphenylchloroarsine, liquid	151	1699
Diphenylchloroarsine, solid	151	1699
Diphenylchloroarsine, solid	151	3450
Diphenyldichlorosilane	156	1769
Diphenylmethyl bromide	153	1770
Diphosgene	125	1076

Name of Material	Guide No.	ID No.
Dipicryl sulfide, wetted with not less than 10% water	113	2852
Dipicryl sulphide, wetted with not less than 10% water	113	2852
Dipropylamine	132	2383
Di-n-propyl ether	127	2384
Dipropyl ether	127	2384
Dipropyl ketone	128	2710
Disinfectant, liquid, corrosive, n.o.s.	153	1903
Disinfectant, liquid, poisonous, n.o.s.	151	3142
Disinfectant, liquid, toxic, n.o.s.	151	3142
Disinfectant, solid, poisonous, n.o.s.	151	1601
Disinfectant, solid, toxic, n.o.s.	151	1601
Disinfectants, corrosive, liquid, n.o.s.	153	1903
Disinfectants, liquid, n.o.s. (poisonous)	151	3142
Disinfectants, solid, n.o.s. (poisonous)	151	1601
Disodium trioxosilicate	154	3253
Disodium trioxosilicate, pentahydrate	154	3253
Dispersant gas, n.o.s.	126	1078
Dispersant gas, n.o.s. (flammable)	115	1954
Dithiocarbamate pesticide, liquid, flammable, poisonous	131	2772
Dithiocarbamate pesticide, liquid, flammable, toxic	131	2772
Dithiocarbamate pesticide, liquid, poisonous	151	3006
Dithiocarbamate pesticide, liquid, poisonous, flammable	131	3005
Dithiocarbamate pesticide, liquid, toxic	151	3006

Name of Material	Guide No.	ID No.
Dithiocarbamate pesticide, liquid, toxic, flammable	131	3005
Dithiocarbamate pesticide, solid, poisonous	151	2771
Dithiocarbamate pesticide, solid, toxic	151	2771
Divinyl ether, stabilized	128P	1167
DM	154	1698
Dodecylbenzenesulfonic acid	153	2584
Dodecylbenzenesulphonic acid	153	2584
Dodecyltrichlorosilane	156	1771
DP	125	1076
Dry ice	120	1845
Dye, liquid, corrosive, n.o.s.	154	2801
Dye, liquid, poisonous, n.o.s.	151	1602
Dye, liquid, toxic, n.o.s.	151	1602
Dye, solid, corrosive, n.o.s.	154	3147
Dye, solid, poisonous, n.o.s.	151	3143
Dye, solid, toxic, n.o.s.	151	3143
Dye intermediate, liquid, corrosive, n.o.s.	154	2801
Dye intermediate, liquid, poisonous, n.o.s.	151	1602
Dye intermediate, liquid, toxic, n.o.s.	151	1602
Dye intermediate, solid, corrosive, n.o.s.	154	3147
Dye intermediate, solid, poisonous, n.o.s.	151	3143
Dye intermediate, solid, toxic, n.o.s.	151	3143
ED	151	1892
Elevated temperature liquid, flammable, n.o.s., with flash point above 37.8°C (100°F), at or above its flash point	128	3256
Elevated temperature liquid, flammable, n.o.s., with flash point above 60.5°C (141°F), at or above its flash point	128	3256
Elevated temperature liquid, n.o.s., at or above 100°C (212°F), and below its flash point	128	3257
Elevated temperature solid, n.o.s., at or above 240°C (464°F)	171	3258
Engine starting fluid	115	1960
Engines, internal combustion, flammable gas powered	128	3166
Engines, internal combustion, flammable liquid powered	128	3166
Engines, internal combustion, including when fitted in machinery or vehicles	128	3166
Environmentally hazardous substances, liquid, n.o.s.	171	3082
Environmentally hazardous substances, solid, n.o.s.	171	3077
Epibromohydrin	131	2558
Epichlorohydrin	131P	2023
1,2-Epoxy-3-ethoxypropane	127	2752
Esters, n.o.s.	127	3272
Ethane	115	1035
Ethane, compressed	115	1035
Ethane, refrigerated liquid	115	1961
Ethane-Propane mixture, refrigerated liquid	115	1961
Ethanol	127	1170
Ethanol and gasoline mixture, with more than 10% ethanol	127	3475
Ethanol and motor spirit mixture, with more than 10% ethanol	127	3475

Name of Material	Guide No.	ID No.	Name of Material	Guide No.	ID No.
Ethanol and petrol mixture, with more than 10% ethanol	127	3475	Ethyl chloroacetate	155	1181
			Ethyl chloroformate	155	1182
Ethanol, solution	127	1170	Ethyl 2-chloropropionate	129	2935
Ethanolamine	153	2491	Ethyl chlorothioformate	155	2826
Ethanolamine, solution	153	2491	Ethyl crotonate	130	1862
Ethers, n.o.s.	127	3271	Ethyl cyanoacetate	156	2666
Ethyl acetate	129	1173	Ethyldichloroarsine	151	1892
Ethylacetylene, stabilized	116P	2452	Ethyldichlorosilane	139	1183
Ethyl acrylate, stabilized	129P	1917	Ethylene	116P	1962
Ethyl alcohol	127	1170	Ethylene, Acetylene and Propylene in mixture, refrigerated liquid containing at least 71.5% Ethylene with not more than 22.5% Acetylene and not more than 6% Propylene	115	3138
Ethyl alcohol, solution	127	1170			
Ethylamine	118	1036			
Ethylamine, aqueous solution, with not less than 50% but not more than 70% Ethylamine	132	2270			
Ethyl amyl ketone	128	2271	Ethylene, compressed	116P	1962
2-Ethylaniline	153	2273	Ethylene, refrigerated liquid (cryogenic liquid)	115	1038
N-Ethylaniline	153	2272			
Ethylbenzene	130	1175	Ethylene chlorohydrin	131	1135
N-Ethyl-N-benzylaniline	153	2274	Ethylenediamine	132	1604
N-Ethylbenzyltoluidines	153	2753	Ethylene dibromide	154	1605
N-Ethylbenzyltoluidines, liquid	153	2753	Ethylene dibromide and Methyl bromide mixture, liquid	151	1647
N-Ethylbenzyltoluidines, solid	153	2753			
N-Ethylbenzyltoluidines, solid	153	3460	Ethylene dichloride	131	1184
Ethyl borate	129	1176	Ethylene glycol diethyl ether	127	1153
Ethyl bromide	131	1891	Ethylene glycol monobutyl ether	152	2369
Ethyl bromoacetate	155	1603	Ethylene glycol monoethyl ether	127	1171
2-Ethylbutanol	129	2275	Ethylene glycol monoethyl ether acetate	129	1172
2-Ethylbutyl acetate	130	1177			
Ethylbutyl acetate	130	1177	Ethylene glycol monomethyl ether	127	1188
Ethyl butyl ether	127	1179	Ethylene glycol monomethyl ether acetate	129	1189
2-Ethylbutyraldehyde	130	1178			
Ethyl butyrate	130	1180	Ethyleneimine, stabilized	131P	1185
Ethyl chloride	115	1037	Ethylene oxide	119P	1040

Name of Material	Guide No.	ID No.	Name of Material	Guide No.	ID No.
Ethylene oxide and Carbon dioxide mixture, with more than 9% but not more than 87% Ethylene oxide	115	1041	Ethyl ether	127	1155
			Ethyl fluoride	115	2453
			Ethyl formate	129	1190
Ethylene oxide and Carbon dioxide mixture, with more than 87% Ethylene oxide	119P	3300	Ethylhexaldehydes	129	1191
			2-Ethylhexylamine	132	2276
			2-Ethylhexyl chloroformate	156	2748
Ethylene oxide and Carbon dioxide mixtures, with more than 6 % Ethylene oxide	115	1041	Ethyl isobutyrate	129	2385
			Ethyl isocyanate	155	2481
Ethylene oxide and Carbon dioxide mixtures, with not more than 6% Ethylene oxide	126	1952	Ethyl lactate	129	1192
			Ethyl mercaptan	129	2363
			Ethyl methacrylate	130P	2277
Ethylene oxide and Carbon dioxide mixtures, with not more than 9% Ethylene oxide	126	1952	Ethyl methacrylate, stabilized	130P	2277
			Ethyl methyl ether	115	1039
Ethylene oxide and Chlorotetrafluoroethane mixture, with not more than 8.8% Ethylene oxide	126	3297	Ethyl methyl ketone	127	1193
			Ethyl nitrite, solution	131	1194
			Ethyl orthoformate	129	2524
Ethylene oxide and Dichlorodifluoromethane mixture, with not more than 12.5% Ethylene oxide	126	3070	Ethyl oxalate	156	2525
			Ethylphenyldichlorosilane	156	2435
			Ethyl phosphonothioic dichloride, anhydrous	154	2927
Ethylene oxide and Dichlorodifluoromethane mixtures, with not more than 12% Ethylene oxide	126	3070	Ethyl phosphonous dichloride, anhydrous	135	2845
			Ethyl phosphorodichloridate	154	2927
Ethylene oxide and Pentafluoroethane mixture, with not more than 7.9% Ethylene oxide	126	3298	1-Ethylpiperidine	132	2386
			Ethyl propionate	129	1195
			Ethyl propyl ether	127	2615
Ethylene oxide and Propylene oxide mixture, with not more than 30% Ethylene oxide	129P	2983	Ethyl silicate	129	1292
			Ethylsulfuric acid	156	2571
			Ethylsulphuric acid	156	2571
Ethylene oxide and Tetrafluoroethane mixture, with not more than 5.6% Ethylene oxide	126	3299	N-Ethyltoluidines	153	2754
			Ethyltrichlorosilane	155	1196
			Explosive A	112	——
Ethylene oxide with Nitrogen	119P	1040	Explosive B	112	——

Name of Material	Guide No.	ID No.	Name of Material	Guide No.	ID No.
Explosive C	114	—	Fibres, animal or vegetable, burnt, wet or damp	133	1372
Explosives, division 1.1, 1.2, 1.3, 1.5 or 1.6	112	—	Fibres, animal or vegetable or synthetic, n.o.s. with oil	133	1373
Explosives, division 1.4	114	—	Fibres, vegetable, dry	133	3360
Extracts, aromatic, liquid	127	1169	Fibres impregnated with weakly nitrated Nitrocellulose, n.o.s.	133	1353
Extracts, flavoring, liquid	127	1197			
Extracts, flavouring, liquid	127	1197	Films, nitrocellulose base	133	1324
Fabrics, animal or vegetable or synthetic, n.o.s. with oil	133	1373	Fire extinguisher charges, corrosive liquid	154	1774
Fabrics impregnated with weakly nitrated Nitrocellulose, n.o.s.	133	1353	Fire extinguishers with compressed gas	126	1044
Ferric arsenate	151	1606	Fire extinguishers with liquefied gas	126	1044
Ferric arsenite	151	1607			
Ferric chloride	157	1773	Firelighters, solid, with flammable liquid	133	2623
Ferric chloride, anhydrous	157	1773			
Ferric chloride, solution	154	2582	First aid kit	171	3316
Ferric nitrate	140	1466	Fish meal, stabilized	171	2216
Ferrocerium	170	1323	Fish meal, unstabilized	133	1374
Ferrosilicon	139	1408	Fish scrap, stabilized	171	2216
Ferrous arsenate	151	1608	Fish scrap, unstabilized	133	1374
Ferrous chloride, solid	154	1759	Flammable liquid, corrosive, n.o.s	132	2924
Ferrous chloride, solution	154	1760			
Ferrous metal borings, shavings, turnings or cuttings	170	2793	Flammable liquid, n.o.s.	128	1993
Fertilizer, ammoniating solution, with free Ammonia	125	1043	Flammable liquid, poisonous, corrosive, n.o.s.	131	3286
Fiber, animal or vegetable, n.o.s., burnt, wet or damp	133	1372	Flammable liquid, poisonous, n.o.s.	131	1992
Fibers, animal or vegetable or synthetic, n.o.s. with oil	133	1373	Flammable liquid, toxic, corrosive, n.o.s.	131	3286
Fibers, animal or vegetable, burnt, wet or damp	133	1372	Flammable liquid, toxic, n.o.s.	131	1992
Fibers, vegetable, dry	133	3360	Flammable solid, corrosive, inorganic, n.o.s.	134	3180
Fibers impregnated with weakly nitrated Nitrocellulose, n.o.s.	133	1353	Flammable solid, corrosive, n.o.s.	134	2925
			Flammable solid, corrosive, organic, n.o.s.	134	2925

Name of Material	Guide No.	ID No.
Flammable solid, inorganic, corrosive, n.o.s.	134	3180
Flammable solid, inorganic, n.o.s.	133	3178
Flammable solid, n.o.s.	133	1325
Flammable solid, organic, molten, n.o.s.	133	3176
Flammable solid, organic, n.o.s.	133	1325
Flammable solid, oxidizing, n.o.s.	140	3097
Flammable solid, poisonous, inorganic, n.o.s.	134	3179
Flammable solid, poisonous, n.o.s.	134	2926
Flammable solid, poisonous, organic, n.o.s.	134	2926
Flammable solid, toxic, inorganic, n.o.s.	134	3179
Flammable solid, toxic, organic, n.o.s.	134	2926
Fluoboric acid	154	1775
Fluorine	124	1045
Fluorine, compressed	124	1045
Fluorine, refrigerated liquid (cryogenic liquid)	167	9192
Fluoroacetic acid	154	2642
Fluoroanilines	153	2941
Fluorobenzene	130	2387
Fluoroboric acid	154	1775
Fluorophosphoric acid, anhydrous	154	1776
Fluorosilicates, n.o.s.	151	2856
Fluorosilicic acid	154	1778
Fluorosulfonic acid	137	1777
Fluorosulphonic acid	137	1777
Fluorotoluenes	130	2388
Fluosilicic acid	154	1778
Formaldehyde, solution, flammable	132	1198
Formaldehyde, solutions (Formalin)	132	1198
Formaldehyde, solutions (Formalin) (corrosive)	132	2209
Formic acid	153	1779
Formic acid, with more than 85% acid	153	1779
Formic acid, with not less than 5% but less than 10% acid	153	3412
Formic acid, with not less than 10% but not more than 85% acid	153	3412
Fuel, aviation, turbine engine	128	1863
Fuel cell cartridges contained in equipment, containing corrosive substances	153	3477
Fuel cell cartridges contained in equipment, containing flammable liquids	128	3473
Fuel cell cartridges contained in equipment, containing hydrogen in metal hydride	115	3479
Fuel cell cartridges contained in equipment, containing liquefied flammable gas	115	3478
Fuel cell cartridges contained in equipment, containing water-reactive substances	138	3476
Fuel cell cartridges, containing corrosive substances	153	3477
Fuel cell cartridges, containing flammable liquids	128	3473
Fuel cell cartridges, containing hydrogen in metal hydride	115	3479
Fuel cell cartridges, containing liquefied flammable gas	115	3478

Name of Material	Guide No.	ID No.	Name of Material	Guide No.	ID No.
Fuel cell cartridges, containing water-reactive substances	138	3476	Gas, refrigerated liquid, oxidizing, n.o.s.	122	3311
Fuel cell cartridges packed with equipment, containing corrosive substances	153	3477	Gas cartridges	115	2037
			Gas generator assemblies	171	8013
			Gas identification set	123	9035
Fuel cell cartridges packed with equipment, containing flammable liquids	128	3473	Gasohol	128	1203
			Gas oil	128	1202
Fuel cell cartridges packed with equipment, containing hydrogen in metal hydride	115	3479	Gasoline	128	1203
			Gasoline and ethanol mixture, with more than 10% ethanol	127	3475
Fuel cell cartridges packed with equipment, containing liquefied flammable gas	115	3478	Gas sample, non-pressurized, flammable, n.o.s., not refrigerated liquid	115	3167
Fuel cell cartridges packed with equipment, containing water-reactive substances	138	3476	Gas sample, non-pressurized, poisonous, flammable, n.o.s., not refrigerated liquid	119	3168
Fuel oil	128	1202	Gas sample, non-pressurized, poisonous, n.o.s., not refrigerated liquid	123	3169
Fuel oil	128	1993			
Fuel oil, no. 1,2,4,5,6	128	1202			
Fumaryl chloride	156	1780	Gas sample, non-pressurized, toxic, flammable, n.o.s., not refrigerated liquid	119	3168
Fumigated unit	171	3359			
Furaldehydes	132P	1199	Gas sample, non-pressurized, toxic, n.o.s., not refrigerated liquid	123	3169
Furan	128	2389			
Furfural	132P	1199			
Furfuraldehydes	132P	1199	GB	153	2810
Furfuryl alcohol	153	2874	GD	153	2810
Furfurylamine	132	2526	Genetically modified micro-organisms	171	3245
Fusee (rail or highway)	133	1325			
Fusel oil	127	1201	Genetically modified organisms	171	3245
GA	153	2810	Germane	119	2192
Gallium	172	2803	GF	153	2810
Gas, refrigerated liquid, flammable, n.o.s.	115	3312	Glycerol alpha-monochlorohydrin	153	2689
			Glycidaldehyde	131P	2622
Gas, refrigerated liquid, n.o.s.	120	3158	Guanidine nitrate	143	1467

Name of Material	Guide No.	ID No.	Name of Material	Guide No.	ID No.
H	153	2810	Hexafluoroacetone hydrate	151	2552
Hafnium powder, dry	135	2545	Hexafluoroacetone hydrate, liquid	151	2552
Hafnium powder, wetted with not less than 25% water	170	1326	Hexafluoroacetone hydrate, solid	151	3436
Halogenated irritating liquid, n.o.s.	159	1610	Hexafluoroethane	126	2193
Hay, wet, damp or contaminated with oil	133	1327	Hexafluoroethane, compressed	126	2193
			Hexafluorophosphoric acid	154	1782
Hazardous waste, liquid, n.o.s.	171	3082	Hexafluoropropylene	126	1858
Hazardous waste, solid, n.o.s.	171	3077	Hexafluoropropylene oxide	126	1956
HD	153	2810	Hexaldehyde	130	1207
Heating oil, light	128	1202	Hexamethylenediamine, solid	153	2280
Heat producing article	171	8038	Hexamethylenediamine, solution	153	1783
Helium	121	1046			
Helium, compressed	121	1046	Hexamethylene diisocyanate	156	2281
Helium, refrigerated liquid (cryogenic liquid)	120	1963	Hexamethyleneimine	132	2493
			Hexamethylenetetramine	133	1328
Heptafluoropropane	126	3296	Hexamine	133	1328
n-Heptaldehyde	129	3056	Hexanes	128	1208
Heptanes	128	1206	Hexanoic acid	153	2829
n-Heptene	128	2278	Hexanols	129	2282
Hexachloroacetone	153	2661	1-Hexene	128	2370
Hexachlorobenzene	152	2729	Hexyltrichlorosilane	156	1784
Hexachlorobutadiene	151	2279	HL	153	2810
Hexachlorocyclopentadiene	151	2646	HN-1	153	2810
Hexachlorophene	151	2875	HN-2	153	2810
Hexadecyltrichlorosilane	156	1781	HN-3	153	2810
Hexadiene	130	2458	Hydrazine, anhydrous	132	2029
Hexaethyl tetraphosphate	151	1611	Hydrazine, aqueous solution, with more than 37% Hydrazine	153	2030
Hexaethyl tetraphosphate, liquid	151	1611			
Hexaethyl tetraphosphate, solid	151	1611	Hydrazine, aqueous solution, with not less than 37% but not more than 64% Hydrazine	153	2030
Hexaethyl tetraphosphate and compressed gas mixture	123	1612			
Hexafluoroacetone	125	2420			

Name of Material	Guide No.	ID No.	Name of Material	Guide No.	ID No.
Hydrazine, aqueous solution, with not more than 37% Hydrazine	152	3293	Hydrofluoric acid and Sulphuric acid mixture	157	1786
Hydrazine, aqueous solutions, with more than 64% Hydrazine	132	2029	Hydrofluorosilicic acid	154	1778
			Hydrogen	115	1049
Hydrazine hydrate	153	2030	Hydrogen absorbed in metal hydride	115	9279
Hydrides, metal, n.o.s.	138	1409	Hydrogen, compressed	115	1049
Hydriodic acid	154	1787	Hydrogen in a metal hydride storage system	115	3468
Hydriodic acid, solution	154	1787			
Hydrobromic acid	154	1788	Hydrogen in a metal hydride storage system contained in equipment	115	3468
Hydrobromic acid, solution	154	1788			
Hydrocarbon gas, compressed, n.o.s.	115	1964	Hydrogen in a metal hydride storage system packed with equipment	115	3468
Hydrocarbon gas, liquefied, n.o.s.	115	1965			
Hydrocarbon gas mixture, compressed, n.o.s.	115	1964	Hydrogen, refrigerated liquid (cryogenic liquid)	115	1966
Hydrocarbon gas mixture, liquefied, n.o.s.	115	1965	Hydrogen and Carbon monoxide mixture	119	2600
Hydrocarbon gas refills for small devices, with release device	115	3150	Hydrogen and Carbon monoxide mixture, compressed	119	2600
Hydrocarbons, liquid, n.o.s.	128	3295	Hydrogen and Methane mixture, compressed	115	2034
Hydrochloric acid	157	1789	Hydrogen bromide, anhydrous	125	1048
Hydrochloric acid, solution	157	1789	Hydrogen chloride, anhydrous	125	1050
Hydrocyanic acid, aqueous solution, with less than 5% Hydrogen cyanide	154	1613	Hydrogen chloride, refrigerated liquid	125	2186
Hydrocyanic acid, aqueous solution, with not more than 20% Hydrogen cyanide	154	1613	Hydrogen cyanide, anhydrous, stabilized	117	1051
			Hydrogen cyanide, aqueous solution, with not more than 20% Hydrogen cyanide	154	1613
Hydrocyanic acid, aqueous solutions, with more than 20% Hydrogen cyanide	117	1051	Hydrogen cyanide, solution in alcohol, with not more than 45% Hydrogen cyanide	131	3294
Hydrofluoric acid	157	1790	Hydrogen cyanide, stabilized	117	1051
Hydrofluoric acid, solution	157	1790	Hydrogen cyanide, stabilized (absorbed)	152	1614
Hydrofluoric acid and Sulfuric acid mixture	157	1786			

Name of Material	Guide No.	ID No.	Name of Material	Guide No.	ID No.
Hydrogendifluorides, n.o.s.	154	1740	Hypochlorite solution, with more than 5% available Chlorine	154	1791
Hydrogendifluorides, solid, n.o.s.	154	1740	Hypochlorites, inorganic, n.o.s.	140	3212
Hydrogendifluorides, solution, n.o.s.	154	3471	3,3'-Iminodipropylamine	153	2269
Hydrogen fluoride, anhydrous	125	1052	Infectious substance, affecting animals only	158	2900
Hydrogen iodide, anhydrous	125	2197	Infectious substance, affecting humans	158	2814
Hydrogen peroxide, aqueous solution, stabilized, with more than 60% Hydrogen peroxide	143	2015	Ink, printer's, flammable	129	1210
			Insecticide gas, flammable, n.o.s.	115	1954
Hydrogen peroxide, aqueous solution, with not less than 8% but less than 20% Hydrogen peroxide	140	2984	Insecticide gas, flammable, n.o.s.	115	3354
			Insecticide gas, n.o.s.	126	1968
			Insecticide gas, poisonous, flammable, n.o.s.	119	3355
Hydrogen peroxide, aqueous solution, with not less than 20% but not more than 60% Hydrogen peroxide (stabilized as necessary)	140	2014	Insecticide gas, poisonous, flammable, n.o.s. (Inhalation Hazard Zone A)	119	3355
			Insecticide gas, poisonous, flammable, n.o.s. (Inhalation Hazard Zone B)	119	3355
Hydrogen peroxide, stabilized	143	2015	Insecticide gas, poisonous, flammable, n.o.s. (Inhalation Hazard Zone C)	119	3355
Hydrogen peroxide and Peroxyacetic acid mixture, with acid(s), water and not more than 5% Peroxyacetic acid, stabilized	140	3149	Insecticide gas, poisonous, flammable, n.o.s. (Inhalation Hazard Zone D)	119	3355
Hydrogen selenide, anhydrous	117	2202	Insecticide gas, poisonous, n.o.s.	123	1967
Hydrogen sulfide	117	1053	Insecticide gas, toxic, flammable, n.o.s.	119	3355
Hydrogen sulphide	117	1053	Insecticide gas, toxic, flammable, n.o.s. (Inhalation Hazard Zone A)	119	3355
Hydroquinone	153	2662			
Hydroquinone, solid	153	2662	Insecticide gas, toxic, flammable, n.o.s. (Inhalation Hazard Zone B)	119	3355
Hydroquinone, solution	153	3435			
1-Hydroxybenzotriazole, anhydrous, wetted with not less than 20% water	113	3474			
Hydroxylamine sulfate	154	2865	Insecticide gas, toxic, flammable, n.o.s. (Inhalation Hazard Zone C)	119	3355
Hydroxylamine sulphate	154	2865			
Hypochlorite solution	154	1791			

Name of Material	Guide No.	ID No.	Name of Material	Guide No.	ID No.
Insecticide gas, toxic, flammable, n.o.s. (Inhalation Hazard Zone D)	119	3355	Isobutyric anhydride	132	2530
			Isobutyronitrile	131	2284
Insecticide gas, toxic, n.o.s.	123	1967	Isobutyryl chloride	132	2395
Iodine monochloride	157	1792	Isocyanate solution, flammable, poisonous, n.o.s.	155	2478
Iodine pentafluoride	144	2495	Isocyanate solution, flammable, toxic, n.o.s.	155	2478
2-Iodobutane	129	2390			
Iodomethylpropanes	129	2391	Isocyanate solution, poisonous, flammable, n.o.s.	155	3080
Iodopropanes	129	2392			
IPDI	156	2290	Isocyanate solution, poisonous, n.o.s.	155	2206
Iron oxide, spent	135	1376			
Iron pentacarbonyl	131	1994	Isocyanate solution, toxic, flammable, n.o.s.	155	3080
Iron sponge, spent	135	1376	Isocyanate solution, toxic, n.o.s.	155	2206
Isobutane	115	1075	Isocyanate solutions, n.o.s.	155	2206
Isobutane	115	1969	Isocyanate solutions, n.o.s.	155	2478
Isobutane mixture	115	1075	Isocyanate solutions, n.o.s.	155	3080
Isobutane mixture	115	1969	Isocyanates, flammable, poisonous, n.o.s.	155	2478
Isobutanol	129	1212			
Isobutyl acetate	129	1213	Isocyanates, flammable, toxic, n.o.s.	155	2478
Isobutyl acrylate, stabilized	129P	2527			
Isobutyl alcohol	129	1212	Isocyanates, n.o.s.	155	2206
Isobutyl aldehyde	130	2045	Isocyanates, n.o.s.	155	2478
Isobutylamine	132	1214	Isocyanates, n.o.s.	155	3080
Isobutyl chloroformate	155	2742	Isocyanates, poisonous, flammable, n.o.s.	155	3080
Isobutylene	115	1055			
Isobutylene	115	1075	Isocyanates, poisonous, n.o.s.	155	2206
Isobutyl formate	129	2393	Isocyanates, toxic, flammable, n.o.s.	155	3080
Isobutyl isobutyrate	130	2528			
Isobutyl isocyanate	155	2486	Isocyanates, toxic, n.o.s.	155	2206
Isobutyl methacrylate, stabilized	130P	2283	Isocyanatobenzotrifluorides	156	2285
Isobutyl propionate	129	2394	Isoheptenes	128	2287
Isobutyraldehyde	130	2045	Isohexenes	128	2288
Isobutyric acid	132	2529	Isooctane	128	1262
			Isooctenes	128	1216

Name of Material	Guide No.	ID No.	Name of Material	Guide No.	ID No.
Isopentane	128	1265	Lead compound, soluble, n.o.s.	151	2291
Isopentenes	128	2371	Lead cyanide	151	1620
Isophoronediamine	153	2289	Lead dioxide	141	1872
Isophorone diisocyanate	156	2290	Lead nitrate	141	1469
Isoprene, stabilized	130P	1218	Lead perchlorate	141	1470
Isopropanol	129	1219	Lead perchlorate, solid	141	1470
Isopropenyl acetate	129P	2403	Lead perchlorate, solution	141	1470
Isopropenylbenzene	128	2303	Lead perchlorate, solution	141	3408
Isopropyl acetate	129	1220	Lead phosphite, dibasic	133	2989
Isopropyl acid phosphate	153	1793	Lead sulfate, with more than 3% free acid	154	1794
Isopropyl alcohol	129	1219			
Isopropylamine	132	1221	Lead sulphate, with more than 3% free acid	154	1794
Isopropylbenzene	130	1918			
Isopropyl butyrate	129	2405	Lewisite	153	2810
Isopropyl chloroacetate	155	2947	Life-saving appliances, not self-inflating	171	3072
Isopropyl chloroformate	155	2407			
Isopropyl 2-chloropropionate	129	2934	Life-saving appliances, self-inflating	171	2990
Isopropyl isobutyrate	127	2406			
Isopropyl isocyanate	155	2483	Lighter refills (cigarettes) (flammable gas)	115	1057
Isopropyl nitrate	130	1222			
Isopropyl propionate	129	2409	Lighters (cigarettes) (flammable gas)	115	1057
Isosorbide dinitrate mixture	133	2907			
Isosorbide-5-mononitrate	133	3251	Lighters for cigars, cigarettes (flammable liquid)	128	1226
Kerosene	128	1223			
Ketones, liquid, n.o.s.	127	1224	Liquefied gas, flammable, n.o.s.	115	3161
Krypton	121	1056	Liquefied gas, n.o.s.	126	3163
Krypton, compressed	121	1056	Liquefied gas, oxidizing, n.o.s.	122	3157
Krypton, refrigerated liquid (cryogenic liquid)	120	1970	Liquefied gas, poisonous, corrosive, n.o.s.	123	3308
			Liquefied gas, poisonous, corrosive, n.o.s. (Inhalation Hazard Zone A)	123	3308
L (Lewisite)	153	2810			
Lead acetate	151	1616	Liquefied gas, poisonous, corrosive, n.o.s. (Inhalation Hazard Zone B)	123	3308
Lead arsenates	151	1617			
Lead arsenites	151	1618			

Name of Material	Guide No.	ID No.	Name of Material	Guide No.	ID No.
Liquefied gas, poisonous, corrosive, n.o.s. (Inhalation Hazard Zone C)	123	3308	Liquefied gas, poisonous, n.o.s. (Inhalation Hazard Zone C)	123	3162
Liquefied gas, poisonous, corrosive, n.o.s. (Inhalation Hazard Zone D)	123	3308	Liquefied gas, poisonous, n.o.s. (Inhalation Hazard Zone D)	123	3162
Liquefied gas, poisonous, flammable, corrosive, n.o.s.	119	3309	Liquefied gas, poisonous, oxidizing, corrosive, n.o.s.	124	3310
Liquefied gas, poisonous, flammable, corrosive, n.o.s. (Inhalation Hazard Zone A)	119	3309	Liquefied gas, poisonous, oxidizing, corrosive, n.o.s. (Inhalation Hazard Zone A)	124	3310
Liquefied gas, poisonous, flammable, corrosive, n.o.s. (Inhalation Hazard Zone B)	119	3309	Liquefied gas, poisonous, oxidizing, corrosive, n.o.s. (Inhalation Hazard Zone B)	124	3310
Liquefied gas, poisonous, flammable, corrosive, n.o.s. (Inhalation Hazard Zone C)	119	3309	Liquefied gas, poisonous, oxidizing, corrosive, n.o.s. (Inhalation Hazard Zone C)	124	3310
Liquefied gas, poisonous, flammable, corrosive, n.o.s. (Inhalation Hazard Zone D)	119	3309	Liquefied gas, poisonous, oxidizing, corrosive, n.o.s. (Inhalation Hazard Zone D)	124	3310
Liquefied gas, poisonous, flammable, n.o.s.	119	3160	Liquefied gas, poisonous, oxidizing, n.o.s.	124	3307
Liquefied gas, poisonous, flammable, n.o.s. (Inhalation Hazard Zone A)	119	3160	Liquefied gas, poisonous, oxidizing, n.o.s. (Inhalation Hazard Zone A)	124	3307
Liquefied gas, poisonous, flammable, n.o.s. (Inhalation Hazard Zone B)	119	3160	Liquefied gas, poisonous, oxidizing, n.o.s. (Inhalation Hazard Zone B)	124	3307
Liquefied gas, poisonous, flammable, n.o.s. (Inhalation Hazard Zone C)	119	3160	Liquefied gas, poisonous, oxidizing, n.o.s. (Inhalation Hazard Zone C)	124	3307
Liquefied gas, poisonous, flammable, n.o.s. (Inhalation Hazard Zone D)	119	3160	Liquefied gas, poisonous, oxidizing, n.o.s. (Inhalation Hazard Zone D)	124	3307
Liquefied gas, poisonous, n.o.s.	123	3162	Liquefied gas, toxic, corrosive, n.o.s.	123	3308
Liquefied gas, poisonous, n.o.s. (Inhalation Hazard Zone A)	123	3162	Liquefied gas, toxic, corrosive, n.o.s. (Inhalation Hazard Zone A)	123	3308
Liquefied gas, poisonous, n.o.s. (Inhalation Hazard Zone B)	123	3162	Liquefied gas, toxic, corrosive, n.o.s. (Inhalation Hazard Zone B)	123	3308

Name of Material	Guide No.	ID No.	Name of Material	Guide No.	ID No.
Liquefied gas, toxic, corrosive, n.o.s. (Inhalation Hazard Zone C)	123	3308	Liquefied gas, toxic, n.o.s. (Inhalation Hazard Zone C)	123	3162
Liquefied gas, toxic, corrosive, n.o.s. (Inhalation Hazard Zone D)	123	3308	Liquefied gas, toxic, n.o.s. (Inhalation Hazard Zone D)	123	3162
Liquefied gas, toxic, flammable, corrosive, n.o.s.	119	3309	Liquefied gas, toxic, oxidizing, corrosive, n.o.s.	124	3310
Liquefied gas, toxic, flammable, corrosive, n.o.s. (Inhalation Hazard Zone A)	119	3309	Liquefied gas, toxic, oxidizing, corrosive, n.o.s. (Inhalation Hazard Zone A)	124	3310
Liquefied gas, toxic, flammable, corrosive, n.o.s. (Inhalation Hazard Zone B)	119	3309	Liquefied gas, toxic, oxidizing, corrosive, n.o.s. (Inhalation Hazard Zone B)	124	3310
Liquefied gas, toxic, flammable, corrosive, n.o.s. (Inhalation Hazard Zone C)	119	3309	Liquefied gas, toxic, oxidizing, corrosive, n.o.s. (Inhalation Hazard Zone C)	124	3310
Liquefied gas, toxic, flammable, corrosive, n.o.s. (Inhalation Hazard Zone D)	119	3309	Liquefied gas, toxic, oxidizing, corrosive, n.o.s. (Inhalation Hazard Zone D)	124	3310
Liquefied gas, toxic, flammable, n.o.s.	119	3160	Liquefied gas, toxic, oxidizing, n.o.s.	124	3307
Liquefied gas, toxic, flammable, n.o.s. (Inhalation Hazard Zone A)	119	3160	Liquefied gas, toxic, oxidizing, n.o.s. (Inhalation Hazard Zone A)	124	3307
Liquefied gas, toxic, flammable, n.o.s. (Inhalation Hazard Zone B)	119	3160	Liquefied gas, toxic, oxidizing, n.o.s. (Inhalation Hazard Zone B)	124	3307
Liquefied gas, toxic, flammable, n.o.s. (Inhalation Hazard Zone C)	119	3160	Liquefied gas, toxic, oxidizing, n.o.s. (Inhalation Hazard Zone C)	124	3307
Liquefied gas, toxic, flammable, n.o.s. (Inhalation Hazard Zone D)	119	3160	Liquefied gas, toxic, oxidizing, n.o.s. (Inhalation Hazard Zone D)	124	3307
Liquefied gas, toxic, n.o.s.	123	3162	Liquefied gases, non-flammable, charged with Nitrogen, Carbon dioxide or Air	120	1058
Liquefied gas, toxic, n.o.s. (Inhalation Hazard Zone A)	123	3162	Liquefied natural gas (cryogenic liquid)	115	1972
Liquefied gas, toxic, n.o.s. (Inhalation Hazard Zone B)	123	3162	Liquefied petroleum gas	115	1075
			Lithium	138	1415

Name of Material	Guide No.	ID No.	Name of Material	Guide No.	ID No.
Lithium alkyls	135	2445	Lithium metal batteries contained in equipment (including lithium alloy batteries)	138	3091
Lithium alkyls, liquid	135	2445			
Lithium alkyls, solid	135	3433			
Lithium aluminum hydride	138	1410	Lithium metal batteries (including lithium alloy batteries)	138	3090
Lithium aluminum hydride, ethereal	138	1411			
Lithium amide	139	1412	Lithium metal batteries packed with equipment (including lithium alloy batteries)	138	3091
Lithium batteries	138	3090			
Lithium batteries, liquid or solid cathode	138	3090	Lithium nitrate	140	2722
			Lithium nitride	138	2806
Lithium batteries contained in equipment	138	3091	Lithium peroxide	143	1472
Lithium batteries packed with equipment	138	3091	Lithium silicon	138	1417
			LNG (cryogenic liquid)	115	1972
Lithium borohydride	138	1413	London purple	151	1621
Lithium ferrosilicon	139	2830	LPG	115	1075
Lithium hydride	138	1414	Magnesium	138	1869
Lithium hydride, fused solid	138	2805	Magnesium, in pellets, turnings or ribbons	138	1869
Lithium hydroxide	154	2680			
Lithium hydroxide, monohydrate	154	2680	Magnesium alkyls	135	3053
Lithium hydroxide, solid	154	2680	Magnesium alloys, with more than 50% Magnesium, in pellets, turnings or ribbons	138	1869
Lithium hydroxide, solution	154	2679			
Lithium hypochlorite, dry	140	1471			
Lithium hypochlorite mixture	140	1471	Magnesium alloys powder	138	1418
Lithium hypochlorite mixtures, dry	140	1471	Magnesium aluminum phosphide	139	1419
			Magnesium arsenate	151	1622
Lithium ion batteries contained in equipment (including lithium ion polymer batteries)	147	3481	Magnesium bromate	140	1473
			Magnesium chlorate	140	2723
			Magnesium chloride and Chlorate mixture	140	1459
Lithium ion batteries (including lithium ion polymer batteries)	147	3480			
			Magnesium chloride and Chlorate mixture, solid	140	1459
Lithium ion batteries packed with equipment (including lithium ion polymer batteries)	147	3481			
			Magnesium chloride and Chlorate mixture, solution	140	3407
			Magnesium diamide	135	2004
			Magnesium diphenyl	135	2005

Name of Material	Guide No.	ID No.	Name of Material	Guide No.	ID No.
Magnesium fluorosilicate	151	2853	Medicine, liquid, toxic, n.o.s.	151	1851
Magnesium granules, coated	138	2950	Medicine, solid, poisonous, n.o.s.	151	3249
Magnesium hydride	138	2010			
Magnesium nitrate	140	1474	Medicine, solid, toxic, n.o.s.	151	3249
Magnesium perchlorate	140	1475	Medicines, corrosive, liquid, n.o.s.	154	1760
Magnesium peroxide	140	1476			
Magnesium phosphide	139	2011	Medicines, corrosive, solid, n.o.s.	154	1759
Magnesium powder	138	1418	Medicines, flammable, liquid, n.o.s.	128	1993
Magnesium silicide	138	2624			
Magnesium silicofluoride	151	2853	Medicines, flammable, solid, n.o.s.	133	1325
Magnetized material	171	2807			
Maleic acid	156	2215	Mercaptan mixture, liquid, flammable, n.o.s.	130	3336
Maleic anhydride	156	2215			
Maleic anhydride, molten	156	2215	Mercaptan mixture, liquid, flammable, poisonous, n.o.s.	131	1228
Malononitrile	153	2647	Mercaptan mixture, liquid, flammable, toxic, n.o.s.	131	1228
Maneb	135	2210			
Maneb, stabilized	135	2968	Mercaptan mixture, liquid, poisonous, flammable, n.o.s.	131	3071
Maneb preparation, stabilized	135	2968			
Maneb preparation, with not less than 60% Maneb	135	2210	Mercaptan mixture, liquid, toxic, flammable, n.o.s.	131	3071
			Mercaptans, liquid, flammable, n.o.s.	130	3336
Manganese nitrate	140	2724			
Manganese resinate	133	1330	Mercaptans, liquid, flammable, poisonous, n.o.s.	131	1228
Matches, fusee	133	2254			
Matches, safety	133	1944	Mercaptans, liquid, flammable, toxic, n.o.s.	131	1228
Matches, "strike anywhere"	133	1331			
Matches, wax "vesta"	133	1945	Mercaptans, liquid, poisonous, flammable, n.o.s.	131	3071
MD	152	1556			
Medical waste, n.o.s.	158	3291	Mercaptans, liquid, toxic, flammable, n.o.s.	131	3071
Medicine, liquid, flammable, poisonous, n.o.s.	131	3248	Mercuric arsenate	151	1623
			Mercuric bromide	154	1634
Medicine, liquid, flammable, toxic, n.o.s.	131	3248	Mercuric chloride	154	1624
			Mercuric cyanide	154	1636
Medicine, liquid, poisonous, n.o.s.	151	1851	Mercuric nitrate	141	1625

Name of Material	Guide No.	ID No.	Name of Material	Guide No.	ID No.
Mercuric oxycyanide	151	1642	Mercury oxide	151	1641
Mercuric potassium cyanide	157	1626	Mercury oxycyanide, desensitized	151	1642
Mercuric sulfate	151	1645			
Mercuric sulphate	151	1645	Mercury potassium iodide	151	1643
Mercurous bromide	154	1634	Mercury salicylate	151	1644
Mercurous nitrate	141	1627	Mercury sulfate	151	1645
Mercury	172	2809	Mercury sulphate	151	1645
Mercury acetate	151	1629	Mercury thiocyanate	151	1646
Mercury ammonium chloride	151	1630	Mesityl oxide	129	1229
Mercury based pesticide, liquid, flammable, poisonous	131	2778	Metal alkyl, solution, n.o.s.	135	9195
			Metal alkyl halides, n.o.s.	138	3049
Mercury based pesticide, liquid, flammable, toxic	131	2778	Metal alkyl halides, water-reactive, n.o.s.	138	3049
Mercury based pesticide, liquid, poisonous	151	3012	Metal alkyl hydrides, n.o.s.	138	3050
Mercury based pesticide, liquid, poisonous, flammable	131	3011	Metal alkyl hydrides, water-reactive, n.o.s.	138	3050
			Metal alkyls, n.o.s.	135	2003
Mercury based pesticide, liquid, toxic	151	3012	Metal alkyls, water-reactive, n.o.s.	135	2003
Mercury based pesticide, liquid, toxic, flammable	131	3011	Metal aryl halides, n.o.s.	138	3049
Mercury based pesticide, solid, poisonous	151	2777	Metal aryl halides, water-reactive, n.o.s.	138	3049
			Metal aryl hydrides, n.o.s.	138	3050
Mercury based pesticide, solid, toxic	151	2777	Metal aryl hydrides, water-reactive, n.o.s.	138	3050
Mercury benzoate	154	1631	Metal aryls, n.o.s	135	2003
Mercury bromides	154	1634	Metal aryls, water-reactive, n.o.s.	135	2003
Mercury compound, liquid, n.o.s.	151	2024			
Mercury compound, solid, n.o.s.	151	2025	Metal carbonyls, liquid, n.o.s.	151	3281
Mercury cyanide	154	1636	Metal carbonyls, n.o.s.	151	3281
Mercury gluconate	151	1637	Metal carbonyls, solid, n.o.s.	151	3466
Mercury iodide	151	1638	Metal catalyst, dry	135	2881
Mercury metal	172	2809	Metal catalyst, wetted	170	1378
Mercury nucleate	151	1639	Metaldehyde	133	1332
Mercury oleate	151	1640	Metal hydrides, flammable, n.o.s.	170	3182

Name of Material	Guide No.	ID No.
Metal hydrides, water-reactive, n.o.s.	138	1409
Metallic substance, water-reactive, n.o.s.	138	3208
Metallic substance, water-reactive, self-heating, n.o.s.	138	3209
Metal powder, flammable, n.o.s.	170	3089
Metal powder, self-heating, n.o.s.	135	3189
Metal salts of organic compounds, flammable, n.o.s.	133	3181
Methacrylaldehyde, stabilized	131P	2396
Methacrylic acid, stabilized	153P	2531
Methacrylonitrile, stabilized	131P	3079
Methallyl alcohol	129	2614
Methane	115	1971
Methane, compressed	115	1971
Methane, refrigerated liquid (cryogenic liquid)	115	1972
Methane and Hydrogen mixture, compressed	115	2034
Methanesulfonyl chloride	156	3246
Methanesulphonyl chloride	156	3246
Methanol	131	1230
Methoxymethyl isocyanate	155	2605
4-Methoxy-4-methyl-pentan-2-one	128	2293
1-Methoxy-2-propanol	129	3092
Methyl acetate	129	1231
Methylacetylene and Propadiene mixture, stabilized	116P	1060
Methyl acrylate, stabilized	129P	1919
Methylal	127	1234
Methyl alcohol	131	1230
Methylallyl chloride	130P	2554

Name of Material	Guide No.	ID No.
Methylamine, anhydrous	118	1061
Methylamine, aqueous solution	132	1235
Methylamyl acetate	130	1233
Methylamyl alcohol	129	2053
Methyl amyl ketone	127	1110
N-Methylaniline	153	2294
Methyl benzoate	152	2938
alpha-Methylbenzyl alcohol	153	2937
alpha-Methylbenzyl alcohol, liquid	153	2937
alpha-Methylbenzyl alcohol, solid	153	3438
Methylbenzyl alcohol (alpha)	153	2937
Methyl bromide	123	1062
Methyl bromide and Chloropicrin mixture	123	1581
Methyl bromide and Ethylene dibromide mixture, liquid	151	1647
Methyl bromoacetate	155	2643
2-Methylbutanal	129	3371
3-Methylbutan-2-one	127	2397
2-Methyl-1-butene	128	2459
2-Methyl-2-butene	128	2460
3-Methyl-1-butene	128	2561
N-Methylbutylamine	132	2945
Methyl tert-butyl ether	127	2398
Methyl butyrate	129	1237
Methyl chloride	115	1063
Methyl chloride and Chloropicrin mixture	119	1582
Methyl chloride and Methylene chloride mixture	115	1912
Methyl chloroacetate	155	2295
Methyl chloroformate	155	1238

Name of Material	Guide No.	ID No.
Methyl chloromethyl ether	131	1239
Methyl 2-chloropropionate	129	2933
Methylchlorosilane	119	2534
Methyl cyanide	127	1648
Methylcyclohexane	128	2296
Methylcyclohexanols	129	2617
Methylcyclohexanone	128	2297
Methylcyclopentane	128	2298
Methyl dichloroacetate	155	2299
Methyldichloroarsine	152	1556
Methyldichlorosilane	139	1242
Methylene chloride	160	1593
Methylene chloride and Methyl chloride mixture	115	1912
Methyl ethyl ether	115	1039
Methyl ethyl ketone	127	1193
2-Methyl-5-ethylpyridine	153	2300
Methyl fluoride	115	2454
Methyl formate	129	1243
2-Methylfuran	128	2301
2-Methyl-2-heptanethiol	131	3023
5-Methylhexan-2-one	127	2302
Methylhydrazine	131	1244
Methyl iodide	151	2644
Methyl isobutyl carbinol	129	2053
Methyl isobutyl ketone	127	1245
Methyl isocyanate	155	2480
Methyl isopropenyl ketone, stabilized	127P	1246
Methyl isothiocyanate	131	2477
Methyl isovalerate	130	2400
Methyl magnesium bromide in Ethyl ether	135	1928

Name of Material	Guide No.	ID No.
Methyl mercaptan	117	1064
Methyl methacrylate monomer, stabilized	129P	1247
4-Methylmorpholine	132	2535
N-Methylmorpholine	132	2535
Methylmorpholine	132	2535
Methyl nitrite	116	2455
Methyl orthosilicate	155	2606
Methyl parathion, liquid	152	3018
Methyl parathion, solid	152	2783
Methylpentadiene	128	2461
2-Methylpentan-2-ol	129	2560
Methylphenyldichlorosilane	156	2437
Methyl phosphonic dichloride	137	9206
Methyl phosphonous dichloride	135	2845
1-Methylpiperidine	132	2399
Methyl propionate	129	1248
Methyl propyl ether	127	2612
Methyl propyl ketone	127	1249
Methyltetrahydrofuran	127	2536
Methyl trichloroacetate	156	2533
Methyltrichlorosilane	155	1250
alpha-Methylvaleraldehyde	130	2367
Methyl valeraldehyde (alpha)	130	2367
Methyl vinyl ketone, stabilized	131P	1251
M.I.B.C.	129	2053
Molybdenum pentachloride	156	2508
Monoethanolamine	153	2491
Mononitrotoluidines	153	2660
Monopropylamine	132	1277
Morpholine	132	2054
Motor fuel anti-knock mixture	131	1649
Motor spirit	128	1203

Name of Material	Guide No.	ID No.	Name of Material	Guide No.	ID No.
Motor spirit and ethanol mixture, with more than 10% ethanol	127	3475	Nicotine compound, liquid, n.o.s.	151	3144
Muriatic acid	157	1789	Nicotine compound, solid, n.o.s.	151	1655
Musk xylene	149	2956	Nicotine hydrochloride	151	1656
Mustard	153	2810	Nicotine hydrochloride, liquid	151	1656
Mustard Lewisite	153	2810	Nicotine hydrochloride, solid	151	1656
Naphthalene, crude	133	1334	Nicotine hydrochloride, solid	151	3444
Naphthalene, molten	133	2304	Nicotine hydrochloride, solution	151	1656
Naphthalene, refined	133	1334	Nicotine preparation, liquid, n.o.s.	151	3144
alpha-Naphthylamine	153	2077	Nicotine preparation, solid, n.o.s.	151	1655
Naphthylamine (alpha)	153	2077	Nicotine salicylate	151	1657
beta-Naphthylamine	153	1650	Nicotine sulfate, solid	151	1658
beta-Naphthylamine, solid	153	1650	Nicotine sulfate, solid	151	3445
beta-Naphthylamine, solution	153	3411	Nicotine sulfate, solution	151	1658
Naphthylamine (beta)	153	1650	Nicotine sulphate, solid	151	1658
Naphthylamine (beta), solid	153	1650	Nicotine sulphate, solid	151	3445
Naphthylamine (beta), solution	153	3411	Nicotine sulphate, solution	151	1658
Naphthylthiourea	153	1651	Nicotine tartrate	151	1659
Naphthylurea	153	1652	Nitrates, inorganic, aqueous solution, n.o.s.	140	3218
Natural gas, compressed	115	1971	Nitrates, inorganic, n.o.s.	140	1477
Natural gas, refrigerated liquid (cryogenic liquid)	115	1972	Nitrating acid mixture	157	1796
Neohexane	128	1208	Nitrating acid mixture, spent	157	1826
Neon	121	1065	Nitric acid, fuming	157	2032
Neon, compressed	121	1065	Nitric acid, other than red fuming	157	2031
Neon, refrigerated liquid (cryogenic liquid)	120	1913	Nitric acid, red fuming	157	2032
Nickel carbonyl	131	1259	Nitric oxide	124	1660
Nickel catalyst, dry	135	2881	Nitric oxide, compressed	124	1660
Nickel cyanide	151	1653	Nitric oxide and Dinitrogen tetroxide mixture	124	1975
Nickel nitrate	140	2725			
Nickel nitrite	140	2726	Nitric oxide and Nitrogen dioxide mixture	124	1975
Nicotine	151	1654			

Name of Material	Guide No.	ID No.	Name of Material	Guide No.	ID No.
Nitric oxide and Nitrogen tetroxide mixture	124	1975	Nitrocellulose mixture, without pigment	133	2557
Nitriles, flammable, poisonous, n.o.s.	131	3273	Nitrocellulose mixture, without plasticizer	133	2557
Nitriles, flammable, toxic, n.o.s.	131	3273	Nitrocellulose mixture, with pigment	133	2557
Nitriles, poisonous, flammable, n.o.s.	131	3275	Nitrocellulose mixture, with pigment and plasticizer	133	2557
Nitriles, poisonous, liquid, n.o.s.	151	3276	Nitrocellulose mixture, with plasticizer	133	2557
Nitriles, poisonous, n.o.s.	151	3276	Nitrocellulose, solution, flammable	127	2059
Nitriles, poisonous, solid, n.o.s.	151	3439	Nitrocellulose, solution, in a flammable liquid	127	2059
Nitriles, toxic, flammable, n.o.s.	131	3275			
Nitriles, toxic, liquid, n.o.s.	151	3276	Nitrocellulose with alcohol	113	2556
Nitriles, toxic, n.o.s.	151	3276	Nitrocellulose with not less than 25% alcohol	113	2556
Nitriles, toxic, solid, n.o.s.	151	3439	Nitrocellulose with water, not less than 25% water	113	2555
Nitrites, inorganic, aqueous solution, n.o.s.	140	3219	3-Nitro-4-chlorobenzotrifluoride	152	2307
Nitrites, inorganic, n.o.s.	140	2627	Nitrocresols	153	2446
Nitroanilines	153	1661	Nitrocresols, liquid	153	3434
Nitroanisoles	152	2730	Nitrocresols, solid	153	2446
Nitroanisoles, liquid	152	2730	Nitroethane	129	2842
Nitroanisoles, solid	152	2730	Nitrogen	121	1066
Nitroanisoles, solid	152	3458	Nitrogen, compressed	121	1066
Nitrobenzene	152	1662	Nitrogen, refrigerated liquid (cryogenic liquid)	120	1977
Nitrobenzenesulfonic acid	153	2305			
Nitrobenzenesulphonic acid	153	2305	Nitrogen and Rare gases mixture	121	1981
Nitrobenzotrifluorides	152	2306	Nitrogen and Rare gases mixture, compressed	121	1981
Nitrobenzotrifluorides, liquid	152	2306			
Nitrobenzotrifluorides, solid	152	3431	Nitrogen dioxide	124	1067
Nitrobromobenzenes	152	2732	Nitrogen dioxide and Nitric oxide mixture	124	1975
Nitrobromobenzenes, liquid	152	2732			
Nitrobromobenzenes, solid	152	2732	Nitrogen tetroxide and Nitric oxide mixture	124	1975
Nitrobromobenzenes, solid	152	3459			
Nitrocellulose	133	2557			
Nitrocellulose membrane filters	133	3270			

Name of Material	Guide No.	ID No.	Name of Material	Guide No.	ID No.
Nitrogen trifluoride	122	2451	Nitrostarch, wetted with not less than 20% water	113	1337
Nitrogen trifluoride, compressed	122	2451	Nitrostarch, wetted with not less than 30% solvent	113	1337
Nitrogen trioxide	124	2421	Nitrosyl chloride	125	1069
Nitroglycerin, solution in alcohol, with more than 1% but not more than 5% Nitroglycerin	127	3064	Nitrosylsulfuric acid	157	2308
			Nitrosylsulfuric acid, liquid	157	2308
Nitroglycerin, solution in alcohol, with not more than 1% Nitroglycerin	127	1204	Nitrosylsulfuric acid, solid	157	2308
			Nitrosylsulfuric acid, solid	157	3456
Nitroglycerin mixture, desensitized, liquid, flammable, n.o.s., with not more than 30% Nitroglycerin	113	3343	Nitrosylsulphuric acid	157	2308
			Nitrosylsulphuric acid, liquid	157	2308
			Nitrosylsulphuric acid, solid	157	2308
Nitroglycerin mixture, desensitized, liquid, n.o.s., with not more than 30% Nitroglycerin	113	3357	Nitrosylsulphuric acid, solid	157	3456
			Nitrotoluenes	152	1664
			Nitrotoluenes, liquid	152	1664
Nitroglycerin mixture, desensitized, solid, n.o.s., with more than 2% but not more than 10% Nitroglycerin	113	3319	Nitrotoluenes, solid	152	1664
			Nitrotoluenes, solid	152	3446
			Nitrotoluidines (mono)	153	2660
			Nitrous oxide	122	1070
Nitroglycerin mixture with more than 2% but not more than 10% Nitroglycerin, desensitized	113	3319	Nitrous oxide, compressed	122	1070
			Nitrous oxide, refrigerated liquid	122	2201
Nitroguanidine (Picrite), wetted with not less than 20% water	113	1336	Nitrous oxide and Carbon dioxide mixture	126	1015
Nitroguanidine, wetted with not less than 20% water	113	1336	Nitroxylenes	152	1665
			Nitroxylenes, liquid	152	1665
Nitrohydrochloric acid	157	1798	Nitroxylenes, solid	152	1665
Nitromethane	129	1261	Nitroxylenes, solid	152	3447
Nitronaphthalene	133	2538	Nonanes	128	1920
Nitrophenols	153	1663	Nonyltrichlorosilane	156	1799
4-Nitrophenylhydrazine, with not less than 30% water	113	3376	2,5-Norbornadiene, stabilized	128P	2251
			Octadecyltrichlorosilane	156	1800
Nitropropanes	129	2608	Octadiene	128P	2309
p-Nitrosodimethylaniline	135	1369	Octafluorobut-2-ene	126	2422

Name of Material	Guide No.	ID No.	Name of Material	Guide No.	ID No.
Octafluorocyclobutane	126	1976	Organic peroxide type F, liquid, temperature controlled	148	3119
Octafluoropropane	126	2424			
Octanes	128	1262	Organic peroxide type F, solid	145	3110
Octyl aldehydes	129	1191	Organic peroxide type F, solid, temperature controlled	148	3120
tert-Octyl mercaptan	131	3023			
Octyltrichlorosilane	156	1801	Organic phosphate compound mixed with compressed gas	123	1955
Oil, petroleum	128	1270			
Oil gas	119	1071	Organic phosphate mixed with compressed gas	123	1955
Oil gas, compressed	119	1071			
Organic peroxide type B, liquid	146	3101	Organic phosphorus compound mixed with compressed gas	123	1955
Organic peroxide type B, liquid, temperature controlled	148	3111			
			Organic pigments, self-heating	135	3313
Organic peroxide type B, solid	146	3102	Organoarsenic compound, liquid, n.o.s.	151	3280
Organic peroxide type B, solid, temperature controlled	148	3112			
			Organoarsenic compound, n.o.s.	151	3280
Organic peroxide type C, liquid	146	3103	Organoarsenic compound, solid, n.o.s.	151	3465
Organic peroxide type C, liquid, temperature controlled	148	3113			
			Organochlorine pesticide, liquid, flammable, poisonous	131	2762
Organic peroxide type C, solid	146	3104			
Organic peroxide type C, solid, temperature controlled	148	3114	Organochlorine pesticide, liquid, flammable, toxic	131	2762
Organic peroxide type D, liquid	145	3105	Organochlorine pesticide, liquid, poisonous	151	2996
Organic peroxide type D, liquid, temperature controlled	148	3115			
			Organochlorine pesticide, liquid, poisonous, flammable	131	2995
Organic peroxide type D, solid	145	3106			
Organic peroxide type D, solid, temperature controlled	148	3116	Organochlorine pesticide, liquid, toxic	151	2996
Organic peroxide type E, liquid	145	3107	Organochlorine pesticide, liquid, toxic, flammable	131	2995
Organic peroxide type E, liquid, temperature controlled	148	3117			
			Organochlorine pesticide, solid, poisonous	151	2761
Organic peroxide type E, solid	145	3108			
Organic peroxide type E, solid, temperature controlled	148	3118	Organochlorine pesticide, solid, toxic	151	2761
Organic peroxide type F, liquid	145	3109	Organometallic compound, poisonous, liquid, n.o.s.	151	3282
			Organometallic compound, poisonous, n.o.s.	151	3282

Name of Material	Guide No.	ID No.
Organometallic compound, poisonous, solid, n.o.s.	151	3467
Organometallic compound, solid water-reactive, flammable, n.o.s.	138	3372
Organometallic compound, toxic, liquid, n.o.s.	151	3282
Organometallic compound, toxic, n.o.s.	151	3282
Organometallic compound, toxic, solid, n.o.s.	151	3467
Organometallic compound, water-reactive, flammable, n.o.s.	138	3207
Organometallic compound dispersion, water-reactive, flammable, n.o.s.	138	3207
Organometallic compound solution, water-reactive, flammable, n.o.s.	138	3207
Organometallic substance, liquid, pyrophoric	135	3392
Organometallic substance, liquid, pyrophoric, water-reactive	135	3394
Organometallic substance, liquid, water-reactive	135	3398
Organometallic substance, liquid, water-reactive, flammable	138	3399
Organometallic substance, solid, pyrophoric	135	3391
Organometallic substance, solid, pyrophoric, water-reactive	135	3393
Organometallic substance, solid, self-heating	138	3400
Organometallic substance, solid, water-reactive	135	3395

Name of Material	Guide No.	ID No.
Organometallic substance, solid, water-reactive, flammable	138	3396
Organometallic substance, solid, water-reactive, self-heating	138	3397
Organophosphorus compound, poisonous, flammable, n.o.s.	131	3279
Organophosphorus compound, poisonous, liquid, n.o.s.	151	3278
Organophosphorus compound, poisonous, n.o.s.	151	3278
Organophosphorus compound, poisonous, solid, n.o.s.	151	3464
Organophosphorus compound, toxic, flammable, n.o.s.	131	3279
Organophosphorus compound, toxic, liquid, n.o.s.	151	3278
Organophosphorus compound, toxic, n.o.s.	151	3278
Organophosphorus compound, toxic, solid, n.o.s.	151	3464
Organophosphorus pesticide, liquid, flammable, poisonous	131	2784
Organophosphorus pesticide, liquid, flammable, toxic	131	2784
Organophosphorus pesticide, liquid, poisonous	152	3018
Organophosphorus pesticide, liquid, poisonous, flammable	131	3017
Organophosphorus pesticide, liquid, toxic	152	3018
Organophosphorus pesticide, liquid, toxic, flammable	131	3017
Organophosphorus pesticide, solid, poisonous	152	2783
Organophosphorus pesticide, solid, toxic	152	2783

Name of Material	Guide No.	ID No.	Name of Material	Guide No.	ID No.
Organotin compound, liquid, n.o.s.	153	2788	Oxidizing solid, toxic, n.o.s.	141	3087
Organotin compound, solid, n.o.s.	153	3146	Oxidizing solid, water-reactive, n.o.s.	144	3121
Organotin pesticide, liquid, flammable, poisonous	131	2787	Oxygen	122	1072
			Oxygen, compressed	122	1072
Organotin pesticide, liquid, flammable, toxic	131	2787	Oxygen, refrigerated liquid (cryogenic liquid)	122	1073
Organotin pesticide, liquid, poisonous	153	3020	Oxygen and Carbon dioxide mixture	122	1014
Organotin pesticide, liquid, poisonous, flammable	131	3019	Oxygen and Carbon dioxide mixture, compressed	122	1014
Organotin pesticide, liquid, toxic	153	3020	Oxygen and Rare gases mixture	121	1980
Organotin pesticide, liquid, toxic, flammable	131	3019	Oxygen and Rare gases mixture, compressed	121	1980
Organotin pesticide, solid, poisonous	153	2786	Oxygen difluoride	124	2190
			Oxygen difluoride, compressed	124	2190
Organotin pesticide, solid, toxic	153	2786	Oxygen generator, chemical	140	3356
Osmium tetroxide	154	2471	Oxygen generator, chemical, spent	140	3356
Other regulated substances, liquid, n.o.s.	171	3082	Paint (corrosive)	153	3066
Other regulated substances, solid, n.o.s.	171	3077	Paint, corrosive, flammable	132	3470
			Paint (flammable)	128	1263
Oxidizing liquid, corrosive, n.o.s.	140	3098	Paint, flammable, corrosive	132	3469
Oxidizing liquid, n.o.s.	140	3139	Paint related material (corrosive)	153	3066
Oxidizing liquid, poisonous, n.o.s.	142	3099	Paint related material, corrosive, flammable	132	3470
Oxidizing liquid, toxic, n.o.s.	142	3099	Paint related material (flammable)	128	1263
Oxidizing solid, corrosive, n.o.s.	140	3085			
Oxidizing solid, flammable, n.o.s.	140	3137	Paint related material, flammable, corrosive	132	3469
Oxidizing solid, n.o.s.	140	1479	Paper, unsaturated oil treated	133	1379
Oxidizing solid, poisonous, n.o.s.	141	3087	Paraformaldehyde	133	2213
			Paraldehyde	129	1264
Oxidizing solid, self-heating, n.o.s.	135	3100	Parathion	152	2783

Name of Material	Guide No.	ID No.
Parathion and compressed gas mixture	123	1967
PCB	171	2315
PD	152	1556
Pentaborane	135	1380
Pentachloroethane	151	1669
Pentachlorophenol	154	3155
Pentaerythrite tetranitrate mixture,desensitized, solid, n.o.s., with more than 10% but not more than 20% PETN	113	3344
Pentaerythritol tetranitrate mixture, desensitized, solid, n.o.s., with more than 10% but not more than 20% PETN	113	3344
Pentafluoroethane	126	3220
Pentafluoroethane and Ethylene oxide mixture, with not more than 7.9% Ethylene oxide	126	3298
Pentamethylheptane	128	2286
Pentan-2,4-dione	131	2310
n-Pentane	128	1265
2,4-Pentanedione	131	2310
Pentane-2,4-dione	131	2310
Pentanes	128	1265
Pentanols	129	1105
1-Pentene	128	1108
1-Pentol	153P	2705
Percarbonates, inorganic, n.o.s.	140	3217
Perchlorates, inorganic, aqueous solution, n.o.s.	140	3211
Perchlorates, inorganic, n.o.s.	140	1481
Perchloric acid, with more than 50% but not more than 72% acid	143	1873
Perchloric acid, with not more than 50% acid	140	1802
Perchloroethylene	160	1897
Perchloromethyl mercaptan	157	1670
Perchloryl fluoride	124	3083
Perfluoroethyl vinyl ether	115	3154
Perfluoro(ethyl vinyl ether)	115	3154
Perfluoromethyl vinyl ether	115	3153
Perfluoro(methyl vinyl ether)	115	3153
Perfumery products, with flammable solvents	127	1266
Permanganates, inorganic, aqueous solution, n.o.s.	140	3214
Permanganates, inorganic, n.o.s.	140	1482
Peroxides, inorganic, n.o.s.	140	1483
Persulfates, inorganic, aqueous solution, n.o.s.	140	3216
Persulfates, inorganic, n.o.s.	140	3215
Persulphates, inorganic, aqueous solution, n.o.s.	140	3216
Persulphates, inorganic, n.o.s.	140	3215
Pesticide, liquid, flammable, poisonous, n.o.s.	131	3021
Pesticide, liquid, flammable, toxic, n.o.s.	131	3021
Pesticide, liquid, poisonous, flammable, n.o.s.	131	2903
Pesticide, liquid, poisonous, n.o.s.	151	2902
Pesticide, liquid, toxic, flammable, n.o.s.	131	2903
Pesticide, liquid, toxic, n.o.s.	151	2902
Pesticide, solid, poisonous	151	2588
Pesticide, solid, poisonous, n.o.s.	151	2588

Name of Material	Guide No.	ID No.	Name of Material	Guide No.	ID No.
Pesticide, solid, toxic, n.o.s.	151	2588	Phenoxyacetic acid derivative pesticide, liquid, toxic, flammable	131	3347
PETN mixture, desensitized, solid, n.o.s., with more than 10% but not more than 20% PETN	113	3344	Phenoxyacetic acid derivative pesticide, solid, poisonous	153	3345
Petrol	128	1203	Phenoxyacetic acid derivative pesticide, solid, toxic	153	3345
Petrol and ethanol mixture, with more than 10% ethanol	127	347	Phenoxy pesticide, liquid, flammable, poisonous	131	2766
Petroleum crude oil	128	1267	Phenoxy pesticide, liquid, flammable, toxic	131	2766
Petroleum distillates, n.o.s.	128	1268			
Petroleum gases, liquefied	115	1075	Phenoxy pesticide, liquid, poisonous	152	3000
Petroleum oil	128	1270	Phenoxy pesticide, liquid, poisonous, flammable	131	2999
Petroleum products, n.o.s.	128	1268			
Phenacyl bromide	153	2645	Phenoxy pesticide, liquid, toxic	152	3000
Phenetidines	153	2311	Phenoxy pesticide, liquid, toxic, flammable	131	2999
Phenol, molten	153	2312	Phenoxy pesticide, solid, poisonous	152	2765
Phenol, solid	153	1671			
Phenol solution	153	2821	Phenoxy pesticide, solid, toxic	152	2765
Phenolates, liquid	154	2904	Phenylacetonitrile, liquid	152	2470
Phenolates, solid	154	2905	Phenylacetyl chloride	156	2577
Phenolsulfonic acid, liquid	153	1803	Phenylcarbylamine chloride	151	1672
Phenolsulphonic acid, liquid	153	1803	Phenyl chloroformate	156	2746
Phenoxyacetic acid derivative pesticide, liquid, flammable, poisonous	131	3346	Phenylenediamines	153	1673
			Phenylhydrazine	153	2572
Phenoxyacetic acid derivative pesticide, liquid, flammable, toxic	131	3346	Phenyl isocyanate	155	2487
			Phenyl mercaptan	131	2337
Phenoxyacetic acid derivative pesticide, liquid, poisonous	153	3348	Phenylmercuric acetate	151	1674
Phenoxyacetic acid derivative pesticide, liquid, poisonous, flammable	131	3347	Phenylmercuric compound, n.o.s.	151	2026
			Phenylmercuric hydroxide	151	1894
Phenoxyacetic acid derivative pesticide, liquid, toxic	153	3348	Phenylmercuric nitrate	151	1895
			Phenylphosphorus dichloride	137	2798

Name of Material	Guide No.	ID No.	Name of Material	Guide No.	ID No.
Phenylphosphorus thiodichloride	137	2799	Phosphorus heptasulfide, free from yellow and white Phosphorus	139	1339
Phenyltrichlorosilane	156	1804	Phosphorus heptasulphide, free from yellow and white Phosphorus	139	1339
Phenyl urea pesticide, liquid, flammable, poisonous	131	2768	Phosphorus oxybromide	137	1939
Phenyl urea pesticide, liquid, flammable, toxic	131	2768	Phosphorus oxybromide, molten	137	2576
Phenyl urea pesticide, liquid, poisonous	151	3002	Phosphorus oxybromide, solid	137	1939
Phenyl urea pesticide, liquid, poisonous, flammable	131	3001	Phosphorus oxychloride	137	1810
			Phosphorus pentabromide	137	2691
Phenyl urea pesticide, liquid, toxic	151	3002	Phosphorus pentachloride	137	1806
			Phosphorus pentafluoride	125	2198
Phenyl urea pesticide, liquid, toxic, flammable	131	3001	Phosphorus pentafluoride, compressed	125	2198
Phenyl urea pesticide, solid, poisonous	151	2767	Phosphorus pentasulfide, free from yellow and white Phosphorus	139	1340
Phenyl urea pesticide, solid, toxic	151	2767	Phosphorus pentasulphide, free from yellow and white Phosphorus	139	1340
Phosgene	125	1076	Phosphorus pentoxide	137	1807
9-Phosphabicyclononanes	135	2940	Phosphorus sesquisulfide, free from yellow and white Phosphorus	139	1341
Phosphine	119	2199			
Phosphoric acid	154	1805	Phosphorus sesquisulphide, free from yellow and white Phosphorus	139	1341
Phosphoric acid, liquid	154	1805			
Phosphoric acid, solid	154	1805	Phosphorus tribromide	137	1808
Phosphoric acid, solid	154	3453	Phosphorus trichloride	137	1809
Phosphoric acid, solution	154	1805	Phosphorus trioxide	157	2578
Phosphorous acid	154	2834	Phosphorus trisulfide, free from yellow and white Phosphorus	139	1343
Phosphorous acid, ortho	154	2834	Phosphorus trisulphide, free from yellow and white Phosphorus	139	1343
Phosphorus, amorphous	133	1338			
Phosphorus, amorphous, red	133	1338			
Phosphorus, white, dry or under water or in solution	136	1381			
Phosphorus, white, molten	136	2447			
Phosphorus, yellow, dry or under water or in solution	136	1381	Phthalic anhydride	156	2214

Name of Material	Guide No.	ID No.
Phthalimide derivative pesticide, liquid, flammable, poisonous	131	2774
Phthalimide derivative pesticide, liquid, flammable, toxic	131	2774
Phthalimide derivative pesticide, liquid, poisonous	151	3008
Phthalimide derivative pesticide, liquid, poisonous, flammable	131	3007
Phthalimide derivative pesticide, liquid, toxic	151	3008
Phthalimide derivative pesticide, liquid, toxic, flammable	131	3007
Phthalimide derivative pesticide, solid, poisonous	151	2773
Phthalimide derivative pesticide, solid, toxic	151	2773
Picolines	129	2313
Picric acid, wet, with not less than 10% water	113	1344
Picric acid, wetted with not less than 10% water	113	3364
Picrite, wetted	113	1336
Picryl chloride, wetted with not less than 10% water	113	3365
Picric acid, wetted with not less than 30% water	113	1344
alpha-Pinene	128	2368
Pinene (alpha)	128	2368
Pine oil	129	1272
Piperazine	153	2579
Piperidine	132	2401
Plastic molding compound	171	3314

Name of Material	Guide No.	ID No.
Plastic, nitrocellulose-based, spontaneously combustible, n.o.s.	135	2006
Plastics moulding compound	171	3314
Plastics, nitrocellulose-based, self-heating, n.o.s.	135	2006
Poison B, liquid, n.o.s.	153	2810
Poisonous by inhalation liquid, corrosive, n.o.s. (Inhalation Hazard Zone A)	154	3389
Poisonous by inhalation liquid, corrosive, n.o.s. (Inhalation Hazard Zone B)	154	3390
Poisonous by inhalation liquid, flammable, n.o.s. (Inhalation Hazard Zone A)	131	3383
Poisonous by inhalation liquid, flammable, n.o.s. (Inhalation Hazard Zone B)	131	3384
Poisonous by inhalation liquid, n.o.s. (Inhalation Hazard Zone A)	151	3381
Poisonous by inhalation liquid, n.o.s. (Inhalation Hazard Zone B)	151	3382
Poisonous by inhalation liquid, oxidizing, n.o.s. (Inhalation Hazard Zone A)	142	3387
Poisonous by inhalation liquid, oxidizing, n.o.s. (Inhalation Hazard Zone B)	142	3388
Poisonous by inhalation liquid, water-reactive, n.o.s. (Inhalation Hazard Zone A)	139	3385
Poisonous by inhalation liquid, water-reactive, n.o.s. (Inhalation Hazard Zone B)	139	3386
Poisonous liquid, corrosive, inorganic, n.o.s.	154	3289

Name of Material	Guide No.	ID No.	Name of Material	Guide No.	ID No.
Poisonous liquid, corrosive, inorganic, n.o.s. (Inhalation Hazard Zone A)	154	3289	Poisonous liquid, inorganic, n.o.s. (Inhalation Hazard Zone A)	151	3287
Poisonous liquid, corrosive, inorganic, n.o.s. (Inhalation Hazard Zone B)	154	3289	Poisonous liquid, inorganic, n.o.s. (Inhalation Hazard Zone B)	151	3287
Poisonous liquid, corrosive, n.o.s.	154	2927	Poisonous liquid, n.o.s.	153	2810
Poisonous liquid, corrosive, n.o.s. (Inhalation Hazard Zone A)	154	2927	Poisonous liquid, n.o.s. (Inhalation Hazard Zone A)	153	2810
Poisonous liquid, corrosive, n.o.s. (Inhalation Hazard Zone B)	154	2927	Poisonous liquid, n.o.s. (Inhalation Hazard Zone B)	153	2810
Poisonous liquid, corrosive, organic, n.o.s.	154	2927	Poisonous liquid, organic, n.o.s.	153	2810
Poisonous liquid, corrosive, organic, n.o.s. (Inhalation Hazard Zone A)	154	2927	Poisonous liquid, organic, n.o.s. (Inhalation Hazard Zone A)	153	2810
Poisonous liquid, corrosive, organic, n.o.s. (Inhalation Hazard Zone B)	154	2927	Poisonous liquid, organic, n.o.s. (Inhalation Hazard Zone B)	153	2810
Poisonous liquid, flammable, n.o.s.	131	2929	Poisonous liquid, oxidizing, n.o.s.	142	3122
Poisonous liquid, flammable, n.o.s. (Inhalation Hazard Zone A)	131	2929	Poisonous liquid, oxidizing, n.o.s. (Inhalation Hazard Zone A)	142	3122
Poisonous liquid, flammable, n.o.s. (Inhalation Hazard Zone B)	131	2929	Poisonous liquid, oxidizing, n.o.s. (Inhalation Hazard Zone B)	142	3122
Poisonous liquid, flammable, organic, n.o.s.	131	2929	Poisonous liquid, water-reactive, n.o.s.	139	3123
Poisonous liquid, flammable, organic, n.o.s. (Inhalation Hazard Zone A)	131	2929	Poisonous liquid, water-reactive, n.o.s. (Inhalation Hazard Zone A)	139	3123
Poisonous liquid, flammable, organic, n.o.s. (Inhalation Hazard Zone B)	131	2929	Poisonous liquid, water-reactive, n.o.s. (Inhalation Hazard Zone B)	139	3123
Poisonous liquid, inorganic, n.o.s.	151	3287	Poisonous liquid, which in contact with water emits flammable gases, n.o.s.	139	3123
			Poisonous liquid, which in contact with water emits flammable gases, n.o.s. (Inhalation Hazard Zone A)	139	3123

Name of Material	Guide No.	ID No.
Poisonous liquid, which in contact with water emits flammable gases, n.o.s. (Inhalation Hazard Zone B)	139	3123
Poisonous solid, corrosive, inorganic, n.o.s.	154	3290
Poisonous solid, corrosive, n.o.s.	154	2928
Poisonous solid, flammable, n.o.s.	134	2930
Poisonous solid, flammable, organic, n.o.s.	134	2930
Poisonous solid, inorganic, n.o.s.	151	3288
Poisonous solid, organic, n.o.s.	154	2811
Poisonous solid, oxidizing, n.o.s.	141	3086
Poisonous solid, self-heating, n.o.s.	136	3124
Poisonous solid, water-reactive, n.o.s.	139	3125
Poisonous solid, which in contact with water emits flammable gases, n.o.s.	139	3125
Polyalkylamines, n.o.s.	132	2733
Polyalkylamines, n.o.s.	132	2734
Polyalkylamines, n.o.s.	153	2735
Polyamines, flammable, corrosive, n.o.s.	132	2733
Polyamines, liquid, corrosive, flammable, n.o.s.	132	2734
Polyamines, liquid, corrosive, n.o.s.	153	2735
Polyamines, solid, corrosive, n.o.s.	154	3259
Polychlorinated biphenyls	171	2315
Polychlorinated biphenyls, liquid	171	2315

Name of Material	Guide No.	ID No.
Polychlorinated biphenyls, solid	171	2315
Polychlorinated biphenyls, solid	171	3432
Polyester resin kit	128	3269
Polyhalogenated biphenyls, liquid	171	3151
Polyhalogenated biphenyls, solid	171	3152
Polyhalogenated terphenyls, liquid	171	3151
Polyhalogenated terphenyls, solid	171	3152
Polymeric beads, expandable	133	2211
Polystyrene beads, expandable	133	2211
Potassium	138	2257
Potassium, metal	138	2257
Potassium, metal alloys	138	1420
Potassium, metal alloys, liquid	138	1420
Potassium, metal alloys, solid	138	3403
Potassium arsenate	151	1677
Potassium arsenite	154	1678
Potassium borohydride	138	1870
Potassium bromate	140	1484
Potassium chlorate	140	1485
Potassium chlorate, aqueous solution	140	2427
Potassium chlorate, solution	140	2427
Potassium cuprocyanide	157	1679
Potassium cyanide	157	1680
Potassium cyanide, solid	157	1680
Potassium cyanide, solution	157	3413
Potassium dithionite	135	1929
Potassium fluoride	154	1812
Potassium fluoride, solid	154	1812
Potassium fluoride, solution	154	3422

Name of Material	Guide No.	ID No.
Potassium fluoroacetate	151	2628
Potassium fluorosilicate	151	2655
Potassium hydrogendifluoride	154	1811
Potassium hydrogen difluoride, solid	154	1811
Potassium hydrogen difluoride, solution	154	3421
Potassium hydrogen sulfate	154	2509
Potassium hydrogen sulphate	154	2509
Potassium hydrosulfite	135	1929
Potassium hydrosulphite	135	1929
Potassium hydroxide, dry, solid	154	1813
Potassium hydroxide, flake	154	1813
Potassium hydroxide, solid	154	1813
Potassium hydroxide, solution	154	1814
Potassium metavanadate	151	2864
Potassium monoxide	154	2033
Potassium nitrate	140	1486
Potassium nitrate and Sodium nitrate mixture	140	1499
Potassium nitrate and Sodium nitrite mixture	140	1487
Potassium nitrite	140	1488
Potassium perchlorate	140	1489
Potassium permanganate	140	1490
Potassium peroxide	144	1491
Potassium persulfate	140	1492
Potassium persulphate	140	1492
Potassium phosphide	139	2012
Potassium silicofluoride	151	2655
Potassium sodium alloys	138	1422
Potassium sodium alloys, liquid	138	1422
Potassium sodium alloys, solid	138	3404
Potassium sulfide, anhydrous	135	1382
Potassium sulfide, hydrated, with not less than 30% water of crystallization	153	1847
Potassium sulfide, hydrated, with not less than 30% water of hydration	153	1847
Potassium sulfide, with less than 30% water of crystallization	135	1382
Potassium sulfide, with less than 30% water of hydration	135	1382
Potassium sulphide, anhydrous	135	1382
Potassium sulphide, hydrated, with not less than 30% water of crystallization	153	1847
Potassium sulphide, hydrated, with not less than 30% water of hydration	153	1847
Potassium sulphide, with less than 30% water of crystallization	135	1382
Potassium sulphide, with less than 30% water of hydration	135	1382
Potassium superoxide	143	2466
Printing ink, flammable	129	1210
Printing ink related material	129	1210
Propadiene, stabilized	116P	2200
Propadiene and Methylacetylene mixture, stabilized	116P	1060
Propane	115	1075
Propane	115	1978
Propane-Ethane mixture, refrigerated liquid	115	1961
Propane mixture	115	1075
Propane mixture	115	1978
Propanethiols	130	2402
n-Propanol	129	1274

Name of Material	Guide No.	ID No.	Name of Material	Guide No.	ID No.
Propargyl alcohol	131	1986	Propylene tetramer	128	2850
Propionaldehyde	129	1275	Propyl formates	129	1281
Propionic acid	132	1848	n-Propyl isocyanate	155	2482
Propionic acid, with not less than 10% and less than 90% acid	132	1848	n-Propyl nitrate	131	1865
			Propyltrichlorosilane	155	1816
Propionic acid, with not less than 90% acid	132	3463	Pyrethroid pesticide, liquid, flammable, poisonous	131	3350
Propionic anhydride	156	2496	Pyrethroid pesticide, liquid, flammable, toxic	131	3350
Propionitrile	131	2404	Pyrethroid pesticide, liquid, poisonous	151	3352
Propionyl chloride	132	1815	Pyrethroid pesticide, liquid, poisonous, flammable	131	3351
n-Propyl acetate	129	1276			
normal Propyl alcohol	129	1274	Pyrethroid pesticide, liquid, toxic	151	3352
Propyl alcohol, normal	129	1274	Pyrethroid pesticide, liquid, toxic, flammable	131	3351
Propylamine	132	1277			
n-Propyl benzene	128	2364	Pyrethroid pesticide, solid, poisonous	151	3349
Propyl chloride	129	1278	Pyrethroid pesticide, solid, toxic	151	3349
n-Propyl chloroformate	155	2740	Pyridine	129	1282
Propylene	115	1075	Pyrophoric alloy, n.o.s.	135	1383
Propylene	115	1077	Pyrophoric liquid, inorganic, n.o.s.	135	3194
Propylene, Ethylene and Acetylene in mixture, refrigerated liquid containing at least 71.5% Ethylene with not more than 22.5% Acetylene and not more than 6% Propylene	115	3138	Pyrophoric liquid, n.o.s.	135	2845
			Pyrophoric liquid, organic, n.o.s.	135	2845
			Pyrophoric metal, n.o.s.	135	1383
			Pyrophoric organometallic compound, n.o.s.	135	3203
Propylene chlorohydrin	131	2611	Pyrophoric organometallic compound, water-reactive, n.o.s.	135	3203
1,2-Propylenediamine	132	2258			
1,3-Propylenediamine	132	2258	Pyrophoric solid, inorganic, n.o.s.	135	3200
Propylene dichloride	130	1279			
Propyleneimine, stabilized	131P	1921	Pyrophoric solid, n.o.s.	135	2846
Propylene oxide	127P	1280	Pyrophoric solid, organic, n.o.s.	135	2846
Propylene oxide and Ethylene oxide mixture, with not more than 30% Ethylene oxide	129P	2983			

Name of Material	Guide No.	ID No.
Pyrosulfuryl chloride	137	1817
Pyrosulphuryl chloride	137	1817
Pyrrolidine	132	1922
Quinoline	154	2656
Radioactive material, excepted package, articles manufactured from depleted Uranium	161	2909
Radioactive material, excepted package, articles manufactured from depleted Uranium	161	2910
Radioactive material, excepted package, articles manufactured from natural Thorium	161	2909
Radioactive material, excepted package, articles manufactured from natural Thorium	161	2910
Radioactive material, excepted package, articles manufactured from natural Uranium	161	2909
Radioactive material, excepted package, articles manufactured from natural Uranium	161	2910
Radioactive material, excepted package, empty packaging	161	2908
Radioactive material, excepted package, empty packaging	161	2910
Radioactive material, excepted package, instruments or articles	161	2910
Radioactive material, excepted package, instruments or articles	161	2911
Radioactive material, excepted package, limited quantity of material	161	2910
Radioactive material, fissile, n.o.s.	165	2918
Radioactive material, low specific activity (LSA), n.o.s.	162	2912
Radioactive material, low specific activity (LSA-I) non fissile or fissile-excepted	162	2912
Radioactive material, low specific activity (LSA-II), fissile	165	3324
Radioactive material, low specific activity (LSA-II), non fissile or fissile-excepted	162	3321
Radioactive material, low specific activity (LSA-III), fissile	165	3325
Radioactive material, low specific activity (LSA-III), non fissile or fissile-excepted	162	3322
Radioactive material, n.o.s.	163	2982
Radioactive material, special form, n.o.s.	164	2974
Radioactive material, surface contaminated objects (SCO)	162	2913
Radioactive material, surface contaminated objects (SCO-I), fissile	165	3326
Radioactive material, surface contaminated objects (SCO-I) non fissile or fissile-excepted	162	2913
Radioactive material, surface contaminated objects (SCO-II), fissile	165	3326
Radioactive material, surface contaminated objects (SCO-II) non fissile or fissile-excepted	162	2913
Radioactive material, transported under special arrangement, fissile	165	3331
Radioactive material, transported under special arrangement non fissile or fissile-excepted	163	2919
Radioactive material, Type A package, fissile, non-special form	165	3327

Name of Material	Guide No.	ID No.	Name of Material	Guide No.	ID No.
Radioactive material, Type A package non-special form, non fissile or fissile-excepted	163	2915	Red phosphorus	133	1338
			Red phosphorus, amorphous	133	1338
			Refrigerant gas, n.o.s.	126	1078
Radioactive material, Type A package, special form, fissile	165	3333	Refrigerant gas, n.o.s. (flammable)	115	1954
Radioactive material, Type A package, special form, non fissile or fissile-excepted	164	3332	Refrigerant gas R-12	126	1028
			Refrigerant gas R-12 and Refrigerant gas R-152a azeotropic mixture with 74% Refrigerant gas R-12	126	2602
Radioactive material, Type B(M) package, fissile	165	3329			
Radioactive material, Type B(M) package non fissile or fissile-excepted	163	2917	Refrigerant gas R-12B1	126	1974
			Refrigerant gas R-13	126	1022
Radioactive material, Type B(U) package, fissile	165	3328	Refrigerant gas R-13 and Refrigerant gas R-23 azeotropic mixture with 60% Refrigerant gas R-13	126	2599
Radioactive material, Type B(U) package non fissile or fissile-excepted	163	2916			
			Refrigerant gas R-13B1	126	1009
Radioactive material, Type C package	163	3323	Refrigerant gas R-14	126	1982
			Refrigerant gas R-14, compressed	126	1982
Radioactive material, Type C package, fissile	165	3330	Refrigerant gas R-21	126	1029
Radioactive material, Uranium hexafluoride	166	2978	Refrigerant gas R-22	126	1018
			Refrigerant gas R-23	126	1984
Radioactive material, Uranium hexafluoride, fissile	166	2977	Refrigerant gas R-23 and Refrigerant gas R-13 azeotropic mixture with 60% Refrigerant gas R-13	126	2599
Rags, oily	133	1856			
Rare gases and Nitrogen mixture	121	1981			
Rare gases and Nitrogen mixture, compressed	121	1981	Refrigerant gas R-32	115	3252
			Refrigerant gas R-40	115	1063
Rare gases and Oxygen mixture	121	1980	Refrigerant gas R-41	115	2454
Rare gases and Oxygen mixture, compressed	121	1980	Refrigerant gas R-114	126	1958
Rare gases mixture	121	1979	Refrigerant gas R-115	126	1020
Rare gases mixture, compressed	121	1979	Refrigerant gas R-116	126	2193
Receptacles, small, containing gas	115	2037	Refrigerant gas R-116, compressed	126	2193
			Refrigerant gas R-124	126	1021

Name of Material	Guide No.	ID No.	Name of Material	Guide No.	ID No.
Refrigerant gas R-125	126	3220	Refrigerating machines, containing Ammonia solutions (UN2672)	126	2857
Refrigerant gas R-133a	126	1983			
Refrigerant gas R-134a	126	3159			
Refrigerant gas R-142b	115	2517	Refrigerating machines, containing flammable, non-poisonous, non-corrosive, liquefied gas	115	1954
Refrigerant gas R-143a	115	2035			
Refrigerant gas R-152a	115	1030			
Refrigerant gas R-152a and Refrigerant gas R-12 azeotropic mixture with 74% Refrigerant gas R-12	126	2602	Refrigerating machines, containing flammable, non-poisonous, liquefied gases	115	3358
			Refrigerating machines, containing flammable, non-toxic, liquefied gases	115	3358
Refrigerant gas R-161	115	2453			
Refrigerant gas R-218	126	2424	Refrigerating machines, containing non-flammable, non-poisonous gases	126	2857
Refrigerant gas R-227	126	3296			
Refrigerant gas R-404A	126	3337			
Refrigerant gas R-407A	126	3338	Refrigerating machines, containing non-flammable, non-toxic gases	126	2857
Refrigerant gas R-407B	126	3339			
Refrigerant gas R-407C	126	3340	Regulated medical waste, n.o.s.	158	3291
Refrigerant gas R-500 (azeotropic mixture of Refrigerant gas R-12 and Refrigerant gas R-152a with approximately 74% Refrigerant gas R-12)	126	2602	Resin solution	127	1866
			Resorcinol	153	2876
			Rosin oil	127	1286
			Rubber scrap, powdered or granulated	133	1345
Refrigerant gas R-502	126	1973	Rubber shoddy, powdered or granulated	133	1345
Refrigerant gas R-503 (azeotropic mixture of Refrigerant gas R-13 and Refrigerant gas R-23 with approximately 60% Refrigerant gas R-13)	126	2599	Rubber solution	127	1287
			Rubidium	138	1423
			Rubidium hydroxide	154	2678
			Rubidium hydroxide, solid	154	2678
Refrigerant gas R-1132a	116P	1959	Rubidium hydroxide, solution	154	2677
Refrigerant gas R-1216	126	1858	Rubidium metal	138	1423
Refrigerant gas R-1318	126	2422	SA	119	2188
Refrigerant gas RC-318	126	1976	Sarin	153	2810
Refrigerating machine	128	1993	Seat-belt modules	171	3268
			Seat-belt pre-tensioners	171	3268

Name of Material	Guide No.	ID No.	Name of Material	Guide No.	ID No.
Seat-belt pre-tensioners, compressed gas	126	3353	Self-heating liquid, poisonous, organic, n.o.s.	136	3184
Seat-belt pre-tensioners, pyrotechnic	171	3268	Self-heating liquid, toxic, inorganic, n.o.s.	136	3187
Seed cake, with more than 1.5% oil and not more than 11% moisture	135	1386	Self-heating liquid, toxic, organic, n.o.s.	136	3184
			Self-heating metal powders, n.o.s.	135	3189
Seed cake, with not more than 1.5% oil and not more than 11% moisture	135	2217	Self-heating solid, corrosive, inorganic, n.o.s.	136	3192
Selenates	151	2630	Self-heating solid, corrosive, organic, n.o.s.	136	3126
Selenic acid	154	1905			
Selenites	151	2630	Self-heating solid, inorganic, n.o.s.	135	3190
Selenium compound, liquid, n.o.s.	151	3440	Self-heating solid, inorganic, poisonous, n.o.s.	136	3191
Selenium compound, n.o.s.	151	3283	Self-heating solid, inorganic, toxic, n.o.s.	136	3191
Selenium compound, solid, n.o.s.	151	3283	Self-heating solid, organic, n.o.s.	135	3088
Selenium disulfide	153	2657			
Selenium disulphide	153	2657	Self-heating solid, oxidizing, n.o.s.	135	3127
Selenium hexafluoride	125	2194	Self-heating solid, poisonous, inorganic, n.o.s.	136	3191
Selenium oxide	154	2811	Self-heating solid, poisonous, organic, n.o.s.	136	3128
Selenium oxychloride	157	2879			
Selenium powder	152	2658	Self-heating solid, toxic, inorganic, n.o.s.	136	3191
Self-defense spray, non-pressurized	171	3334	Self-heating solid, toxic, organic, n.o.s.	136	3128
Self-heating liquid, corrosive, inorganic, n.o.s.	136	3188	Self-reactive liquid type B	149	3221
Self-heating liquid, corrosive, organic, n.o.s.	136	3185	Self-reactive liquid type B, temperature controlled	150	3231
Self-heating liquid, inorganic, n.o.s.	135	3186	Self-reactive liquid type C	149	3223
Self-heating liquid, organic, n.o.s.	135	3183	Self-reactive liquid type C, temperature controlled	150	3233
Self-heating liquid, poisonous, inorganic, n.o.s.	136	3187	Self-reactive liquid type D	149	3225

Name of Material	Guide No.	ID No.
Self-reactive liquid type D, temperature controlled	150	3235
Self-reactive liquid type E	149	3227
Self-reactive liquid type E, temperature controlled	150	3237
Self-reactive liquid type F	149	3229
Self-reactive liquid type F, temperature controlled	150	3239
Self-reactive solid type B	149	3222
Self-reactive solid type B, temperature controlled	150	3232
Self-reactive solid type C	149	3224
Self-reactive solid type C, temperature controlled	150	3234
Self-reactive solid type D	149	3226
Self-reactive solid type D, temperature controlled	150	3236
Self-reactive solid type E	149	3228
Self-reactive solid type E, temperature controlled	150	3238
Self-reactive solid type F	149	3230
Self-reactive solid type F, temperature controlled	150	3240
Shale oil	128	1288
Silane	116	2203
Silicofluorides, n.o.s.	151	2856
Silane, compressed	116	2203
Silicon powder, amorphous	170	1346
Silicon tetrachloride	157	1818
Silicon tetrafluoride	125	1859
Silicon tetrafluoride, compressed	125	1859
Silver arsenite	151	1683
Silver cyanide	151	1684
Silver nitrate	140	1493

Name of Material	Guide No.	ID No.
Silver picrate, wetted with not less than 30% water	113	1347
Sludge acid	153	1906
Smokeless powder for small arms	133	3178
Soda lime, with more than 4% Sodium hydroxide	154	1907
Sodium	138	1428
Sodium aluminate, solid	154	2812
Sodium aluminate, solution	154	1819
Sodium aluminum hydride	138	2835
Sodium ammonium vanadate	154	2863
Sodium arsanilate	154	2473
Sodium arsenate	151	1685
Sodium arsenite, aqueous solution	154	1686
Sodium arsenite, solid	151	2027
Sodium azide	153	1687
Sodium bisulfate, solution	154	2837
Sodium bisulphate, solution	154	2837
Sodium borohydride	138	1426
Sodium borohydride and Sodium hydroxide solution, with not more than 12% Sodium borohydride and not more than 40% Sodium hydroxide	157	3320
Sodium bromate	141	1494
Sodium cacodylate	152	1688
Sodium carbonate peroxyhydrate	140	3378
Sodium chlorate	140	1495
Sodium chlorate, aqueous solution	140	2428
Sodium chlorite	143	1496
Sodium chlorite, solution, with more than 5% available Chlorine	154	1908

Name of Material	Guide No.	ID No.	Name of Material	Guide No.	ID No.
Sodium chloroacetate	151	2659	Sodium hydrosulfide, with not less than 25% water of crystallization	154	2949
Sodium cuprocyanide, solid	157	2316			
Sodium cuprocyanide, solution	157	2317			
Sodium cyanide	157	1689	Sodium hydrosulfite	135	1384
Sodium cyanide, solid	157	1689	Sodium hydrosulphide, solid, with less than 25% water of crystallization	135	2318
Sodium cyanide, solution	157	3414			
Sodium dichloroisocyanurate	140	2465	Sodium hydrosulphide, solution	154	2922
Sodium dichloro-s-triazinetrione	140	2465	Sodium hydrosulphide, with less than 25% water of crystallization	135	2318
Sodium dinitro-o-cresolate, wetted with not less than 10% water	113	3369			
Sodium dinitro-o-cresolate, wetted with not less than 15% water	113	1348	Sodium hydrosulphide, with not less than 25% water of crystallization	154	2949
Sodium dinitro-ortho-cresolate, wetted	113	1348	Sodium hydrosulphite	135	1384
			Sodium hydroxide, bead	154	1823
Sodium dithionite	135	1384	Sodium hydroxide, dry	154	1823
Sodium fluoride	154	1690	Sodium hydroxide, flake	154	1823
Sodium fluoride, solid	154	1690	Sodium hydroxide, granular	154	1823
Sodium fluoride, solution	154	3415	Sodium hydroxide, solid	154	1823
Sodium fluoroacetate	151	2629	Sodium hydroxide, solution	154	1824
Sodium fluorosilicate	154	2674	Sodium methylate	138	1431
Sodium hydride	138	1427	Sodium methylate, dry	138	1431
Sodium hydrogendifluoride	154	2439	Sodium methylate, solution in alcohol	132	1289
Sodium hydrogen sulfate, solution	154	2837			
Sodium hydrogen sulphate, solution	154	2837	Sodium monoxide	157	1825
			Sodium nitrate	140	1498
Sodium hydrosulfide, solid, with less than 25% water of crystallization	135	2318	Sodium nitrate and Potassium nitrate mixture	140	1499
			Sodium nitrite	140	1500
Sodium hydrosulfide, solution	154	2922	Sodium nitrite and Potassium nitrate mixture	140	1487
Sodium hydrosulfide, with less than 25% water of crystallization	135	2318	Sodium pentachlorophenate	154	2567
			Sodium perborate monohydrate	140	3377

Name of Material	Guide No.	ID No.	Name of Material	Guide No.	ID No.
Sodium percarbonates	140	2467	Stannic chloride, anhydrous	137	1827
Sodium perchlorate	140	1502	Stannic chloride, pentahydrate	154	2440
Sodium permanganate	140	1503	Stannic phosphides	139	1433
Sodium peroxide	144	1504	Stibine	119	2676
Sodium peroxoborate, anhydrous	140	3247	Straw, wet, damp or contaminated with oil	133	1327
Sodium persulfate	140	1505	Strontium arsenite	151	1691
Sodium persulphate	140	1505	Strontium chlorate	143	1506
Sodium phosphide	139	1432	Strontium chlorate, solid	143	1506
Sodium picramate, wetted with not less than 20% water	113	1349	Strontium chlorate, solution	143	1506
			Strontium nitrate	140	1507
Sodium potassium alloys	138	1422	Strontium perchlorate	140	1508
Sodium potassium alloys, liquid	138	1422	Strontium peroxide	143	1509
Sodium potassium alloys, solid	138	3404	Strontium phosphide	139	2013
Sodium selenite	151	2630	Strychnine	151	1692
Sodium silicofluoride	154	2674	Strychnine salts	151	1692
Sodium sulfide, anhydrous	135	1385	Styrene monomer, stabilized	128P	2055
Sodium sulfide, hydrated, with not less than 30% water	153	1849	Substituted nitrophenol pesticide, liquid, flammable, poisonous	131	2780
Sodium sulfide, with less than 30% water of crystallization	135	1385	Substituted nitrophenol pesticide, liquid, flammable, toxic	131	2780
Sodium sulphide, anhydrous	135	1385			
Sodium sulphide, hydrated, with not less than 30% water	153	1849	Substituted nitrophenol pesticide, liquid, poisonous	153	3014
Sodium sulphide, with less than 30% water of crystallization	135	1385	Substituted nitrophenol pesticide, liquid, poisonous, flammable	131	3013
Sodium superoxide	143	2547	Substituted nitrophenol pesticide, liquid, toxic	153	3014
Solids containing corrosive liquid, n.o.s.	154	3244	Substituted nitrophenol pesticide, liquid, toxic, flammable	131	3013
Solids containing flammable liquid, n.o.s.	133	3175			
Solids containing poisonous liquid, n.o.s.	151	3243	Substituted nitrophenol pesticide, solid, poisonous	153	2779
Solids containing toxic liquid, n.o.s.	151	3243			
Soman	153	2810			

Name of Material	Guide No.	ID No.
Substituted nitrophenol pesticide, solid, toxic	153	2779
Sulfamic acid	154	2967
Sulfur	133	1350
Sulfur, molten	133	2448
Sulfur chlorides	137	1828
Sulfur dioxide	125	1079
Sulfur hexafluoride	126	1080
Sulfuric acid	137	1830
Sulfuric acid, fuming	137	1831
Sulfuric acid, fuming, with less than 30% free Sulfur trioxide	137	1831
Sulfuric acid, fuming, with not less than 30% free Sulfur trioxide	137	1831
Sulfuric acid, spent	137	1832
Sulfuric acid, with more than 51% acid	137	1830
Sulfuric acid, with not more than 51% acid	157	2796
Sulfuric acid and Hydrofluoric acid mixture	157	1786
Sulfurous acid	154	1833
Sulfur tetrafluoride	125	2418
Sulfur trioxide, inhibited	137	1829
Sulfur trioxide, stabilized	137	1829
Sulfur trioxide, uninhibited	137	1829
Sulfur trioxide and Chlorosulfonic acid mixture	137	1754
Sulfuryl chloride	137	1834
Sulfuryl fluoride	123	2191
Sulphamic acid	154	2967
Sulphur	133	1350
Sulphur, molten	133	2448
Sulphur chlorides	137	1828

Name of Material	Guide No.	ID No.
Sulphur dioxide	125	1079
Sulphur hexafluoride	126	1080
Sulphuric acid	137	1830
Sulphuric acid, fuming	137	1831
Sulphuric acid, fuming, with less than 30% free Sulphur trioxide	137	1831
Sulphuric acid, fuming, with not less than 30% free Sulphur trioxide	137	1831
Sulphuric acid, spent	137	1832
Sulphuric acid, with more than 51% acid	137	1830
Sulphuric acid, with not more than 51% acid	157	2796
Sulphuric acid and Hydrofluoric acid mixture	157	1786
Sulphurous acid	154	1833
Sulphur tetrafluoride	125	2418
Sulphur trioxide, inhibited	137	1829
Sulphur trioxide, stabilized	137	1829
Sulphur trioxide, uninhibited	137	1829
Sulphur trioxide and Chlorosulphonic acid mixture	137	1754
Sulphuryl chloride	137	1834
Sulphuryl fluoride	123	2191
Tabun	153	2810
Tars, liquid	130	1999
Tear gas candles	159	1700
Tear gas devices	159	1693
Tear gas grenades	159	1700
Tear gas substance, liquid, n.o.s.	159	1693
Tear gas substance, solid, n.o.s.	159	1693
Tear gas substance, solid, n.o.s.	159	3448

Name of Material	Guide No.	ID No.
Tellurium compound, n.o.s.	151	3284
Tellurium hexafluoride	125	2195
Terpene hydrocarbons, n.o.s.	128	2319
Terpinolene	128	2541
Tetrabromoethane	159	2504
1,1,2,2-Tetrachloroethane	151	1702
Tetrachloroethane	151	1702
Tetrachloroethylene	160	1897
Tetraethyl dithiopyrophosphate	153	1704
Tetraethyl dithiopyrophosphate, mixture, dry or liquid	153	1704
Tetraethylenepentamine	153	2320
Tetraethyl lead, liquid	131	1649
Tetraethyl pyrophosphate, liquid	152	3018
Tetraethyl pyrophosphate, solid	152	2783
Tetraethyl silicate	129	1292
1,1,1,2-Tetrafluoroethane	126	3159
Tetrafluoroethane and Ethylene oxide mixture, with not more than 5.6% Ethylene oxide	126	3299
Tetrafluoroethylene, stabilized	116P	1081
Tetrafluoromethane	126	1982
Tetrafluoromethane, compressed	126	1982
1,2,3,6-Tetrahydro-benzaldehyde	129	2498
Tetrahydrofuran	127	2056
Tetrahydrofurfurylamine	129	2943
Tetrahydrophthalic anhydrides	156	2698
1,2,3,6-Tetrahydropyridine	129	2410
1,2,5,6-Tetrahydropyridine	129	2410
Tetrahydrothiophene	130	2412
Tetramethylammonium hydroxide	153	1835
Tetramethylammonium hydroxide, solid	153	3423
Tetramethylammonium hydroxide, solution	153	1835
Tetramethylsilane	130	2749
Tetranitromethane	143	1510
Tetrapropyl orthotitanate	128	2413
Textile waste, wet	133	1857
Thallium chlorate	141	2573
Thallium compound, n.o.s.	151	1707
Thallium nitrate	141	2727
Thallium sulfate, solid	151	1707
Thallium sulphate, solid	151	1707
4-Thiapentanal	152	2785
Thia-4-pentanal	152	2785
Thickened GD	153	2810
Thioacetic acid	129	2436
Thiocarbamate pesticide, liquid, flammable, poisonous	131	2772
Thiocarbamate pesticide, liquid, flammable, toxic	131	2772
Thiocarbamate pesticide, liquid, poisonous	151	3006
Thiocarbamate pesticide, liquid, poisonous, flammable	131	3005
Thiocarbamate pesticide, liquid, toxic	151	3006
Thiocarbamate pesticide, liquid, toxic, flammable	131	3005
Thiocarbamate pesticide, solid, poisonous	151	2771
Thiocarbamate pesticide, solid, toxic	151	2771
Thioglycol	153	2966
Thioglycolic acid	153	1940

Name of Material	Guide No.	ID No.	Name of Material	Guide No.	ID No.
Thiolactic acid	153	2936	Toluene diisocyanate	156	2078
Thionyl chloride	137	1836	Toluidines	153	1708
Thiophene	130	2414	Toluidines, liquid	153	1708
Thiophosgene	157	2474	Toluidines, solid	153	1708
Thiophosphoryl chloride	157	1837	Toluidines, solid	153	3451
Thiourea dioxide	135	3341	2,4-Toluylenediamine	151	1709
Thorium metal, pyrophoric	162	2975	2,4-Toluylenediamine, solid	151	1709
Thorium nitrate, solid	162	2976	2,4-Toluylenediamine, solution	151	3418
Tinctures, medicinal	127	1293	Toxic by inhalation liquid, corrosive, n.o.s. (Inhalation Hazard Zone A)	154	3389
Tin tetrachloride	137	1827			
Tin tetrachloride, pentahydrate	154	2440	Toxic by inhalation liquid, corrosive, n.o.s. (Inhalation Hazard Zone B)	154	3390
Titanium disulfide	135	3174			
Titanium disulphide	135	3174	Toxic by inhalation liquid, flammable, n.o.s. (Inhalation Hazard Zone A)	131	3383
Titanium hydride	170	1871			
Titanium powder, dry	135	2546	Toxic by inhalation liquid, flammable, n.o.s. (Inhalation Hazard Zone B)	131	3384
Titanium powder, wetted with not less than 25% water	170	1352			
Titanium sponge granules	170	2878	Toxic by inhalation liquid, n.o.s. (Inhalation Hazard Zone A)	151	3381
Titanium sponge powders	170	2878	Toxic by inhalation liquid, n.o.s. (Inhalation Hazard Zone B)	151	3382
Titanium sulfate, solution	154	1760			
Titanium sulphate, solution	154	1760	Toxic by inhalation liquid, oxidizing, n.o.s. (Inhalation Hazard Zone A)	142	3387
Titanium tetrachloride	137	1838			
Titanium trichloride, pyrophoric	135	2441	Toxic by inhalation liquid, oxidizing, n.o.s. (Inhalation Hazard Zone B)	142	3388
Titanium trichloride mixture	157	2869			
Titanium trichloride mixture, pyrophoric	135	2441	Toxic by inhalation liquid, water-reactive, n.o.s. (Inhalation Hazard Zone A)	139	3385
TNT, wetted with not less than 10% water	113	3366			
TNT, wetted with not less than 30% water	113	1356	Toxic by inhalation liquid, water-reactive, n.o.s. (Inhalation Hazard Zone B)	139	3386
Toe puffs, nitrocellulose base	133	1353			
Toluene	130	1294	Toxic liquid, corrosive, inorganic, n.o.s.	154	3289
2,4-Toluenediamine	151	1709			

Name of Material	Guide No.	ID No.	Name of Material	Guide No.	ID No.
Toxic liquid, corrosive, inorganic, n.o.s. (Inhalation Hazard Zone A)	154	3289	Toxic liquid, n.o.s.	153	2810
Toxic liquid, corrosive, inorganic, n.o.s. (Inhalation Hazard Zone B)	154	3289	Toxic liquid, n.o.s. (Inhalation Hazard Zone A)	153	2810
Toxic liquid, corrosive, n.o.s.	154	2927	Toxic liquid, n.o.s. (Inhalation Hazard Zone B)	153	2810
Toxic liquid, corrosive, n.o.s. (Inhalation Hazard Zone A)	154	2927	Toxic liquid, organic, n.o.s.	153	2810
Toxic liquid, corrosive, n.o.s. (Inhalation Hazard Zone B)	154	2927	Toxic liquid, organic, n.o.s. (Inhalation Hazard Zone A)	153	2810
Toxic liquid, corrosive, organic, n.o.s.	154	2927	Toxic liquid, organic, n.o.s. (Inhalation Hazard Zone B)	153	2810
Toxic liquid, corrosive, organic, n.o.s. (Inhalation Hazard Zone A)	154	2927	Toxic liquid, oxidizing, n.o.s.	142	3122
Toxic liquid, corrosive, organic, n.o.s. (Inhalation Hazard Zone B)	154	2927	Toxic liquid, oxidizing, n.o.s. (Inhalation Hazard Zone A)	142	3122
Toxic liquid, flammable, n.o.s.	131	2929	Toxic liquid, oxidizing, n.o.s. (Inhalation Hazard Zone B)	142	3122
Toxic liquid, flammable, n.o.s. (Inhalation Hazard Zone A)	131	2929	Toxic liquid, water-reactive, n.o.s.	139	3123
Toxic liquid, flammable, n.o.s. (Inhalation Hazard Zone B)	131	2929	Toxic liquid, water-reactive, n.o.s. (Inhalation Hazard Zone A)	139	3123
Toxic liquid, flammable, organic, n.o.s.	131	2929	Toxic liquid, water-reactive, n.o.s. (Inhalation Hazard Zone B)	139	3123
Toxic liquid, flammable, organic, n.o.s. (Inhalation Hazard Zone A)	131	2929	Toxic liquid, which in contact with water emits flammable gases, n.o.s.	139	3123
Toxic liquid, flammable, organic, n.o.s. (Inhalation Hazard Zone B)	131	2929	Toxic liquid, which in contact with water emits flammable gases, n.o.s. (Inhalation Hazard Zone A)	139	3123
Toxic liquid, inorganic, n.o.s.	151	3287	Toxic liquid, which in contact with water emits flammable gases, n.o.s. (Inhalation Hazard Zone B)	139	3123
Toxic liquid, inorganic, n.o.s. (Inhalation Hazard Zone A)	151	3287	Toxic solid, corrosive, inorganic, n.o.s.	154	3290
Toxic liquid, inorganic, n.o.s. (Inhalation Hazard Zone B)	151	3287	Toxic solid, corrosive, organic, n.o.s.	154	2928
			Toxic solid, flammable, n.o.s.	134	2930

Name of Material	Guide No.	ID No.	Name of Material	Guide No.	ID No.
Toxic solid, flammable, organic, n.o.s.	134	2930	Tri-(1-aziridinyl)phosphine oxide, solution	152	2501
Toxic solid, inorganic, n.o.s.	151	3288	Tributylamine	153	2542
Toxic solid, organic, n.o.s.	154	2811	Tributylphosphane	135	3254
Toxic solid, oxidizing, n.o.s.	141	3086	Tributylphosphine	135	3254
Toxic solid, self-heating, n.o.s.	136	3124	Trichloroacetic acid	153	1839
Toxic solid, water-reactive, n.o.s.	139	3125	Trichloroacetic acid, solution	153	2564
Toxic solid, which in contact with water emits flammable gases, n.o.s.	139	3125	Trichloroacetyl chloride	156	2442
			Trichlorobenzenes, liquid	153	2321
Toxins	153	——	Trichlorobutene	152	2322
Toxins, extracted from living sources, liquid, n.o.s.	153	3172	1,1,1-Trichloroethane	160	2831
			Trichloroethylene	160	1710
Toxins, extracted from living sources, n.o.s.	153	3172	Trichloroisocyanuric acid, dry	140	2468
Toxins, extracted from living sources, solid, n.o.s.	153	3172	Trichlorosilane	139	1295
			(mono)-(Trichloro)-tetra-(monopotassium dichloro)-penta-s-triazinetrione, dry	140	2468
Toxins, extracted from living sources, solid, n.o.s.	153	3462			
Triallylamine	132	2610	Tricresyl phosphate	151	2574
Triallyl borate	156	2609	Triethylamine	132	1296
Triazine pesticide, liquid, flammable, poisonous	131	2764	Triethylenetetramine	153	2259
			Triethyl phosphite	130	2323
Triazine pesticide, liquid, flammable, toxic	131	2764	Trifluoroacetic acid	154	2699
Triazine pesticide, liquid, poisonous	151	2998	Trifluoroacetyl chloride	125	3057
Triazine pesticide, liquid, poisonous, flammable	131	2997	Trifluorochloroethylene, stabilized	119P	1082
			1,1,1-Trifluoroethane	115	2035
Triazine pesticide, liquid, toxic	151	2998	Trifluoroethane, compressed	115	2035
Triazine pesticide, liquid, toxic, flammable	131	2997	Trifluoromethane	126	1984
Triazine pesticide, solid, poisonous	151	2763	Trifluoromethane, refrigerated liquid	120	3136
Triazine pesticide, solid, toxic	151	2763	Trifluoromethane and Chlorotrifluoromethane azeotropic mixture with approximately 60% Chlorotrifluoromethane	126	2599

Name of Material	Guide No.	ID No.
2-Trifluoromethylaniline	153	2942
3-Trifluoromethylaniline	153	2948
Triisobutylene	128	2324
Triisopropyl borate	129	2616
Trimethoxysilane	132	9269
Trimethylacetyl chloride	132	2438
Trimethylamine, anhydrous	118	1083
Trimethylamine, aqueous solution	132	1297
1,3,5-Trimethylbenzene	129	2325
Trimethyl borate	129	2416
Trimethylchlorosilane	155	1298
Trimethylcyclohexylamine	153	2326
Trimethylhexamethylenediamines	153	2327
Trimethylhexamethylene diisocyanate	156	2328
Trimethyl phosphite	130	2329
Trinitrobenzene, wetted with not less than 10% water	113	3367
Trinitrobenzene, wetted with not less than 30% water	113	1354
Trinitrobenzoic acid, wetted with not less than 10% water	113	3368
Trinitrobenzoic acid, wetted with not less than 30% water	113	1355
Trinitrochlorobenzene, wetted with not less than 10% water	113	3365
Trinitrophenol, wetted with not less than 10% water	113	3364
Trinitrophenol, wetted with not less than 30% water	113	1344
Trinitrotoluene, wetted with not less than 10% water	113	3366
Trinitrotoluene, wetted with not less than 30% water	113	1356
Tripropylamine	132	2260
Tripropylene	128	2057
Tris-(1-aziridinyl)phosphine oxide, solution	152	2501
Tungsten hexafluoride	125	2196
Turpentine	128	1299
Turpentine substitute	128	1300
Undecane	128	2330
Uranium hexafluoride	166	2978
Uranium hexafluoride, fissile containing more than 1% Uranium-235	166	2977
Uranium hexafluoride, non fissile or fissile-excepted	166	2978
Uranium metal, pyrophoric	162	2979
Uranyl nitrate, hexahydrate, solution	162	2980
Uranyl nitrate, solid	162	2981
Urea hydrogen peroxide	140	1511
Urea nitrate, wetted with not less than 10% water	113	3370
Urea nitrate, wetted with not less than 20% water	113	1357
Valeraldehyde	129	2058
Valeryl chloride	132	2502
Vanadium compound, n.o.s.	151	3285
Vanadium oxytrichloride	137	2443
Vanadium pentoxide	151	2862
Vanadium tetrachloride	137	2444
Vanadium trichloride	157	2475
Vanadyl sulfate	151	2931
Vanadyl sulphate	151	2931
Vehicle, flammable gas powered	128	3166
Vehicle, flammable liquid powered	128	3166
Vinyl acetate, stabilized	129P	1301

Name of Material	Guide No.	ID No.	Name of Material	Guide No.	ID No.
Vinyl bromide, stabilized	116P	1085	White asbestos	171	2590
Vinyl butyrate, stabilized	129P	2838	White phosphorus, dry	136	1381
Vinyl chloride, stabilized	116P	1086	White phosphorus, in solution	136	1381
Vinyl chloroacetate	155	2589	White phosphorus, molten	136	2447
Vinyl ethyl ether, stabilized	127P	1302	White phosphorus, under water	136	1381
Vinyl fluoride, stabilized	116P	1860	Wood preservatives, liquid	129	1306
Vinylidene chloride, stabilized	130P	1303	Wool waste, wet	133	1387
Vinyl isobutyl ether, stabilized	127P	1304	Xanthates	135	3342
Vinyl methyl ether, stabilized	116P	1087	Xenon	121	2036
Vinylpyridines, stabilized	131P	3073	Xenon, compressed	121	2036
Vinyltoluenes, stabilized	130P	2618	Xenon, refrigerated liquid (cryogenic liquid)	120	2591
Vinyltrichlorosilane	155P	1305	Xylenes	130	1307
Vinyltrichlorosilane, stabilized	155P	1305	Xylenols	153	2261
VX	153	2810	Xylenols, liquid	153	3430
Water-reactive liquid, corrosive, n.o.s.	138	3129	Xylenols, solid	153	2261
Water-reactive liquid, n.o.s.	138	3148	Xylidines	153	1711
Water-reactive liquid, poisonous, n.o.s.	139	3130	Xylidines, liquid	153	1711
Water-reactive liquid, toxic, n.o.s.	139	3130	Xylidines, solid	153	1711
Water-reactive solid, corrosive, n.o.s.	138	3131	Xylidines, solid	153	3452
Water-reactive solid, flammable, n.o.s.	138	3132	Xylyl bromide	152	1701
Water-reactive solid, n.o.s.	138	2813	Xylyl bromide, liquid	152	1701
Water-reactive solid, oxidizing, n.o.s.	138	3133	Xylyl bromide, solid	152	3417
Water-reactive solid, poisonous, n.o.s.	139	3134	Yellow phosphorus, dry	136	1381
Water-reactive solid, self-heating, n.o.s.	138	3135	Yellow phosphorus, in solution	136	1381
			Yellow phosphorus, molten	136	2447
Water-reactive solid, toxic, n.o.s.	139	3134	Yellow phosphorus, under water	136	1381
Wheelchair, electric, with batteries	154	3171	Zinc ammonium nitrite	140	1512
			Zinc arsenate	151	1712
			Zinc arsenate and Zinc arsenite mixture	151	1712
			Zinc arsenite	151	1712
			Zinc arsenite and Zinc arsenate mixture	151	1712

Name of Material	Guide No.	ID No.
Zinc ashes	138	1435
Zinc bromate	140	2469
Zinc chlorate	140	1513
Zinc chloride, anhydrous	154	2331
Zinc chloride, solution	154	1840
Zinc cyanide	151	1713
Zinc dithionite	171	1931
Zinc dross	138	1435
Zinc dust	138	1436
Zinc fluorosilicate	151	2855
Zinc hydrosulfite	171	1931
Zinc hydrosulphite	171	1931
Zinc nitrate	140	1514
Zinc permanganate	140	1515
Zinc peroxide	143	1516
Zinc phosphide	139	1714
Zinc powder	138	1436
Zinc residue	138	1435
Zinc resinate	133	2714
Zinc silicofluoride	151	2855
Zinc skimmings	138	1435
Zirconium, dry, coiled wire, finished metal sheets or strips	170	2858
Zirconium, dry, finished sheets, strips or coiled wire	135	2009
Zirconium hydride	138	1437
Zirconium metal, liquid suspension	170	1308
Zirconium metal, powder, wet	170	1358
Zirconium nitrate	140	2728
Zirconium picramate, wetted with not less than 20% water	113	1517
Zirconium powder, dry	135	2008

Name of Material	Guide No.	ID No.
Zirconium powder, wetted with not less than 25% water	170	1358
Zirconium scrap	135	1932
Zirconium sulfate	171	9163
Zirconium sulphate	171	9163
Zirconium suspended in a flammable liquid	170	1308
Zirconium suspended in a liquid (flammable)	170	1308
Zirconium tetrachloride	137	2503

NOTES

GUIDES

POTENTIAL HAZARDS

FIRE OR EXPLOSION
- May explode from heat, shock, friction or contamination.
- May react violently or explosively on contact with air, water or foam.
- May be ignited by heat, sparks or flames.
- Vapors may travel to source of ignition and flash back.
- Containers may explode when heated.
- Ruptured cylinders may rocket.

HEALTH
- Inhalation, ingestion or contact with substance may cause severe injury, infection, disease or death.
- High concentration of gas may cause asphyxiation without warning.
- Contact may cause burns to skin and eyes.
- Fire or contact with water may produce irritating, toxic and/or corrosive gases.
- Runoff from fire control may cause pollution.

PUBLIC SAFETY

- **CALL Emergency Response Telephone Number on Shipping Paper first. If Shipping Paper not available or no answer, refer to appropriate telephone number listed on the inside back cover.**
- As an immediate precautionary measure, isolate spill or leak area for at least 100 meters (330 feet) in all directions.
- Keep unauthorized personnel away.
- Stay upwind.
- Keep out of low areas.

PROTECTIVE CLOTHING
- Wear positive pressure self-contained breathing apparatus (SCBA).
- Structural firefighters' protective clothing provides limited protection in fire situations ONLY; it may not be effective in spill situations.

EVACUATION
Fire
- If tank, rail car or tank truck is involved in a fire, ISOLATE for 800 meters (1/2 mile) in all directions; also, consider initial evacuation for 800 meters (1/2 mile) in all directions.

EMERGENCY RESPONSE

FIRE

CAUTION: Material may react with extinguishing agent.

Small Fire

- Dry chemical, CO_2, water spray or regular foam.

Large Fire

- Water spray, fog or regular foam.
- Move containers from fire area if you can do it without risk.

Fire involving Tanks

- Cool containers with flooding quantities of water until well after fire is out.
- Do not get water inside containers.
- Withdraw immediately in case of rising sound from venting safety devices or discoloration of tank.
- ALWAYS stay away from tanks engulfed in fire.

SPILL OR LEAK

- Do not touch or walk through spilled material.
- ELIMINATE all ignition sources (no smoking, flares, sparks or flames in immediate area).
- All equipment used when handling the product must be grounded.
- Keep combustibles (wood, paper, oil, etc.) away from spilled material.
- Use water spray to reduce vapors or divert vapor cloud drift. Avoid allowing water runoff to contact spilled material.
- Prevent entry into waterways, sewers, basements or confined areas.

Small Spill • Take up with sand or other non-combustible absorbent material and place into containers for later disposal.

Large Spill • Dike far ahead of liquid spill for later disposal.

FIRST AID

- Move victim to fresh air.   • Call 911 or emergency medical service.
- Give artificial respiration if victim is not breathing.
- **Do not use mouth-to-mouth method if victim ingested or inhaled the substance; give artificial respiration with the aid of a pocket mask equipped with a one-way valve or other proper respiratory medical device.**
- Administer oxygen if breathing is difficult.
- Remove and isolate contaminated clothing and shoes.
- In case of contact with substance, immediately flush skin or eyes with running water for at least 20 minutes.
- Shower and wash with soap and water.
- Keep victim warm and quiet.
- Effects of exposure (inhalation, ingestion or skin contact) to substance may be delayed.
- Ensure that medical personnel are aware of the material(s) involved and take precautions to protect themselves.

POTENTIAL HAZARDS

FIRE OR EXPLOSION
- MAY EXPLODE AND THROW FRAGMENTS 1600 meters (1 MILE) OR MORE IF FIRE REACHES CARGO.
- For information on "Compatibility Group" letters, refer to Glossary section.

HEALTH
- Fire may produce irritating, corrosive and/or toxic gases.

PUBLIC SAFETY

- CALL Emergency Response Telephone Number on Shipping Paper first. If Shipping Paper not available or no answer, refer to appropriate telephone number listed on the inside back cover.
- Isolate spill or leak area immediately for at least 500 meters (1/3 mile) in all directions.
- Move people out of line of sight of the scene and away from windows.
- Keep unauthorized personnel away.
- Stay upwind.
- Ventilate closed spaces before entering.

PROTECTIVE CLOTHING
- Wear positive pressure self-contained breathing apparatus (SCBA).
- Structural firefighters' protective clothing will only provide limited protection.

EVACUATION
Large Spill
- Consider initial evacuation for 800 meters (1/2 mile) in all directions.
Fire
- If rail car or trailer is involved in a fire and heavily encased explosives such as bombs or artillery projectiles are suspected, ISOLATE for 1600 meters (1 mile) in all directions; also, initiate evacuation including emergency responders for 1600 meters (1 mile) in all directions.
- When heavily encased explosives are not involved, evacuate the area for 800 meters (1/2 mile) in all directions.

* For information on "Compatibility Group" letters, refer to the Glossary section.

EMERGENCY RESPONSE

FIRE

CARGO Fire

- **DO NOT fight fire when fire reaches cargo! Cargo may EXPLODE!**
- Stop all traffic and clear the area for at least 1600 meters (1 mile) in all directions and let burn.
- **Do not move cargo or vehicle if cargo has been exposed to heat.**

TIRE or VEHICLE Fire

- **Use plenty of water - FLOOD it! If water is not available, use CO_2, dry chemical or dirt.**
- If possible, and WITHOUT RISK, use unmanned hose holders or monitor nozzles from maximum distance to prevent fire from spreading to cargo area.
- Pay special attention to tire fires as re-ignition may occur. Stand by with extinguisher ready.

SPILL OR LEAK

- ELIMINATE all ignition sources (no smoking, flares, sparks or flames in immediate area).
- All equipment used when handling the product must be grounded.
- Do not touch or walk through spilled material.
- DO NOT OPERATE RADIO TRANSMITTERS WITHIN 100 meters (330 feet) OF ELECTRIC DETONATORS.
- **DO NOT CLEAN-UP OR DISPOSE OF, EXCEPT UNDER SUPERVISION OF A SPECIALIST.**

FIRST AID

- Move victim to fresh air.   • Call 911 or emergency medical service.
- Give artificial respiration if victim is not breathing.
- Administer oxygen if breathing is difficult.
- Remove and isolate contaminated clothing and shoes.
- In case of contact with substance, immediately flush skin or eyes with running water for at least 20 minutes.
- Ensure that medical personnel are aware of the material(s) involved and take precautions to protect themselves.

* For information on "Compatibility Group" letters, refer to the Glossary section.

POTENTIAL HAZARDS

FIRE OR EXPLOSION
- Flammable/combustible material.
- May be ignited by heat, sparks or flames.
- **DRIED OUT material may explode if exposed to heat, flame, friction or shock; Treat as an explosive (GUIDE 112).**
- **Keep material wet with water or treat as an explosive (GUIDE 112).**
- Runoff to sewer may create fire or explosion hazard.

HEALTH
- Some are toxic and may be fatal if inhaled, swallowed or absorbed through skin.
- Contact may cause burns to skin and eyes.
- Fire may produce irritating, corrosive and/or toxic gases.
- Runoff from fire control or dilution water may cause pollution.

PUBLIC SAFETY
- **CALL Emergency Response Telephone Number on Shipping Paper first. If Shipping Paper not available or no answer, refer to appropriate telephone number listed on the inside back cover.**
- Isolate spill or leak area immediately for at least 100 meters (330 feet) in all directions.
- Keep unauthorized personnel away.
- Stay upwind.
- Ventilate closed spaces before entering.

PROTECTIVE CLOTHING
- Wear positive pressure self-contained breathing apparatus (SCBA).
- Structural firefighters' protective clothing will only provide limited protection.

EVACUATION
Large Spill
- **Consider initial evacuation for 500 meters (1/3 mile) in all directions.**
Fire
- If tank, rail car or tank truck is involved in a fire, ISOLATE for 800 meters (1/2 mile) in all directions; also, consider initial evacuation for 800 meters (1/2 mile) in all directions.

EMERGENCY RESPONSE

FIRE

CARGO Fire

- **DO NOT fight fire when fire reaches cargo! Cargo may EXPLODE!**
- Stop all traffic and clear the area for at least 800 meters (1/2 mile) in all directions and let burn.
- **Do not move cargo or vehicle if cargo has been exposed to heat.**

TIRE or VEHICLE Fire

- **Use plenty of water - FLOOD it! If water is not available, use CO_2, dry chemical or dirt.**
- If possible, and WITHOUT RISK, use unmanned hose holders or monitor nozzles from maximum distance to prevent fire from spreading to cargo area.
- Pay special attention to tire fires as re-ignition may occur. Stand by with extinguisher ready.

SPILL OR LEAK

- ELIMINATE all ignition sources (no smoking, flares, sparks or flames in immediate area).
- All equipment used when handling the product must be grounded.
- Do not touch or walk through spilled material.

Small Spill

- Flush area with flooding quantities of water.

Large Spill

- Wet down with water and dike for later disposal.
- KEEP "WETTED" PRODUCT WET BY SLOWLY ADDING FLOODING QUANTITIES OF WATER.

FIRST AID

- Move victim to fresh air. • Call 911 or emergency medical service.
- Give artificial respiration if victim is not breathing.
- Administer oxygen if breathing is difficult.
- Remove and isolate contaminated clothing and shoes.
- In case of contact with substance, immediately flush skin or eyes with running water for at least 20 minutes.
- Ensure that medical personnel are aware of the material(s) involved and take precautions to protect themselves.

POTENTIAL HAZARDS

FIRE OR EXPLOSION
- **MAY EXPLODE AND THROW FRAGMENTS 500 meters (1/3 MILE) OR MORE IF FIRE REACHES CARGO.**
- **For information on "Compatibility Group" letters, refer to Glossary section.**

HEALTH
- Fire may produce irritating, corrosive and/or toxic gases.

PUBLIC SAFETY

- **CALL Emergency Response Telephone Number on Shipping Paper first. If Shipping Paper not available or no answer, refer to appropriate telephone number listed on the inside back cover.**
- Isolate spill or leak area immediately for at least 100 meters (330 feet) in all directions.
- Move people out of line of sight of the scene and away from windows.
- Keep unauthorized personnel away.
- Stay upwind.
- Ventilate closed spaces before entering.

PROTECTIVE CLOTHING
- Wear positive pressure self-contained breathing apparatus (SCBA).
- Structural firefighters' protective clothing will only provide limited protection.

EVACUATION
Large Spill
- **Consider initial evacuation for 250 meters (800 feet) in all directions.**

Fire
- If rail car or trailer is involved in a fire, ISOLATE for 500 meters (1/3 mile) in all directions; also initiate evacuation including emergency responders for 500 meters (1/3 mile) in all directions.

* For information on "Compatibility Group" letters, refer to the Glossary section.

EMERGENCY RESPONSE

FIRE

CARGO Fire

- **DO NOT fight fire when fire reaches cargo! Cargo may EXPLODE!**
- Stop all traffic and clear the area for at least 500 meters (1/3 mile) in all directions and let burn.
- **Do not move cargo or vehicle if cargo has been exposed to heat.**

TIRE or VEHICLE Fire

- **Use plenty of water - FLOOD it! If water is not available, use CO_2, dry chemical or dirt.**
- If possible, and WITHOUT RISK, use unmanned hose holders or monitor nozzles from maximum distance to prevent fire from spreading to cargo area.
- Pay special attention to tire fires as re-ignition may occur. Stand by with extinguisher ready.

SPILL OR LEAK

- ELIMINATE all ignition sources (no smoking, flares, sparks or flames in immediate area).
- All equipment used when handling the product must be grounded.
- Do not touch or walk through spilled material.
- DO NOT OPERATE RADIO TRANSMITTERS WITHIN 100 meters (330 feet) OF ELECTRIC DETONATORS.
- **DO NOT CLEAN-UP OR DISPOSE OF, EXCEPT UNDER SUPERVISION OF A SPECIALIST.**

FIRST AID

- Move victim to fresh air.   • Call 911 or emergency medical service.
- Give artificial respiration if victim is not breathing.
- Administer oxygen if breathing is difficult.
- Remove and isolate contaminated clothing and shoes.
- In case of contact with substance, immediately flush skin or eyes with running water for at least 20 minutes.
- Ensure that medical personnel are aware of the material(s) involved and take precautions to protect themselves.

SUPPLEMENTAL INFORMATION

- Packages bearing the 1.4S label or packages containing material classified as 1.4S are designed or packaged in such a manner that when involved in a fire, may burn vigorously with localized detonations and projection of fragments.
- Effects are usually confined to immediate vicinity of packages.
- If fire threatens cargo area containing packages bearing the 1.4S label or packages containing material classified as 1.4S, consider isolating at least 15 meters (50 feet) in all directions. Fight fire with normal precautions from a reasonable distance.

* For information on "Compatibility Group" letters, refer to the Glossary section.

POTENTIAL HAZARDS

FIRE OR EXPLOSION

- **EXTREMELY FLAMMABLE.**
- Will be easily ignited by heat, sparks or flames.
- Will form explosive mixtures with air.
- Vapors from liquefied gas are initially heavier than air and spread along ground.

CAUTION:Hydrogen (UN1049), Deuterium (UN1957), Hydrogen, refrigerated liquid (UN1966) and Methane (UN1971) are lighter than air and will rise. Hydrogen and Deuterium fires are difficult to detect since they burn with an invisible flame. Use an alternate method of detection (thermal camera, broom handle, etc.)

- Vapors may travel to source of ignition and flash back.
- Cylinders exposed to fire may vent and release flammable gas through pressure relief devices.
- Containers may explode when heated.
- Ruptured cylinders may rocket.

HEALTH

- Vapors may cause dizziness or asphyxiation without warning.
- Some may be irritating if inhaled at high concentrations.
- Contact with gas or liquefied gas may cause burns, severe injury and/or frostbite.
- Fire may produce irritating and/or toxic gases.

PUBLIC SAFETY

- **CALL Emergency Response Telephone Number on Shipping Paper first. If Shipping Paper not available or no answer, refer to appropriate telephone number listed on the inside back cover.**
- As an immediate precautionary measure, isolate spill or leak area for at least 100 meters (330 feet) in all directions.
- Keep unauthorized personnel away.
- Stay upwind.
- Many gases are heavier than air and will spread along ground and collect in low or confined areas (sewers, basements, tanks).
- Keep out of low areas.

PROTECTIVE CLOTHING

- Wear positive pressure self-contained breathing apparatus (SCBA).
- Structural firefighters' protective clothing will only provide limited protection.
- Always wear thermal protective clothing when handling refrigerated/cryogenic liquids.

EVACUATION

Large Spill

- Consider initial downwind evacuation for at least 800 meters (1/2 mile).

Fire

- If tank, rail car or tank truck is involved in a fire, ISOLATE for 1600 meters (1 mile) in all directions; also, consider initial evacuation for 1600 meters (1 mile) in all directions.

EMERGENCY RESPONSE

FIRE

- **DO NOT EXTINGUISH A LEAKING GAS FIRE UNLESS LEAK CAN BE STOPPED.**

CAUTION: Hydrogen (UN1049), Deuterium (UN1957) and Hydrogen, refrigerated liquid (UN1966) burn with an invisible flame. Hydrogen and Methane mixture, compressed (UN2034) may burn with an invisible flame.

Small Fire

- Dry chemical or CO_2.

Large Fire

- Water spray or fog.
- Move containers from fire area if you can do it without risk.

Fire involving Tanks

- Fight fire from maximum distance or use unmanned hose holders or monitor nozzles.
- Cool containers with flooding quantities of water until well after fire is out.
- Do not direct water at source of leak or safety devices; icing may occur.
- Withdraw immediately in case of rising sound from venting safety devices or discoloration of tank.
- ALWAYS stay away from tanks engulfed in fire.
- For massive fire, use unmanned hose holders or monitor nozzles; if this is impossible, withdraw from area and let fire burn.

SPILL OR LEAK

- ELIMINATE all ignition sources (no smoking, flares, sparks or flames in immediate area).
- All equipment used when handling the product must be grounded.
- Do not touch or walk through spilled material.
- Stop leak if you can do it without risk.
- If possible, turn leaking containers so that gas escapes rather than liquid.
- Use water spray to reduce vapors or divert vapor cloud drift. Avoid allowing water runoff to contact spilled material.
- Do not direct water at spill or source of leak.
- Prevent spreading of vapors through sewers, ventilation systems and confined areas.
- Isolate area until gas has dispersed.

CAUTION: When in contact with refrigerated/cryogenic liquids, many materials become brittle and are likely to break without warning.

FIRST AID

- Move victim to fresh air.   • Call 911 or emergency medical service.
- Give artificial respiration if victim is not breathing.
- Administer oxygen if breathing is difficult.
- Remove and isolate contaminated clothing and shoes.
- Clothing frozen to the skin should be thawed before being removed.
- In case of contact with liquefied gas, thaw frosted parts with lukewarm water.
- In case of burns, immediately cool affected skin for as long as possible with cold water. Do not remove clothing if adhering to skin.   • Keep victim warm and quiet.
- Ensure that medical personnel are aware of the material(s) involved and take precautions to protect themselves.

POTENTIAL HAZARDS

FIRE OR EXPLOSION

- **EXTREMELY FLAMMABLE.**
- Will be easily ignited by heat, sparks or flames.
- Will form explosive mixtures with air.
- Silane will ignite spontaneously in air.
- Those substances designated with a **"P"** may polymerize explosively when heated or involved in a fire.
- Vapors from liquefied gas are initially heavier than air and spread along ground.
- Vapors may travel to source of ignition and flash back.
- Cylinders exposed to fire may vent and release flammable gas through pressure relief devices.
- Containers may explode when heated.
- Ruptured cylinders may rocket.

HEALTH

- Vapors may cause dizziness or asphyxiation without warning.
- Some may be toxic if inhaled at high concentrations.
- Contact with gas or liquefied gas may cause burns, severe injury and/or frostbite.
- Fire may produce irritating and/or toxic gases.

PUBLIC SAFETY

- **CALL Emergency Response Telephone Number on Shipping Paper first. If Shipping Paper not available or no answer, refer to appropriate telephone number listed on the inside back cover.**
- As an immediate precautionary measure, isolate spill or leak area for at least 100 meters (330 feet) in all directions.
- Keep unauthorized personnel away.
- Stay upwind.
- Many gases are heavier than air and will spread along ground and collect in low or confined areas (sewers, basements, tanks).
- Keep out of low areas.

PROTECTIVE CLOTHING

- Wear positive pressure self-contained breathing apparatus (SCBA).
- Structural firefighters' protective clothing will only provide limited protection.

EVACUATION

Large Spill

- Consider initial downwind evacuation for at least 800 meters (1/2 mile).

Fire

- If tank, rail car or tank truck is involved in a fire, ISOLATE for 1600 meters (1 mile) in all directions; also, consider initial evacuation for 1600 meters (1 mile) in all directions.

EMERGENCY RESPONSE

FIRE
- **DO NOT EXTINGUISH A LEAKING GAS FIRE UNLESS LEAK CAN BE STOPPED.**

Small Fire
- Dry chemical or CO_2.

Large Fire
- Water spray or fog.
- Move containers from fire area if you can do it without risk.

Fire involving Tanks
- Fight fire from maximum distance or use unmanned hose holders or monitor nozzles.
- Cool containers with flooding quantities of water until well after fire is out.
- Do not direct water at source of leak or safety devices; icing may occur.
- Withdraw immediately in case of rising sound from venting safety devices or discoloration of tank.
- ALWAYS stay away from tanks engulfed in fire.
- For massive fire, use unmanned hose holders or monitor nozzles; if this is impossible, withdraw from area and let fire burn.

SPILL OR LEAK
- ELIMINATE all ignition sources (no smoking, flares, sparks or flames in immediate area).
- All equipment used when handling the product must be grounded.
- Stop leak if you can do it without risk.
- Do not touch or walk through spilled material.
- Do not direct water at spill or source of leak.
- Use water spray to reduce vapors or divert vapor cloud drift. Avoid allowing water runoff to contact spilled material.
- If possible, turn leaking containers so that gas escapes rather than liquid.
- Prevent entry into waterways, sewers, basements or confined areas.
- Isolate area until gas has dispersed.

FIRST AID
- Move victim to fresh air. • Call 911 or emergency medical service.
- Give artificial respiration if victim is not breathing.
- Administer oxygen if breathing is difficult.
- Remove and isolate contaminated clothing and shoes.
- In case of contact with liquefied gas, thaw frosted parts with lukewarm water.
- In case of burns, immediately cool affected skin for as long as possible with cold water. Do not remove clothing if adhering to skin.
- Keep victim warm and quiet.
- Ensure that medical personnel are aware of the material(s) involved and take precautions to protect themselves.

POTENTIAL HAZARDS

HEALTH

- **TOXIC; Extremely Hazardous.**
- May be fatal if inhaled or absorbed through skin.
- Initial odor may be irritating or foul and may deaden your sense of smell.
- Contact with gas or liquefied gas may cause burns, severe injury and/or frostbite.
- Fire will produce irritating, corrosive and/or toxic gases.
- Runoff from fire control may cause pollution.

FIRE OR EXPLOSION

- These materials are extremely flammable.
- May form explosive mixtures with air.
- May be ignited by heat, sparks or flames.
- Vapors from liquefied gas are initially heavier than air and spread along ground.
- Vapors may travel to source of ignition and flash back.
- Runoff may create fire or explosion hazard.
- Cylinders exposed to fire may vent and release toxic and flammable gas through pressure relief devices.
- Containers may explode when heated.
- Ruptured cylinders may rocket.

PUBLIC SAFETY

- **CALL Emergency Response Telephone Number on Shipping Paper first. If Shipping Paper not available or no answer, refer to appropriate telephone number listed on the inside back cover.**
- As an immediate precautionary measure, isolate spill or leak area for at least 100 meters (330 feet) in all directions.
- Keep unauthorized personnel away.
- Stay upwind.
- Many gases are heavier than air and will spread along ground and collect in low or confined areas (sewers, basements, tanks).
- Keep out of low areas.
- Ventilate closed spaces before entering.

PROTECTIVE CLOTHING

- Wear positive pressure self-contained breathing apparatus (SCBA).
- Wear chemical protective clothing that is specifically recommended by the manufacturer. It may provide little or no thermal protection.
- Structural firefighters' protective clothing provides limited protection in fire situations ONLY; it is not effective in spill situations where direct contact with the substance is possible.

EVACUATION

Spill

- See Table 1 - Initial Isolation and Protective Action Distances.

Fire

- If tank, rail car or tank truck is involved in a fire, ISOLATE for 1600 meters (1 mile) in all directions; also, consider initial evacuation for 1600 meters (1 mile) in all directions.

EMERGENCY RESPONSE

FIRE

- **DO NOT EXTINGUISH A LEAKING GAS FIRE UNLESS LEAK CAN BE STOPPED.**

Small Fire

- Dry chemical, CO_2, water spray or regular foam.

Large Fire

- Water spray, fog or regular foam.
- Move containers from fire area if you can do it without risk.
- Damaged cylinders should be handled only by specialists.

Fire involving Tanks

- Fight fire from maximum distance or use unmanned hose holders or monitor nozzles.
- Cool containers with flooding quantities of water until well after fire is out.
- Do not direct water at source of leak or safety devices; icing may occur.
- Withdraw immediately in case of rising sound from venting safety devices or discoloration of tank.
- ALWAYS stay away from tanks engulfed in fire.

SPILL OR LEAK

- ELIMINATE all ignition sources (no smoking, flares, sparks or flames in immediate area).
- All equipment used when handling the product must be grounded.
- Fully encapsulating, vapor protective clothing should be worn for spills and leaks with no fire.   • Do not touch or walk through spilled material.
- Stop leak if you can do it without risk.
- Use water spray to reduce vapors or divert vapor cloud drift. Avoid allowing water runoff to contact spilled material.   • Do not direct water at spill or source of leak.
- If possible, turn leaking containers so that gas escapes rather than liquid.
- Prevent entry into waterways, sewers, basements or confined areas.
- Isolate area until gas has dispersed.
- Consider igniting spill or leak to eliminate toxic gas concerns.

FIRST AID

- Move victim to fresh air.   • Call 911 or emergency medical service.
- Give artificial respiration if victim is not breathing.
- **Do not use mouth-to-mouth method if victim ingested or inhaled the substance; give artificial respiration with the aid of a pocket mask equipped with a one-way valve or other proper respiratory medical device.**
- Administer oxygen if breathing is difficult.
- Remove and isolate contaminated clothing and shoes.
- In case of contact with substance, immediately flush skin or eyes with running water for at least 20 minutes.
- In case of contact with liquefied gas, thaw frosted parts with lukewarm water.
- In case of burns, immediately cool affected skin for as long as possible with cold water. Do not remove clothing if adhering to skin.
- Keep victim warm and quiet.   • Keep victim under observation.
- Effects of contact or inhalation may be delayed.
- Ensure that medical personnel are aware of the material(s) involved and take precautions to protect themselves.

POTENTIAL HAZARDS

FIRE OR EXPLOSION
- **EXTREMELY FLAMMABLE.**
- May be ignited by heat, sparks or flames.
- May form explosive mixtures with air.
- Vapors from liquefied gas are initially heavier than air and spread along ground.
- Vapors may travel to source of ignition and flash back.
- Some of these materials may react violently with water.
- Cylinders exposed to fire may vent and release flammable gas through pressure relief devices.
- Containers may explode when heated.
- Ruptured cylinders may rocket.

HEALTH
- May cause toxic effects if inhaled.
- Vapors are extremely irritating.
- Contact with gas or liquefied gas may cause burns, severe injury and/or frostbite.
- Fire will produce irritating, corrosive and/or toxic gases.
- Runoff from fire control may cause pollution.

PUBLIC SAFETY
- **CALL Emergency Response Telephone Number on Shipping Paper first. If Shipping Paper not available or no answer, refer to appropriate telephone number listed on the inside back cover.**
- As an immediate precautionary measure, isolate spill or leak area for at least 100 meters (330 feet) in all directions.
- Keep unauthorized personnel away.
- Stay upwind.
- Many gases are heavier than air and will spread along ground and collect in low or confined areas (sewers, basements, tanks).
- Keep out of low areas.   • Ventilate closed spaces before entering.

PROTECTIVE CLOTHING
- Wear positive pressure self-contained breathing apparatus (SCBA).
- Wear chemical protective clothing that is specifically recommended by the manufacturer. It may provide little or no thermal protection.
- Structural firefighters' protective clothing provides limited protection in fire situations ONLY; it is not effective in spill situations where direct contact with the substance is possible.

EVACUATION
Large Spill
- Consider initial downwind evacuation for at least 800 meters (1/2 mile).

Fire
- If tank, rail car or tank truck is involved in a fire, ISOLATE for 1600 meters (1 mile) in all directions; also, consider initial evacuation for 1600 meters (1 mile) in all directions.

EMERGENCY RESPONSE

FIRE
- **DO NOT EXTINGUISH A LEAKING GAS FIRE UNLESS LEAK CAN BE STOPPED.**

Small Fire
- Dry chemical or CO_2.

Large Fire
- Water spray, fog or regular foam.
- Move containers from fire area if you can do it without risk.
- Damaged cylinders should be handled only by specialists.

Fire involving Tanks
- Fight fire from maximum distance or use unmanned hose holders or monitor nozzles.
- Cool containers with flooding quantities of water until well after fire is out.
- Do not direct water at source of leak or safety devices; icing may occur.
- Withdraw immediately in case of rising sound from venting safety devices or discoloration of tank.
- ALWAYS stay away from tanks engulfed in fire.

SPILL OR LEAK
- ELIMINATE all ignition sources (no smoking, flares, sparks or flames in immediate area).
- All equipment used when handling the product must be grounded.
- Fully encapsulating, vapor protective clothing should be worn for spills and leaks with no fire.
- Do not touch or walk through spilled material.
- Stop leak if you can do it without risk.
- If possible, turn leaking containers so that gas escapes rather than liquid.
- Use water spray to reduce vapors or divert vapor cloud drift. Avoid allowing water runoff to contact spilled material.
- Do not direct water at spill or source of leak.
- Isolate area until gas has dispersed.

FIRST AID
- Move victim to fresh air. • Call 911 or emergency medical service.
- Give artificial respiration if victim is not breathing.
- **Do not use mouth-to-mouth method if victim ingested or inhaled the substance; give artificial respiration with the aid of a pocket mask equipped with a one-way valve or other proper respiratory medical device.**
- Administer oxygen if breathing is difficult.
- Remove and isolate contaminated clothing and shoes.
- In case of contact with liquefied gas, thaw frosted parts with lukewarm water.
- In case of burns, immediately cool affected skin for as long as possible with cold water. Do not remove clothing if adhering to skin.
- Keep victim warm and quiet. • Keep victim under observation.
- Effects of contact or inhalation may be delayed.
- Ensure that medical personnel are aware of the material(s) involved and take precautions to protect themselves.

POTENTIAL HAZARDS

HEALTH
- **TOXIC; may be fatal if inhaled or absorbed through skin.**
- Contact with gas or liquefied gas may cause burns, severe injury and/or frostbite.
- Fire will produce irritating, corrosive and/or toxic gases.
- Runoff from fire control may cause pollution.

FIRE OR EXPLOSION
- Flammable; may be ignited by heat, sparks or flames.
- May form explosive mixtures with air.
- Those substances designated with a **"P"** may polymerize explosively when heated or involved in a fire.
- Vapors from liquefied gas are initially heavier than air and spread along ground.
- Vapors may travel to source of ignition and flash back.
- Some of these materials may react violently with water.
- Cylinders exposed to fire may vent and release toxic and flammable gas through pressure relief devices.
- Containers may explode when heated.
- Ruptured cylinders may rocket.
- Runoff may create fire or explosion hazard.

PUBLIC SAFETY
- **CALL Emergency Response Telephone Number on Shipping Paper first. If Shipping Paper not available or no answer, refer to appropriate telephone number listed on the inside back cover.**
- As an immediate precautionary measure, isolate spill or leak area for at least 100 meters (330 feet) in all directions.
- Keep unauthorized personnel away. • Stay upwind.
- Many gases are heavier than air and will spread along ground and collect in low or confined areas (sewers, basements, tanks).
- Keep out of low areas. • Ventilate closed spaces before entering.

PROTECTIVE CLOTHING
- Wear positive pressure self-contained breathing apparatus (SCBA).
- Wear chemical protective clothing that is specifically recommended by the manufacturer. It may provide little or no thermal protection.
- Structural firefighters' protective clothing provides limited protection in fire situations ONLY; it is not effective in spill situations where direct contact with the substance is possible.

EVACUATION
Spill
- See Table 1 - Initial Isolation and Protective Action Distances for highlighted materials. For non-highlighted materials, increase, in the downwind direction, as necessary, the isolation distance shown under "PUBLIC SAFETY".

Fire
- If tank, rail car or tank truck is involved in a fire, ISOLATE for 1600 meters (1 mile) in all directions; also, consider initial evacuation for 1600 meters (1 mile) in all directions.

EMERGENCY RESPONSE

FIRE
- **DO NOT EXTINGUISH A LEAKING GAS FIRE UNLESS LEAK CAN BE STOPPED.**

Small Fire
- Dry chemical, CO_2, water spray or alcohol-resistant foam.

Large Fire
- Water spray, fog or alcohol-resistant foam.
- **FOR CHLOROSILANES, DO NOT USE WATER**; use AFFF alcohol-resistant medium expansion foam.   • Move containers from fire area if you can do it without risk.
- Damaged cylinders should be handled only by specialists.

Fire involving Tanks
- Fight fire from maximum distance or use unmanned hose holders or monitor nozzles.
- Cool containers with flooding quantities of water until well after fire is out.
- Do not direct water at source of leak or safety devices; icing may occur.
- Withdraw immediately in case of rising sound from venting safety devices or discoloration of tank.   • ALWAYS stay away from tanks engulfed in fire.

SPILL OR LEAK
- ELIMINATE all ignition sources (no smoking, flares, sparks or flames in immediate area).
- All equipment used when handling the product must be grounded.
- Fully encapsulating, vapor protective clothing should be worn for spills and leaks with no fire.
- Do not touch or walk through spilled material.
- Stop leak if you can do it without risk.
- Do not direct water at spill or source of leak.
- Use water spray to reduce vapors or divert vapor cloud drift. Avoid allowing water runoff to contact spilled material.
- **FOR CHLOROSILANES**, use AFFF alcohol-resistant medium expansion foam to reduce vapors.
- If possible, turn leaking containers so that gas escapes rather than liquid.
- Prevent entry into waterways, sewers, basements or confined areas.
- Isolate area until gas has dispersed.

FIRST AID
- Move victim to fresh air.   • Call 911 or emergency medical service.
- Give artificial respiration if victim is not breathing.
- **Do not use mouth-to-mouth method if victim ingested or inhaled the substance; give artificial respiration with the aid of a pocket mask equipped with a one-way valve or other proper respiratory medical device.**
- Administer oxygen if breathing is difficult.
- Remove and isolate contaminated clothing and shoes.
- In case of contact with substance, immediately flush skin or eyes with running water for at least 20 minutes.
- In case of contact with liquefied gas, thaw frosted parts with lukewarm water.
- In case of burns, immediately cool affected skin for as long as possible with cold water. Do not remove clothing if adhering to skin.
- Keep victim warm and quiet.   • Keep victim under observation.
- Effects of contact or inhalation may be delayed.
- Ensure that medical personnel are aware of the material(s) involved and take precautions to protect themselves.

POTENTIAL HAZARDS

HEALTH
- Vapors may cause dizziness or asphyxiation without warning.
- Vapors from liquefied gas are initially heavier than air and spread along ground.
- Contact with gas or liquefied gas may cause burns, severe injury and/or frostbite.

FIRE OR EXPLOSION
- **Non-flammable gases.**
- Containers may explode when heated.
- Ruptured cylinders may rocket.

PUBLIC SAFETY
- **CALL Emergency Response Telephone Number on Shipping Paper first. If Shipping Paper not available or no answer, refer to appropriate telephone number listed on the inside back cover.**
- As an immediate precautionary measure, isolate spill or leak area for at least 100 meters (330 feet) in all directions.
- Keep unauthorized personnel away.
- Stay upwind.
- Many gases are heavier than air and will spread along ground and collect in low or confined areas (sewers, basements, tanks).
- Keep out of low areas.
- Ventilate closed spaces before entering.

PROTECTIVE CLOTHING
- Wear positive pressure self-contained breathing apparatus (SCBA).
- Structural firefighters' protective clothing will only provide limited protection.
- Always wear thermal protective clothing when handling refrigerated/cryogenic liquids or solids.

EVACUATION
Large Spill
- Consider initial downwind evacuation for at least 100 meters (330 feet).

Fire
- If tank, rail car or tank truck is involved in a fire, ISOLATE for 800 meters (1/2 mile) in all directions; also, consider initial evacuation for 800 meters (1/2 mile) in all directions.

EMERGENCY RESPONSE

FIRE

- Use extinguishing agent suitable for type of surrounding fire.
- Move containers from fire area if you can do it without risk.
- Damaged cylinders should be handled only by specialists.

Fire involving Tanks

- Fight fire from maximum distance or use unmanned hose holders or monitor nozzles.
- Cool containers with flooding quantities of water until well after fire is out.
- Do not direct water at source of leak or safety devices; icing may occur.
- Withdraw immediately in case of rising sound from venting safety devices or discoloration of tank.
- ALWAYS stay away from tanks engulfed in fire.

SPILL OR LEAK

- Do not touch or walk through spilled material.
- Stop leak if you can do it without risk.
- Use water spray to reduce vapors or divert vapor cloud drift. Avoid allowing water runoff to contact spilled material.
- Do not direct water at spill or source of leak.
- If possible, turn leaking containers so that gas escapes rather than liquid.
- Prevent entry into waterways, sewers, basements or confined areas.
- Allow substance to evaporate.
- Ventilate the area.

CAUTION: When in contact with refrigerated/cryogenic liquids, many materials become brittle and are likely to break without warning.

FIRST AID

- Move victim to fresh air.   • Call 911 or emergency medical service.
- Give artificial respiration if victim is not breathing.
- Administer oxygen if breathing is difficult.
- Clothing frozen to the skin should be thawed before being removed.
- In case of contact with liquefied gas, thaw frosted parts with lukewarm water.
- Keep victim warm and quiet.
- Ensure that medical personnel are aware of the material(s) involved and take precautions to protect themselves.

POTENTIAL HAZARDS

HEALTH

- Vapors may cause dizziness or asphyxiation without warning.
- Vapors from liquefied gas are initially heavier than air and spread along ground.

FIRE OR EXPLOSION

- **Non-flammable gases.**
- Containers may explode when heated.
- Ruptured cylinders may rocket.

PUBLIC SAFETY

- **CALL Emergency Response Telephone Number on Shipping Paper first. If Shipping Paper not available or no answer, refer to appropriate telephone number listed on the inside back cover.**
- As an immediate precautionary measure, isolate spill or leak area for at least 100 meters (330 feet) in all directions.
- Keep unauthorized personnel away.
- Stay upwind.
- Many gases are heavier than air and will spread along ground and collect in low or confined areas (sewers, basements, tanks).
- Keep out of low areas.
- Ventilate closed spaces before entering.

PROTECTIVE CLOTHING

- Wear positive pressure self-contained breathing apparatus (SCBA).
- Structural firefighters' protective clothing will only provide limited protection.

EVACUATION

Large Spill

- Consider initial downwind evacuation for at least 100 meters (330 feet).

Fire

- If tank, rail car or tank truck is involved in a fire, ISOLATE for 800 meters (1/2 mile) in all directions; also, consider initial evacuation for 800 meters (1/2 mile) in all directions.

EMERGENCY RESPONSE

FIRE
- Use extinguishing agent suitable for type of surrounding fire.
- Move containers from fire area if you can do it without risk.
- Damaged cylinders should be handled only by specialists.

Fire involving Tanks
- Fight fire from maximum distance or use unmanned hose holders or monitor nozzles.
- Cool containers with flooding quantities of water until well after fire is out.
- Do not direct water at source of leak or safety devices; icing may occur.
- Withdraw immediately in case of rising sound from venting safety devices or discoloration of tank.
- ALWAYS stay away from tanks engulfed in fire.

SPILL OR LEAK
- Do not touch or walk through spilled material.
- Stop leak if you can do it without risk.
- Use water spray to reduce vapors or divert vapor cloud drift. Avoid allowing water runoff to contact spilled material.
- Do not direct water at spill or source of leak.
- If possible, turn leaking containers so that gas escapes rather than liquid.
- Prevent entry into waterways, sewers, basements or confined areas.
- Allow substance to evaporate.
- Ventilate the area.

FIRST AID
- Move victim to fresh air.   • Call 911 or emergency medical service.
- Give artificial respiration if victim is not breathing.
- Administer oxygen if breathing is difficult.
- Keep victim warm and quiet.
- Ensure that medical personnel are aware of the material(s) involved and take precautions to protect themselves.

POTENTIAL HAZARDS

FIRE OR EXPLOSION

- Substance does not burn but will support combustion.
- Some may react explosively with fuels.
- May ignite combustibles (wood, paper, oil, clothing, etc.).
- Vapors from liquefied gas are initially heavier than air and spread along ground.
- Runoff may create fire or explosion hazard.
- Containers may explode when heated.
- Ruptured cylinders may rocket.

HEALTH

- Vapors may cause dizziness or asphyxiation without warning.
- Contact with gas or liquefied gas may cause burns, severe injury and/or frostbite.
- Fire may produce irritating and/or toxic gases.

PUBLIC SAFETY

- **CALL Emergency Response Telephone Number on Shipping Paper first. If Shipping Paper not available or no answer, refer to appropriate telephone number listed on the inside back cover.**
- As an immediate precautionary measure, isolate spill or leak area for at least 100 meters (330 feet) in all directions.
- Keep unauthorized personnel away.
- Stay upwind.
- Many gases are heavier than air and will spread along ground and collect in low or confined areas (sewers, basements, tanks).
- Keep out of low areas.
- Ventilate closed spaces before entering.

PROTECTIVE CLOTHING

- Wear positive pressure self-contained breathing apparatus (SCBA).
- Wear chemical protective clothing that is specifically recommended by the manufacturer. It may provide little or no thermal protection.
- Structural firefighters' protective clothing provides limited protection in fire situations ONLY; it is not effective in spill situations where direct contact with the substance is possible.
- Always wear thermal protective clothing when handling refrigerated/cryogenic liquids.

EVACUATION

Large Spill

- Consider initial downwind evacuation for at least 500 meters (1/3 mile).

Fire

- If tank, rail car or tank truck is involved in a fire, ISOLATE for 800 meters (1/2 mile) in all directions; also, consider initial evacuation for 800 meters (1/2 mile) in all directions.

EMERGENCY RESPONSE

FIRE

- Use extinguishing agent suitable for type of surrounding fire.

Small Fire

- Dry chemical or CO_2.

Large Fire

- Water spray, fog or regular foam.
- Move containers from fire area if you can do it without risk.
- Damaged cylinders should be handled only by specialists.

Fire involving Tanks

- Fight fire from maximum distance or use unmanned hose holders or monitor nozzles.
- Cool containers with flooding quantities of water until well after fire is out.
- Do not direct water at source of leak or safety devices; icing may occur.
- Withdraw immediately in case of rising sound from venting safety devices or discoloration of tank.
- ALWAYS stay away from tanks engulfed in fire.
- For massive fire, use unmanned hose holders or monitor nozzles; if this is impossible, withdraw from area and let fire burn.

SPILL OR LEAK

- Keep combustibles (wood, paper, oil, etc.) away from spilled material.
- Do not touch or walk through spilled material.
- Stop leak if you can do it without risk.
- If possible, turn leaking containers so that gas escapes rather than liquid.
- Do not direct water at spill or source of leak.
- Use water spray to reduce vapors or divert vapor cloud drift. Avoid allowing water runoff to contact spilled material.
- Prevent entry into waterways, sewers, basements or confined areas.
- Allow substance to evaporate.
- Isolate area until gas has dispersed.

CAUTION: When in contact with refrigerated/cryogenic liquids, many materials become brittle and are likely to break without warning.

FIRST AID

- Move victim to fresh air.   • Call 911 or emergency medical service.
- Give artificial respiration if victim is not breathing.
- Administer oxygen if breathing is difficult.
- Remove and isolate contaminated clothing and shoes.
- Clothing frozen to the skin should be thawed before being removed.
- In case of contact with liquefied gas, thaw frosted parts with lukewarm water.
- Keep victim warm and quiet.
- Ensure that medical personnel are aware of the material(s) involved and take precautions to protect themselves.

POTENTIAL HAZARDS

HEALTH

- **TOXIC; may be fatal if inhaled or absorbed through skin.**
- Vapors may be irritating.
- Contact with gas or liquefied gas may cause burns, severe injury and/or frostbite.
- Fire will produce irritating, corrosive and/or toxic gases.
- Runoff from fire control may cause pollution.

FIRE OR EXPLOSION

- Some may burn but none ignite readily.
- Vapors from liquefied gas are initially heavier than air and spread along ground.
- Cylinders exposed to fire may vent and release toxic and/or corrosive gas through pressure relief devices.
- Containers may explode when heated.
- Ruptured cylinders may rocket.

PUBLIC SAFETY

- **CALL Emergency Response Telephone Number on Shipping Paper first. If Shipping Paper not available or no answer, refer to appropriate telephone number listed on the inside back cover.**
- As an immediate precautionary measure, isolate spill or leak area for at least 100 meters (330 feet) in all directions.
- Keep unauthorized personnel away.
- Stay upwind.
- Many gases are heavier than air and will spread along ground and collect in low or confined areas (sewers, basements, tanks).
- Keep out of low areas.
- Ventilate closed spaces before entering.

PROTECTIVE CLOTHING

- Wear positive pressure self-contained breathing apparatus (SCBA).
- Wear chemical protective clothing that is specifically recommended by the manufacturer. It may provide little or no thermal protection.
- Structural firefighters' protective clothing provides limited protection in fire situations ONLY; it is not effective in spill situations where direct contact with the substance is possible.

EVACUATION

Spill

- See Table 1 - Initial Isolation and Protective Action Distances for highlighted materials. For non-highlighted materials, increase, in the downwind direction, as necessary, the isolation distance shown under "PUBLIC SAFETY".

Fire

- If tank, rail car or tank truck is involved in a fire, ISOLATE for 800 meters (1/2 mile) in all directions; also, consider initial evacuation for 800 meters (1/2 mile) in all directions.

EMERGENCY RESPONSE

FIRE

Small Fire

- Dry chemical or CO_2.

Large Fire

- Water spray, fog or regular foam.
- Do not get water inside containers.
- Move containers from fire area if you can do it without risk.
- Damaged cylinders should be handled only by specialists.

Fire involving Tanks

- Fight fire from maximum distance or use unmanned hose holders or monitor nozzles.
- Cool containers with flooding quantities of water until well after fire is out.
- Do not direct water at source of leak or safety devices; icing may occur.
- Withdraw immediately in case of rising sound from venting safety devices or discoloration of tank.
- ALWAYS stay away from tanks engulfed in fire.

SPILL OR LEAK

- Fully encapsulating, vapor protective clothing should be worn for spills and leaks with no fire.
- Do not touch or walk through spilled material.
- Stop leak if you can do it without risk.
- If possible, turn leaking containers so that gas escapes rather than liquid.
- Prevent entry into waterways, sewers, basements or confined areas.
- Use water spray to reduce vapors or divert vapor cloud drift. Avoid allowing water runoff to contact spilled material.
- Do not direct water at spill or source of leak.
- Isolate area until gas has dispersed.

FIRST AID

- Move victim to fresh air.   • Call 911 or emergency medical service.
- Give artificial respiration if victim is not breathing.
- **Do not use mouth-to-mouth method if victim ingested or inhaled the substance; give artificial respiration with the aid of a pocket mask equipped with a one-way valve or other proper respiratory medical device.**
- Administer oxygen if breathing is difficult.
- Remove and isolate contaminated clothing and shoes.
- In case of contact with liquefied gas, thaw frosted parts with lukewarm water.
- In case of contact with substance, immediately flush skin or eyes with running water for at least 20 minutes.
- Keep victim warm and quiet.   • Keep victim under observation.
- Effects of contact or inhalation may be delayed.
- Ensure that medical personnel are aware of the material(s) involved and take precautions to protect themselves.

POTENTIAL HAZARDS

HEALTH
- **TOXIC; may be fatal if inhaled or absorbed through skin.**
- Fire will produce irritating, corrosive and/or toxic gases.
- Contact with gas or liquefied gas may cause burns, severe injury and/or frostbite.
- Runoff from fire control may cause pollution.

FIRE OR EXPLOSION
- Substance does not burn but will support combustion.
- Vapors from liquefied gas are initially heavier than air and spread along ground.
- These are strong oxidizers and will react vigorously or explosively with many materials including fuels.
- May ignite combustibles (wood, paper, oil, clothing, etc.).
- Some will react violently with air, moist air and/or water.
- Cylinders exposed to fire may vent and release toxic and/or corrosive gas through pressure relief devices.
- Containers may explode when heated.
- Ruptured cylinders may rocket.

PUBLIC SAFETY

- **CALL Emergency Response Telephone Number on Shipping Paper first. If Shipping Paper not available or no answer, refer to appropriate telephone number listed on the inside back cover.**
- As an immediate precautionary measure, isolate spill or leak area for at least 100 meters (330 feet) in all directions.
- Keep unauthorized personnel away.
- Stay upwind.
- Many gases are heavier than air and will spread along ground and collect in low or confined areas (sewers, basements, tanks).
- Keep out of low areas.
- Ventilate closed spaces before entering.

PROTECTIVE CLOTHING
- Wear positive pressure self-contained breathing apparatus (SCBA).
- Wear chemical protective clothing that is specifically recommended by the manufacturer. It may provide little or no thermal protection.
- Structural firefighters' protective clothing provides limited protection in fire situations ONLY; it is not effective in spill situations where direct contact with the substance is possible.

EVACUATION
Spill
- See Table 1 - Initial Isolation and Protective Action Distances.

Fire
- If tank, rail car or tank truck is involved in a fire, ISOLATE for 800 meters (1/2 mile) in all directions; also, consider initial evacuation for 800 meters (1/2 mile) in all directions.

EMERGENCY RESPONSE

FIRE

Small Fire: Water only; no dry chemical, CO_2 or Halon®.

- Contain fire and let burn. If fire must be fought, water spray or fog is recommended.
- Do not get water inside containers.
- Move containers from fire area if you can do it without risk.
- Damaged cylinders should be handled only by specialists.

Fire involving Tanks

- Fight fire from maximum distance or use unmanned hose holders or monitor nozzles.
- Cool containers with flooding quantities of water until well after fire is out.
- Do not direct water at source of leak or safety devices; icing may occur.
- Withdraw immediately in case of rising sound from venting safety devices or discoloration of tank.
- ALWAYS stay away from tanks engulfed in fire.
- For massive fire, use unmanned hose holders or monitor nozzles; if this is impossible, withdraw from area and let fire burn.

SPILL OR LEAK

- Fully encapsulating, vapor protective clothing should be worn for spills and leaks with no fire.
- Do not touch or walk through spilled material.
- Keep combustibles (wood, paper, oil, etc.) away from spilled material.
- Stop leak if you can do it without risk.
- Use water spray to reduce vapors or divert vapor cloud drift. Avoid allowing water runoff to contact spilled material.
- Do not direct water at spill or source of leak.
- If possible, turn leaking containers so that gas escapes rather than liquid.
- Prevent entry into waterways, sewers, basements or confined areas.
- Isolate area until gas has dispersed.
- Ventilate the area.

FIRST AID

- Move victim to fresh air. • Call 911 or emergency medical service.
- Give artificial respiration if victim is not breathing.
- **Do not use mouth-to-mouth method if victim ingested or inhaled the substance; give artificial respiration with the aid of a pocket mask equipped with a one-way valve or other proper respiratory medical device.**
- Administer oxygen if breathing is difficult.
- Clothing frozen to the skin should be thawed before being removed.
- Remove and isolate contaminated clothing and shoes.
- In case of contact with substance, immediately flush skin or eyes with running water for at least 20 minutes.
- Keep victim warm and quiet. • Keep victim under observation.
- Effects of contact or inhalation may be delayed.
- Ensure that medical personnel are aware of the material(s) involved and take precautions to protect themselves.

POTENTIAL HAZARDS

HEALTH

- **TOXIC; may be fatal if inhaled, ingested or absorbed through skin.**
- Vapors are extremely irritating and corrosive.
- Contact with gas or liquefied gas may cause burns, severe injury and/or frostbite.
- Fire will produce irritating, corrosive and/or toxic gases.
- Runoff from fire control may cause pollution.

FIRE OR EXPLOSION

- Some may burn but none ignite readily.
- Vapors from liquefied gas are initially heavier than air and spread along ground.
- Some of these materials may react violently with water.
- Cylinders exposed to fire may vent and release toxic and/or corrosive gas through pressure relief devices.
- Containers may explode when heated.
- Ruptured cylinders may rocket.

PUBLIC SAFETY

- **CALL Emergency Response Telephone Number on Shipping Paper first. If Shipping Paper not available or no answer, refer to appropriate telephone number listed on the inside back cover.**
- As an immediate precautionary measure, isolate spill or leak area for at least 100 meters (330 feet) in all directions.
- Keep unauthorized personnel away.
- Stay upwind.
- Many gases are heavier than air and will spread along ground and collect in low or confined areas (sewers, basements, tanks).
- Keep out of low areas.
- Ventilate closed spaces before entering.

PROTECTIVE CLOTHING

- Wear positive pressure self-contained breathing apparatus (SCBA).
- Wear chemical protective clothing that is specifically recommended by the manufacturer. It may provide little or no thermal protection.
- Structural firefighters' protective clothing provides limited protection in fire situations ONLY; it is not effective in spill situations where direct contact with the substance is possible.

EVACUATION

Spill

- See Table 1 - Initial Isolation and Protective Action Distances for highlighted materials. For non-highlighted materials, increase, in the downwind direction, as necessary, the isolation distance shown under "PUBLIC SAFETY".

Fire

- If tank, rail car or tank truck is involved in a fire, ISOLATE for 1600 meters (1 mile) in all directions; also, consider initial evacuation for 1600 meters (1 mile) in all directions.

EMERGENCY RESPONSE

FIRE

Small Fire
- Dry chemical or CO_2.

Large Fire
- Water spray, fog or regular foam.
- Move containers from fire area if you can do it without risk.
- Do not get water inside containers.
- Damaged cylinders should be handled only by specialists.

Fire involving Tanks
- Fight fire from maximum distance or use unmanned hose holders or monitor nozzles.
- Cool containers with flooding quantities of water until well after fire is out.
- Do not direct water at source of leak or safety devices; icing may occur.
- Withdraw immediately in case of rising sound from venting safety devices or discoloration of tank.   • ALWAYS stay away from tanks engulfed in fire.

SPILL OR LEAK

- Fully encapsulating, vapor protective clothing should be worn for spills and leaks with no fire.
- Do not touch or walk through spilled material.
- Stop leak if you can do it without risk.
- If possible, turn leaking containers so that gas escapes rather than liquid.
- Prevent entry into waterways, sewers, basements or confined areas.
- Do not direct water at spill or source of leak.
- Use water spray to reduce vapors or divert vapor cloud drift. Avoid allowing water runoff to contact spilled material.   • Isolate area until gas has dispersed.

FIRST AID

- Move victim to fresh air.   • Call 911 or emergency medical service.
- Give artificial respiration if victim is not breathing.
- **Do not use mouth-to-mouth method if victim ingested or inhaled the substance; give artificial respiration with the aid of a pocket mask equipped with a one-way valve or other proper respiratory medical device.**
- Administer oxygen if breathing is difficult.
- Remove and isolate contaminated clothing and shoes.
- In case of contact with liquefied gas, thaw frosted parts with lukewarm water.
- In case of contact with substance, immediately flush skin or eyes with running water for at least 20 minutes.
- **In case of contact with Hydrogen fluoride, anhydrous (UN1052)**, flush skin and eyes with water for 5 minutes; then, for skin exposures rub on a calcium/jelly combination; for eyes flush with a water/calcium solution for 15 minutes.
- Keep victim warm and quiet.   • Keep victim under observation.
- Effects of contact or inhalation may be delayed.
- Ensure that medical personnel are aware of the material(s) involved and take precautions to protect themselves.

POTENTIAL HAZARDS

FIRE OR EXPLOSION
- Some may burn but none ignite readily.
- Containers may explode when heated.
- Ruptured cylinders may rocket.

HEALTH
- Vapors may cause dizziness or asphyxiation without warning.
- Vapors from liquefied gas are initially heavier than air and spread along ground.
- Contact with gas or liquefied gas may cause burns, severe injury and/or frostbite.
- Fire may produce irritating, corrosive and/or toxic gases.

PUBLIC SAFETY

- **CALL Emergency Response Telephone Number on Shipping Paper first. If Shipping Paper not available or no answer, refer to appropriate telephone number listed on the inside back cover.**
- As an immediate precautionary measure, isolate spill or leak area for at least 100 meters (330 feet) in all directions.
- Keep unauthorized personnel away.
- Stay upwind.
- Many gases are heavier than air and will spread along ground and collect in low or confined areas (sewers, basements, tanks).
- Keep out of low areas.
- Ventilate closed spaces before entering.

PROTECTIVE CLOTHING
- Wear positive pressure self-contained breathing apparatus (SCBA).
- Wear chemical protective clothing that is specifically recommended by the manufacturer. It may provide little or no thermal protection.
- Structural firefighters' protective clothing will only provide limited protection.

EVACUATION
Large Spill
- Consider initial downwind evacuation for at least 500 meters (1/3 mile).

Fire
- If tank, rail car or tank truck is involved in a fire, ISOLATE for 800 meters (1/2 mile) in all directions; also, consider initial evacuation for 800 meters (1/2 mile) in all directions.

EMERGENCY RESPONSE

FIRE
- Use extinguishing agent suitable for type of surrounding fire.

Small Fire
- Dry chemical or CO_2.

Large Fire
- Water spray, fog or regular foam.
- Move containers from fire area if you can do it without risk.
- Damaged cylinders should be handled only by specialists.

Fire involving Tanks
- Fight fire from maximum distance or use unmanned hose holders or monitor nozzles.
- Cool containers with flooding quantities of water until well after fire is out.
- Do not direct water at source of leak or safety devices; icing may occur.
- Withdraw immediately in case of rising sound from venting safety devices or discoloration of tank.
- ALWAYS stay away from tanks engulfed in fire.
- Some of these materials, if spilled, may evaporate leaving a flammable residue.

SPILL OR LEAK
- Do not touch or walk through spilled material.
- Stop leak if you can do it without risk.
- Do not direct water at spill or source of leak.
- Use water spray to reduce vapors or divert vapor cloud drift. Avoid allowing water runoff to contact spilled material.
- If possible, turn leaking containers so that gas escapes rather than liquid.
- Prevent entry into waterways, sewers, basements or confined areas.
- Allow substance to evaporate.
- Ventilate the area.

FIRST AID
- Move victim to fresh air.   • Call 911 or emergency medical service.
- Give artificial respiration if victim is not breathing.
- Administer oxygen if breathing is difficult.
- Remove and isolate contaminated clothing and shoes.
- In case of contact with liquefied gas, thaw frosted parts with lukewarm water.
- Keep victim warm and quiet.
- Ensure that medical personnel are aware of the material(s) involved and take precautions to protect themselves.

POTENTIAL HAZARDS

FIRE OR EXPLOSION

- **HIGHLY FLAMMABLE: Will be easily ignited by heat, sparks or flames.**
- Vapors may form explosive mixtures with air.
- Vapors may travel to source of ignition and flash back.
- Most vapors are heavier than air. They will spread along ground and collect in low or confined areas (sewers, basements, tanks).
- Vapor explosion hazard indoors, outdoors or in sewers.
- Those substances designated with a **"P"** may polymerize explosively when heated or involved in a fire.
- Runoff to sewer may create fire or explosion hazard.
- Containers may explode when heated.
- Many liquids are lighter than water.

HEALTH

- Inhalation or contact with material may irritate or burn skin and eyes.
- Fire may produce irritating, corrosive and/or toxic gases.
- Vapors may cause dizziness or suffocation.
- Runoff from fire control may cause pollution.

PUBLIC SAFETY

- **CALL Emergency Response Telephone Number on Shipping Paper first. If Shipping Paper not available or no answer, refer to appropriate telephone number listed on the inside back cover.**
- As an immediate precautionary measure, isolate spill or leak area for at least 50 meters (150 feet) in all directions.
- Keep unauthorized personnel away.
- Stay upwind.
- Keep out of low areas.
- Ventilate closed spaces before entering.

PROTECTIVE CLOTHING

- Wear positive pressure self-contained breathing apparatus (SCBA).
- Structural firefighters' protective clothing will only provide limited protection.

EVACUATION

Large Spill

- Consider initial downwind evacuation for at least 300 meters (1000 feet).

Fire

- If tank, rail car or tank truck is involved in a fire, ISOLATE for 800 meters (1/2 mile) in all directions; also, consider initial evacuation for 800 meters (1/2 mile) in all directions.

EMERGENCY RESPONSE

FIRE

CAUTION: All these products have a very low flash point: Use of water spray when fighting fire may be inefficient.

Small Fire

• Dry chemical, CO_2, water spray or alcohol-resistant foam.

Large Fire

• Water spray, fog or alcohol-resistant foam.
• Use water spray or fog; do not use straight streams.
• Move containers from fire area if you can do it without risk.

Fire involving Tanks or Car/Trailer Loads

• Fight fire from maximum distance or use unmanned hose holders or monitor nozzles.
• Cool containers with flooding quantities of water until well after fire is out.
• Withdraw immediately in case of rising sound from venting safety devices or discoloration of tank.
• ALWAYS stay away from tanks engulfed in fire.
• For massive fire, use unmanned hose holders or monitor nozzles; if this is impossible, withdraw from area and let fire burn.

SPILL OR LEAK

• ELIMINATE all ignition sources (no smoking, flares, sparks or flames in immediate area).
• All equipment used when handling the product must be grounded.
• Do not touch or walk through spilled material.
• Stop leak if you can do it without risk.
• Prevent entry into waterways, sewers, basements or confined areas.
• A vapor suppressing foam may be used to reduce vapors.
• Absorb or cover with dry earth, sand or other non-combustible material and transfer to containers.
• Use clean non-sparking tools to collect absorbed material.

Large Spill

• Dike far ahead of liquid spill for later disposal.
• Water spray may reduce vapor; but may not prevent ignition in closed spaces.

FIRST AID

• Move victim to fresh air.   • Call 911 or emergency medical service.
• Give artificial respiration if victim is not breathing.
• Administer oxygen if breathing is difficult.
• Remove and isolate contaminated clothing and shoes.
• In case of contact with substance, immediately flush skin or eyes with running water for at least 20 minutes.   • Wash skin with soap and water.
• In case of burns, immediately cool affected skin for as long as possible with cold water. Do not remove clothing if adhering to skin.
• Keep victim warm and quiet.
• Ensure that medical personnel are aware of the material(s) involved and take precautions to protect themselves.

POTENTIAL HAZARDS

FIRE OR EXPLOSION

- **HIGHLY FLAMMABLE: Will be easily ignited by heat, sparks or flames.**
- Vapors may form explosive mixtures with air.
- Vapors may travel to source of ignition and flash back.
- Most vapors are heavier than air. They will spread along ground and collect in low or confined areas (sewers, basements, tanks).
- Vapor explosion hazard indoors, outdoors or in sewers.
- Those substances designated with a **"P"** may polymerize explosively when heated or involved in a fire.
- Runoff to sewer may create fire or explosion hazard.
- Containers may explode when heated.
- Many liquids are lighter than water.
- Substance may be transported hot.
- **If molten aluminum is involved, refer to GUIDE 169.**

HEALTH

- Inhalation or contact with material may irritate or burn skin and eyes.
- Fire may produce irritating, corrosive and/or toxic gases.
- Vapors may cause dizziness or suffocation.
- Runoff from fire control or dilution water may cause pollution.

PUBLIC SAFETY

- **CALL Emergency Response Telephone Number on Shipping Paper first. If Shipping Paper not available or no answer, refer to appropriate telephone number listed on the inside back cover.**
- As an immediate precautionary measure, isolate spill or leak area for at least 50 meters (150 feet) in all directions.
- Keep unauthorized personnel away.
- Stay upwind.
- Keep out of low areas.
- Ventilate closed spaces before entering.

PROTECTIVE CLOTHING

- Wear positive pressure self-contained breathing apparatus (SCBA).
- Structural firefighters' protective clothing will only provide limited protection.

EVACUATION

Large Spill

- Consider initial downwind evacuation for at least 300 meters (1000 feet).

Fire

- If tank, rail car or tank truck is involved in a fire, ISOLATE for 800 meters (1/2 mile) in all directions; also, consider initial evacuation for 800 meters (1/2 mile) in all directions.

EMERGENCY RESPONSE

FIRE

CAUTION: All these products have a very low flash point: Use of water spray when fighting fire may be inefficient.

CAUTION: For mixtures containing alcohol or polar solvent, alcohol-resistant foam may be more effective.

Small Fire

- Dry chemical, CO_2, water spray or regular foam.

Large Fire

- Water spray, fog or regular foam.
- Use water spray or fog; do not use straight streams.
- Move containers from fire area if you can do it without risk.

Fire involving Tanks or Car/Trailer Loads

- Fight fire from maximum distance or use unmanned hose holders or monitor nozzles.
- Cool containers with flooding quantities of water until well after fire is out.
- Withdraw immediately in case of rising sound from venting safety devices or discoloration of tank.
- ALWAYS stay away from tanks engulfed in fire.
- For massive fire, use unmanned hose holders or monitor nozzles; if this is impossible, withdraw from area and let fire burn.

SPILL OR LEAK

- ELIMINATE all ignition sources (no smoking, flares, sparks or flames in immediate area).
- All equipment used when handling the product must be grounded.
- Do not touch or walk through spilled material. • Stop leak if you can do it without risk.
- Prevent entry into waterways, sewers, basements or confined areas.
- A vapor suppressing foam may be used to reduce vapors.
- Absorb or cover with dry earth, sand or other non-combustible material and transfer to containers. • Use clean non-sparking tools to collect absorbed material.

Large Spill

- Dike far ahead of liquid spill for later disposal.
- Water spray may reduce vapor; but may not prevent ignition in closed spaces.

FIRST AID

- Move victim to fresh air. • Call 911 or emergency medical service.
- Give artificial respiration if victim is not breathing.
- Administer oxygen if breathing is difficult.
- Remove and isolate contaminated clothing and shoes.
- In case of contact with substance, immediately flush skin or eyes with running water for at least 20 minutes.
- Wash skin with soap and water.
- In case of burns, immediately cool affected skin for as long as possible with cold water. Do not remove clothing if adhering to skin. • Keep victim warm and quiet.
- Ensure that medical personnel are aware of the material(s) involved and take precautions to protect themselves.

POTENTIAL HAZARDS

FIRE OR EXPLOSION

- **HIGHLY FLAMMABLE: Will be easily ignited by heat, sparks or flames.**
- Vapors may form explosive mixtures with air.
- Vapors may travel to source of ignition and flash back.
- Most vapors are heavier than air. They will spread along ground and collect in low or confined areas (sewers, basements, tanks).
- Vapor explosion hazard indoors, outdoors or in sewers.
- Those substances designated with a **"P"** may polymerize explosively when heated or involved in a fire.
- Runoff to sewer may create fire or explosion hazard.
- Containers may explode when heated.
- Many liquids are lighter than water.

HEALTH

- May cause toxic effects if inhaled or absorbed through skin.
- Inhalation or contact with material may irritate or burn skin and eyes.
- Fire will produce irritating, corrosive and/or toxic gases.
- Vapors may cause dizziness or suffocation.
- Runoff from fire control or dilution water may cause pollution.

PUBLIC SAFETY

- **CALL Emergency Response Telephone Number on Shipping Paper first. If Shipping Paper not available or no answer, refer to appropriate telephone number listed on the inside back cover.**
- As an immediate precautionary measure, isolate spill or leak area for at least 50 meters (150 feet) in all directions.
- Keep unauthorized personnel away.
- Stay upwind.
- Keep out of low areas.
- Ventilate closed spaces before entering.

PROTECTIVE CLOTHING

- Wear positive pressure self-contained breathing apparatus (SCBA).
- Structural firefighters' protective clothing will only provide limited protection.

EVACUATION

Large Spill

- Consider initial downwind evacuation for at least 300 meters (1000 feet).

Fire

- If tank, rail car or tank truck is involved in a fire, ISOLATE for 800 meters (1/2 mile) in all directions; also, consider initial evacuation for 800 meters (1/2 mile) in all directions.

EMERGENCY RESPONSE

FIRE

CAUTION: All these products have a very low flash point: Use of water spray when fighting fire may be inefficient.

Small Fire • Dry chemical, CO_2, water spray or alcohol-resistant foam.

- **Do not use dry chemical extinguishers to control fires involving nitromethane or nitroethane.**

Large Fire

- Water spray, fog or alcohol-resistant foam.
- **Do not use straight streams.**
- Move containers from fire area if you can do it without risk.

Fire involving Tanks or Car/Trailer Loads

- Fight fire from maximum distance or use unmanned hose holders or monitor nozzles.
- Cool containers with flooding quantities of water until well after fire is out.
- Withdraw immediately in case of rising sound from venting safety devices or discoloration of tank.
- ALWAYS stay away from tanks engulfed in fire.
- For massive fire, use unmanned hose holders or monitor nozzles; if this is impossible, withdraw from area and let fire burn.

SPILL OR LEAK

- ELIMINATE all ignition sources (no smoking, flares, sparks or flames in immediate area).
- All equipment used when handling the product must be grounded.
- Do not touch or walk through spilled material. • Stop leak if you can do it without risk.
- Prevent entry into waterways, sewers, basements or confined areas.
- A vapor suppressing foam may be used to reduce vapors.
- Absorb or cover with dry earth, sand or other non-combustible material and transfer to containers.
- Use clean non-sparking tools to collect absorbed material.

Large Spill • Dike far ahead of liquid spill for later disposal.

- Water spray may reduce vapor; but may not prevent ignition in closed spaces.

FIRST AID

- Move victim to fresh air. • Call 911 or emergency medical service.
- Give artificial respiration if victim is not breathing.
- Administer oxygen if breathing is difficult.
- Remove and isolate contaminated clothing and shoes.
- In case of contact with substance, immediately flush skin or eyes with running water for at least 20 minutes.
- Wash skin with soap and water.
- In case of burns, immediately cool affected skin for as long as possible with cold water. Do not remove clothing if adhering to skin. • Keep victim warm and quiet.
- Effects of exposure (inhalation, ingestion or skin contact) to substance may be delayed.
- Ensure that medical personnel are aware of the material(s) involved and take precautions to protect themselves.

POTENTIAL HAZARDS

FIRE OR EXPLOSION

- **HIGHLY FLAMMABLE: Will be easily ignited by heat, sparks or flames.**
- Vapors may form explosive mixtures with air.
- Vapors may travel to source of ignition and flash back.
- Most vapors are heavier than air. They will spread along ground and collect in low or confined areas (sewers, basements, tanks).
- Vapor explosion hazard indoors, outdoors or in sewers.
- Those substances designated with a **"P"** may polymerize explosively when heated or involved in a fire.
- Runoff to sewer may create fire or explosion hazard.
- Containers may explode when heated.
- Many liquids are lighter than water.

HEALTH

- May cause toxic effects if inhaled or absorbed through skin.
- Inhalation or contact with material may irritate or burn skin and eyes.
- Fire will produce irritating, corrosive and/or toxic gases.
- Vapors may cause dizziness or suffocation.
- Runoff from fire control or dilution water may cause pollution.

PUBLIC SAFETY

- **CALL Emergency Response Telephone Number on Shipping Paper first. If Shipping Paper not available or no answer, refer to appropriate telephone number listed on the inside back cover.**
- As an immediate precautionary measure, isolate spill or leak area for at least 50 meters (150 feet) in all directions.
- Keep unauthorized personnel away.
- Stay upwind.
- Keep out of low areas.
- Ventilate closed spaces before entering.

PROTECTIVE CLOTHING

- Wear positive pressure self-contained breathing apparatus (SCBA).
- Structural firefighters' protective clothing will only provide limited protection.

EVACUATION

Large Spill

- Consider initial downwind evacuation for at least 300 meters (1000 feet).

Fire

- If tank, rail car or tank truck is involved in a fire, ISOLATE for 800 meters (1/2 mile) in all directions; also, consider initial evacuation for 800 meters (1/2 mile) in all directions.

EMERGENCY RESPONSE

FIRE

CAUTION: All these products have a very low flash point: Use of water spray when fighting fire may be inefficient.

Small Fire

• Dry chemical, CO_2, water spray or regular foam.

Large Fire

• Water spray, fog or regular foam.
• **Do not use straight streams.**
• Move containers from fire area if you can do it without risk.

Fire involving Tanks or Car/Trailer Loads

• Fight fire from maximum distance or use unmanned hose holders or monitor nozzles.
• Cool containers with flooding quantities of water until well after fire is out.
• Withdraw immediately in case of rising sound from venting safety devices or discoloration of tank.
• ALWAYS stay away from tanks engulfed in fire.
• For massive fire, use unmanned hose holders or monitor nozzles; if this is impossible, withdraw from area and let fire burn.

SPILL OR LEAK

• ELIMINATE all ignition sources (no smoking, flares, sparks or flames in immediate area).
• All equipment used when handling the product must be grounded.
• Do not touch or walk through spilled material.
• Stop leak if you can do it without risk.
• Prevent entry into waterways, sewers, basements or confined areas.
• A vapor suppressing foam may be used to reduce vapors.
• Absorb or cover with dry earth, sand or other non-combustible material and transfer to containers.
• Use clean non-sparking tools to collect absorbed material.

Large Spill • Dike far ahead of liquid spill for later disposal.

• Water spray may reduce vapor; but may not prevent ignition in closed spaces.

FIRST AID

• Move victim to fresh air.   • Call 911 or emergency medical service.
• Give artificial respiration if victim is not breathing.
• Administer oxygen if breathing is difficult.
• Remove and isolate contaminated clothing and shoes.
• In case of contact with substance, immediately flush skin or eyes with running water for at least 20 minutes.
• Wash skin with soap and water.
• In case of burns, immediately cool affected skin for as long as possible with cold water. Do not remove clothing if adhering to skin.   • Keep victim warm and quiet.
• Effects of exposure (inhalation, ingestion or skin contact) to substance may be delayed.
• Ensure that medical personnel are aware of the material(s) involved and take precautions to protect themselves.

POTENTIAL HAZARDS

HEALTH

- **TOXIC; may be fatal if inhaled, ingested or absorbed through skin.**
- Inhalation or contact with some of these materials will irritate or burn skin and eyes.
- Fire will produce irritating, corrosive and/or toxic gases.
- Vapors may cause dizziness or suffocation.
- Runoff from fire control or dilution water may cause pollution.

FIRE OR EXPLOSION

- **HIGHLY FLAMMABLE: Will be easily ignited by heat, sparks or flames.**
- Vapors may form explosive mixtures with air.
- Vapors may travel to source of ignition and flash back.
- Most vapors are heavier than air. They will spread along ground and collect in low or confined areas (sewers, basements, tanks).
- Vapor explosion and poison hazard indoors, outdoors or in sewers.
- Those substances designated with a **"P"** may polymerize explosively when heated or involved in a fire.
- Runoff to sewer may create fire or explosion hazard.
- Containers may explode when heated.
- Many liquids are lighter than water.

PUBLIC SAFETY

- **CALL Emergency Response Telephone Number on Shipping Paper first. If Shipping Paper not available or no answer, refer to appropriate telephone number listed on the inside back cover.**
- As an immediate precautionary measure, isolate spill or leak area for at least 50 meters (150 feet) in all directions.
- Keep unauthorized personnel away.
- Stay upwind.   • Keep out of low areas.
- Ventilate closed spaces before entering.

PROTECTIVE CLOTHING

- Wear positive pressure self-contained breathing apparatus (SCBA).
- Wear chemical protective clothing that is specifically recommended by the manufacturer. It may provide little or no thermal protection.
- Structural firefighters' protective clothing provides limited protection in fire situations ONLY; it is not effective in spill situations where direct contact with the substance is possible.

EVACUATION

Spill

- See Table 1 - Initial Isolation and Protective Action Distances for highlighted materials. For non-highlighted materials, increase, in the downwind direction, as necessary, the isolation distance shown under "PUBLIC SAFETY".

Fire

- If tank, rail car or tank truck is involved in a fire, ISOLATE for 800 meters (1/2 mile) in all directions; also, consider initial evacuation for 800 meters (1/2 mile) in all directions.

EMERGENCY RESPONSE

FIRE
CAUTION: All these products have a very low flash point: Use of water spray when fighting fire may be inefficient.
Small Fire • Dry chemical, CO_2, water spray or alcohol-resistant foam.
Large Fire
- Water spray, fog or alcohol-resistant foam.
- Move containers from fire area if you can do it without risk.
- Dike fire-control water for later disposal; do not scatter the material.
- Use water spray or fog; do not use straight streams.
Fire involving Tanks or Car/Trailer Loads
- Fight fire from maximum distance or use unmanned hose holders or monitor nozzles.
- Cool containers with flooding quantities of water until well after fire is out.
- Withdraw immediately in case of rising sound from venting safety devices or discoloration of tank.
- ALWAYS stay away from tanks engulfed in fire.
- For massive fire, use unmanned hose holders or monitor nozzles; if this is impossible, withdraw from area and let fire burn.

SPILL OR LEAK
- Fully encapsulating, vapor protective clothing should be worn for spills and leaks with no fire.
- ELIMINATE all ignition sources (no smoking, flares, sparks or flames in immediate area).
- All equipment used when handling the product must be grounded.
- Do not touch or walk through spilled material. • Stop leak if you can do it without risk.
- Prevent entry into waterways, sewers, basements or confined areas.
- A vapor suppressing foam may be used to reduce vapors.
Small Spill • Absorb with earth, sand or other non-combustible material and transfer to containers for later disposal.
- Use clean non-sparking tools to collect absorbed material.
Large Spill • Dike far ahead of liquid spill for later disposal.
- Water spray may reduce vapor; but may not prevent ignition in closed spaces.

FIRST AID
- Move victim to fresh air. • Call 911 or emergency medical service.
- Give artificial respiration if victim is not breathing.
- **Do not use mouth-to-mouth method if victim ingested or inhaled the substance; give artificial respiration with the aid of a pocket mask equipped with a one-way valve or other proper respiratory medical device.**
- Administer oxygen if breathing is difficult.
- Remove and isolate contaminated clothing and shoes.
- In case of contact with substance, immediately flush skin or eyes with running water for at least 20 minutes.
- Wash skin with soap and water.
- In case of burns, immediately cool affected skin for as long as possible with cold water. Do not remove clothing if adhering to skin. • Keep victim warm and quiet.
- Effects of exposure (inhalation, ingestion or skin contact) to substance may be delayed.
- Ensure that medical personnel are aware of the material(s) involved and take precautions to protect themselves.

POTENTIAL HAZARDS

FIRE OR EXPLOSION
- Flammable/combustible material.
- May be ignited by heat, sparks or flames.
- Vapors may form explosive mixtures with air.
- Vapors may travel to source of ignition and flash back.
- Most vapors are heavier than air. They will spread along ground and collect in low or confined areas (sewers, basements, tanks).
- Vapor explosion hazard indoors, outdoors or in sewers.
- Those substances designated with a **"P"** may polymerize explosively when heated or involved in a fire.
- Runoff to sewer may create fire or explosion hazard.
- Containers may explode when heated.
- Many liquids are lighter than water.

HEALTH
- May cause toxic effects if inhaled or ingested/swallowed.
- Contact with substance may cause severe burns to skin and eyes.
- Fire will produce irritating, corrosive and/or toxic gases.
- Vapors may cause dizziness or suffocation.
- Runoff from fire control or dilution water may cause pollution.

PUBLIC SAFETY

- **CALL Emergency Response Telephone Number on Shipping Paper first. If Shipping Paper not available or no answer, refer to appropriate telephone number listed on the inside back cover.**
- As an immediate precautionary measure, isolate spill or leak area for at least 50 meters (150 feet) in all directions.
- Keep unauthorized personnel away.
- Stay upwind.
- Keep out of low areas.
- Ventilate closed spaces before entering.

PROTECTIVE CLOTHING
- Wear positive pressure self-contained breathing apparatus (SCBA).
- Wear chemical protective clothing that is specifically recommended by the manufacturer. It may provide little or no thermal protection.
- Structural firefighters' protective clothing provides limited protection in fire situations ONLY; it is not effective in spill situations where direct contact with the substance is possible.

EVACUATION
Large Spill
- See Table 1 - Initial Isolation and Protective Action Distances for highlighted materials. For non-highlighted materials, increase, in the downwind direction, as necessary, the isolation distance shown under "PUBLIC SAFETY".
Fire
- If tank, rail car or tank truck is involved in a fire, ISOLATE for 800 meters (1/2 mile) in all directions; also, consider initial evacuation for 800 meters (1/2 mile) in all directions.

EMERGENCY RESPONSE

FIRE
- **Some of these materials may react violently with water.**

Small Fire • Dry chemical, CO_2, water spray or alcohol-resistant foam.

Large Fire • Water spray, fog or alcohol-resistant foam.
- Move containers from fire area if you can do it without risk.
- Dike fire-control water for later disposal; do not scatter the material.
- Do not get water inside containers.

Fire involving Tanks or Car/Trailer Loads
- Fight fire from maximum distance or use unmanned hose holders or monitor nozzles.
- Cool containers with flooding quantities of water until well after fire is out.
- Withdraw immediately in case of rising sound from venting safety devices or discoloration of tank.
- ALWAYS stay away from tanks engulfed in fire.
- For massive fire, use unmanned hose holders or monitor nozzles; if this is impossible, withdraw from area and let fire burn.

SPILL OR LEAK
- Fully encapsulating, vapor protective clothing should be worn for spills and leaks with no fire.
- ELIMINATE all ignition sources (no smoking, flares, sparks or flames in immediate area).
- All equipment used when handling the product must be grounded.
- Do not touch or walk through spilled material. • Stop leak if you can do it without risk.
- Prevent entry into waterways, sewers, basements or confined areas.
- A vapor suppressing foam may be used to reduce vapors.
- Absorb with earth, sand or other non-combustible material and transfer to containers (except for Hydrazine).
- Use clean non-sparking tools to collect absorbed material.

Large Spill • Dike far ahead of liquid spill for later disposal.
- Water spray may reduce vapor; but may not prevent ignition in closed spaces.

FIRST AID
- Move victim to fresh air. • Call 911 or emergency medical service.
- Give artificial respiration if victim is not breathing.
- **Do not use mouth-to-mouth method if victim ingested or inhaled the substance; give artificial respiration with the aid of a pocket mask equipped with a one-way valve or other proper respiratory medical device.**
- Administer oxygen if breathing is difficult.
- Remove and isolate contaminated clothing and shoes.
- In case of contact with substance, immediately flush skin or eyes with running water for at least 20 minutes.
- In case of burns, immediately cool affected skin for as long as possible with cold water. Do not remove clothing if adhering to skin.
- Keep victim warm and quiet.
- Effects of exposure (inhalation, ingestion or skin contact) to substance may be delayed.
- Ensure that medical personnel are aware of the material(s) involved and take precautions to protect themselves.

GUIDE 133   FLAMMABLE SOLIDS   ERG2008

POTENTIAL HAZARDS

FIRE OR EXPLOSION
- Flammable/combustible material.
- May be ignited by friction, heat, sparks or flames.
- Some may burn rapidly with flare burning effect.
- Powders, dusts, shavings, borings, turnings or cuttings may explode or burn with explosive violence.
- Substance may be transported in a molten form at a temperature that may be above its flash point.
- May re-ignite after fire is extinguished.

HEALTH
- Fire may produce irritating and/or toxic gases.
- Contact may cause burns to skin and eyes.
- Contact with molten substance may cause severe burns to skin and eyes.
- Runoff from fire control may cause pollution.

PUBLIC SAFETY
- **CALL Emergency Response Telephone Number on Shipping Paper first. If Shipping Paper not available or no answer, refer to appropriate telephone number listed on the inside back cover.**
- As an immediate precautionary measure, isolate spill or leak area for at least 25 meters (75 feet) in all directions.
- Keep unauthorized personnel away.
- Stay upwind.
- Keep out of low areas.

PROTECTIVE CLOTHING
- Wear positive pressure self-contained breathing apparatus (SCBA).
- Structural firefighters' protective clothing will only provide limited protection.

EVACUATION
Large Spill
- Consider initial downwind evacuation for at least 100 meters (330 feet).

Fire
- If tank, rail car or tank truck is involved in a fire, ISOLATE for 800 meters (1/2 mile) in all directions; also, consider initial evacuation for 800 meters (1/2 mile) in all directions.

EMERGENCY RESPONSE

FIRE

Small Fire

- Dry chemical, CO_2, sand, earth, water spray or regular foam.

Large Fire

- Water spray, fog or regular foam.
- Move containers from fire area if you can do it without risk.

Fire Involving Metal Pigments or Pastes (e.g. "Aluminum Paste")

- Aluminum Paste fires should be treated as a combustible metal fire. Use DRY sand, graphite powder, dry sodium chloride based extinguishers, G-1® or Met-L-X® powder. Also, see GUIDE 170.

Fire involving Tanks or Car/Trailer Loads

- Cool containers with flooding quantities of water until well after fire is out.
- For massive fire, use unmanned hose holders or monitor nozzles; if this is impossible, withdraw from area and let fire burn.
- Withdraw immediately in case of rising sound from venting safety devices or discoloration of tank.
- ALWAYS stay away from tanks engulfed in fire.

SPILL OR LEAK

- ELIMINATE all ignition sources (no smoking, flares, sparks or flames in immediate area).
- Do not touch or walk through spilled material.

Small Dry Spill

- With clean shovel place material into clean, dry container and cover loosely; move containers from spill area.

Large Spill

- Wet down with water and dike for later disposal.
- Prevent entry into waterways, sewers, basements or confined areas.

FIRST AID

- Move victim to fresh air.   • Call 911 or emergency medical service.
- Give artificial respiration if victim is not breathing.
- Administer oxygen if breathing is difficult.
- Remove and isolate contaminated clothing and shoes.
- In case of contact with substance, immediately flush skin or eyes with running water for at least 20 minutes.
- Removal of solidified molten material from skin requires medical assistance.
- Keep victim warm and quiet.
- Ensure that medical personnel are aware of the material(s) involved and take precautions to protect themselves.

POTENTIAL HAZARDS

FIRE OR EXPLOSION

- Flammable/combustible material.
- May be ignited by heat, sparks or flames.
- When heated, vapors may form explosive mixtures with air: indoors, outdoors and sewers explosion hazards.
- Contact with metals may evolve flammable hydrogen gas.
- Containers may explode when heated.

HEALTH

- **TOXIC**; inhalation, ingestion or skin contact with material may cause severe injury or death.
- Fire will produce irritating, corrosive and/or toxic gases.
- Runoff from fire control or dilution water may be corrosive and/or toxic and cause pollution.

PUBLIC SAFETY

- **CALL Emergency Response Telephone Number on Shipping Paper first. If Shipping Paper not available or no answer, refer to appropriate telephone number listed on the inside back cover.**
- As an immediate precautionary measure, isolate spill or leak area for at least 25 meters (75 feet) in all directions.
- Stay upwind.
- Keep unauthorized personnel away.
- Keep out of low areas.
- Ventilate enclosed areas.

PROTECTIVE CLOTHING

- Wear positive pressure self-contained breathing apparatus (SCBA).
- Wear chemical protective clothing that is specifically recommended by the manufacturer. It may provide little or no thermal protection.
- Structural firefighters' protective clothing provides limited protection in fire situations ONLY; it is not effective in spill situations where direct contact with the substance is possible.

EVACUATION

Large Spill

- Consider initial downwind evacuation for at least 100 meters (330 feet).

Fire

- If tank, rail car or tank truck is involved in a fire, ISOLATE for 800 meters (1/2 mile) in all directions; also, consider initial evacuation for 800 meters (1/2 mile) in all directions.

EMERGENCY RESPONSE

FIRE

Small Fire

- Dry chemical, CO_2, water spray or alcohol-resistant foam.

Large Fire

- Water spray, fog or alcohol-resistant foam.
- Move containers from fire area if you can do it without risk.
- Use water spray or fog; do not use straight streams.
- Do not get water inside containers.
- Dike fire-control water for later disposal; do not scatter the material.

Fire involving Tanks or Car/Trailer Loads

- Fight fire from maximum distance or use unmanned hose holders or monitor nozzles.
- Cool containers with flooding quantities of water until well after fire is out.
- Withdraw immediately in case of rising sound from venting safety devices or discoloration of tank.
- ALWAYS stay away from tanks engulfed in fire.

SPILL OR LEAK

- Fully encapsulating, vapor protective clothing should be worn for spills and leaks with no fire.
- ELIMINATE all ignition sources (no smoking, flares, sparks or flames in immediate area).
- Stop leak if you can do it without risk.
- Do not touch damaged containers or spilled material unless wearing appropriate protective clothing.
- Prevent entry into waterways, sewers, basements or confined areas.
- Use clean non-sparking tools to collect material and place it into loosely covered plastic containers for later disposal.

FIRST AID

- Move victim to fresh air.   • Call 911 or emergency medical service.
- Give artificial respiration if victim is not breathing.
- **Do not use mouth-to-mouth method if victim ingested or inhaled the substance; give artificial respiration with the aid of a pocket mask equipped with a one-way valve or other proper respiratory medical device.**
- Administer oxygen if breathing is difficult.
- Remove and isolate contaminated clothing and shoes.
- In case of contact with substance, immediately flush skin or eyes with running water for at least 20 minutes.
- For minor skin contact, avoid spreading material on unaffected skin.
- Keep victim warm and quiet.
- Effects of exposure (inhalation, ingestion or skin contact) to substance may be delayed.
- Ensure that medical personnel are aware of the material(s) involved and take precautions to protect themselves.

POTENTIAL HAZARDS

FIRE OR EXPLOSION
- Flammable/combustible material.
- May ignite on contact with moist air or moisture.
- May burn rapidly with flare-burning effect.
- Some react vigorously or explosively on contact with water.
- Some may decompose explosively when heated or involved in a fire.
- May re-ignite after fire is extinguished.
- Runoff may create fire or explosion hazard.
- Containers may explode when heated.

HEALTH
- Fire will produce irritating, corrosive and/or toxic gases.
- Inhalation of decomposition products may cause severe injury or death.
- Contact with substance may cause severe burns to skin and eyes.
- Runoff from fire control may cause pollution.

PUBLIC SAFETY

- **CALL Emergency Response Telephone Number on Shipping Paper first. If Shipping Paper not available or no answer, refer to appropriate telephone number listed on the inside back cover.**
- As an immediate precautionary measure, isolate spill or leak area in all directions for at least 50 meters (150 feet) for liquids and at least 25 meters (75 feet) for solids.
- Stay upwind.
- Keep unauthorized personnel away.
- Keep out of low areas.

PROTECTIVE CLOTHING
- Wear positive pressure self-contained breathing apparatus (SCBA).
- Wear chemical protective clothing that is specifically recommended by the manufacturer. It may provide little or no thermal protection.
- Structural firefighters' protective clothing will only provide limited protection.

EVACUATION
Spill
- See Table 1 - Initial Isolation and Protective Action Distances for highlighted materials. For non-highlighted materials, increase, in the downwind direction, as necessary, the isolation distance shown under "PUBLIC SAFETY".

Fire
- If tank, rail car or tank truck is involved in a fire, ISOLATE for 800 meters (1/2 mile) in all directions; also, consider initial evacuation for 800 meters (1/2 mile) in all directions.

EMERGENCY RESPONSE

FIRE

- **DO NOT USE WATER, CO_2 OR FOAM ON MATERIAL ITSELF.**
- Some of these materials may react violently with water.

EXCEPTION: For Xanthates, UN3342 and for Dithionite (Hydrosulfite/ Hydrosulphite) UN1384, UN1923 and UN1929, USE FLOODING AMOUNTS OF WATER for SMALL AND LARGE fires to stop the reaction. Smothering will not work for these materials, they do not need air to burn.

Small Fire

- Dry chemical, soda ash, lime or DRY sand, **EXCEPT for UN1384, UN1923 and UN1929**.

Large Fire

- DRY sand, dry chemical, soda ash or lime, **EXCEPT for UN1384, UN1923 and UN1929**, or withdraw from area and let fire burn.
- Move containers from fire area if you can do it without risk.

Fire involving Tanks or Car/Trailer Loads

- Fight fire from maximum distance or use unmanned hose holders or monitor nozzles.
- Do not get water inside containers or in contact with substance.
- Cool containers with flooding quantities of water until well after fire is out.
- Withdraw immediately in case of rising sound from venting safety devices or discoloration of tank.
- ALWAYS stay away from tanks engulfed in fire.

SPILL OR LEAK

- Fully encapsulating, vapor protective clothing should be worn for spills and leaks with no fire.
- ELIMINATE all ignition sources (no smoking, flares, sparks or flames in immediate area).
- Do not touch or walk through spilled material.   • Stop leak if you can do it without risk.

Small Spill

EXCEPTION: For spills of Xanthates, UN3342 and for Dithionite (Hydrosulfite/ Hydrosulphite), UN1384, UN1923 and UN1929, dissolve in 5 parts water and collect for proper disposal.

- Cover with DRY earth, DRY sand or other non-combustible material followed with plastic sheet to minimize spreading or contact with rain.
- Use clean non-sparking tools to collect material and place it into loosely covered plastic containers for later disposal.
- Prevent entry into waterways, sewers, basements or confined areas.

FIRST AID

- Move victim to fresh air.   • Call 911 or emergency medical service.
- Give artificial respiration if victim is not breathing.
- Administer oxygen if breathing is difficult.
- Remove and isolate contaminated clothing and shoes.
- In case of contact with substance, immediately flush skin or eyes with running water for at least 20 minutes.   • Keep victim warm and quiet.
- Ensure that medical personnel are aware of the material(s) involved and take precautions to protect themselves.

POTENTIAL HAZARDS

FIRE OR EXPLOSION
- Extremely flammable; will ignite itself if exposed to air.
- Burns rapidly, releasing dense, white, irritating fumes.
- Substance may be transported in a molten form.
- May re-ignite after fire is extinguished.
- Corrosive substances in contact with metals may produce flammable hydrogen gas.
- Containers may explode when heated.

HEALTH
- Fire will produce irritating, corrosive and/or toxic gases.
- TOXIC; ingestion of substance or inhalation of decomposition products will cause severe injury or death.
- Contact with substance may cause severe burns to skin and eyes.
- Some effects may be experienced due to skin absorption.
- Runoff from fire control may be corrosive and/or toxic and cause pollution.

PUBLIC SAFETY

- **CALL Emergency Response Telephone Number on Shipping Paper first. If Shipping Paper not available or no answer, refer to appropriate telephone number listed on the inside back cover.**
- As an immediate precautionary measure, isolate spill or leak area in all directions for at least 50 meters (150 feet) for liquids and at least 25 meters (75 feet) for solids.
- Stay upwind.
- Keep unauthorized personnel away.
- Keep out of low areas.

PROTECTIVE CLOTHING
- Wear positive pressure self-contained breathing apparatus (SCBA).
- Wear chemical protective clothing that is specifically recommended by the manufacturer. It may provide little or no thermal protection.
- Structural firefighters' protective clothing provides limited protection in fire situations ONLY; it is not effective in spill situations where direct contact with the substance is possible.
- **For Phosphorus (UN1381): Special aluminized protective clothing should be worn when direct contact with the substance is possible.**

EVACUATION
Spill
- Consider initial downwind evacuation for at least 300 meters (1000 feet).
Fire
- If tank, rail car or tank truck is involved in a fire, ISOLATE for 800 meters (1/2 mile) in all directions; also, consider initial evacuation for 800 meters (1/2 mile) in all directions.

EMERGENCY RESPONSE

FIRE
Small Fire
- Water spray, wet sand or wet earth.

Large Fire
- Water spray or fog.
- **Do not scatter spilled material with high pressure water streams.**
- Move containers from fire area if you can do it without risk.

Fire involving Tanks or Car/Trailer Loads
- Fight fire from maximum distance or use unmanned hose holders or monitor nozzles.
- Cool containers with flooding quantities of water until well after fire is out.
- Withdraw immediately in case of rising sound from venting safety devices or discoloration of tank.
- ALWAYS stay away from tanks engulfed in fire.

SPILL OR LEAK
- Fully encapsulating, vapor protective clothing should be worn for spills and leaks with no fire.
- ELIMINATE all ignition sources (no smoking, flares, sparks or flames in immediate area).
- Do not touch or walk through spilled material.
- Do not touch damaged containers or spilled material unless wearing appropriate protective clothing.
- Stop leak if you can do it without risk.

Small Spill
- Cover with water, sand or earth. Shovel into metal container and keep material under water.

Large Spill
- Dike for later disposal and cover with wet sand or earth.
- Prevent entry into waterways, sewers, basements or confined areas.

FIRST AID
- Move victim to fresh air.   • Call 911 or emergency medical service.
- Give artificial respiration if victim is not breathing.
- Administer oxygen if breathing is difficult.
- In case of contact with substance, keep exposed skin areas immersed in water or covered with wet bandages until medical attention is received.
- Removal of solidified molten material from skin requires medical assistance.
- Remove and isolate contaminated clothing and shoes at the site and place in metal container filled with water. Fire hazard if allowed to dry.
- Effects of exposure (inhalation, ingestion or skin contact) to substance may be delayed.
- Keep victim warm and quiet.
- Ensure that medical personnel are aware of the material(s) involved and take precautions to protect themselves.

POTENTIAL HAZARDS

HEALTH
- CORROSIVE and/or TOXIC; inhalation, ingestion or contact (skin, eyes) with vapors, dusts or substance may cause severe injury, burns or death.
- Fire will produce irritating, corrosive and/or toxic gases.
- Reaction with water may generate much heat that will increase the concentration of fumes in the air.
- Contact with molten substance may cause severe burns to skin and eyes.
- Runoff from fire control or dilution water may cause pollution.

FIRE OR EXPLOSION
- **EXCEPT FOR ACETIC ANHYDRIDE (UN1715), THAT IS FLAMMABLE**, some of these materials may burn, but none ignite readily.
- May ignite combustibles (wood, paper, oil, clothing, etc.).
- Substance will react with water (some violently), releasing corrosive and/or toxic gases and runoff.
- Flammable/toxic gases may accumulate in confined areas (basement, tanks, hopper/tank cars, etc.).
- Contact with metals may evolve flammable hydrogen gas.
- Containers may explode when heated or if contaminated with water.
- Substance may be transported in a molten form.

PUBLIC SAFETY
- **CALL Emergency Response Telephone Number on Shipping Paper first. If Shipping Paper not available or no answer, refer to appropriate telephone number listed on the inside back cover.**
- As an immediate precautionary measure, isolate spill or leak area in all directions for at least 50 meters (150 feet) for liquids and at least 25 meters (75 feet) for solids.
- Keep unauthorized personnel away.
- Stay upwind.   • Keep out of low areas.   • Ventilate enclosed areas.

PROTECTIVE CLOTHING
- Wear positive pressure self-contained breathing apparatus (SCBA).
- Wear chemical protective clothing that is specifically recommended by the manufacturer. It may provide little or no thermal protection.
- Structural firefighters' protective clothing provides limited protection in fire situations ONLY; it is not effective in spill situations where direct contact with the substance is possible.

EVACUATION
Spill
- See Table 1 - Initial Isolation and Protective Action Distances for highlighted materials. For non-highlighted materials, increase, in the downwind direction, as necessary, the isolation distance shown under "PUBLIC SAFETY".

Fire
- If tank, rail car or tank truck is involved in a fire, ISOLATE for 800 meters (1/2 mile) in all directions; also, consider initial evacuation for 800 meters (1/2 mile) in all directions.

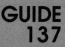

EMERGENCY RESPONSE

FIRE
- **When material is not involved in fire, do not use water on material itself.**

Small Fire
- Dry chemical or CO_2.
- Move containers from fire area if you can do it without risk.

Large Fire
- Flood fire area with large quantities of water, while knocking down vapors with water fog. If insufficient water supply: knock down vapors only.

Fire involving Tanks or Car/Trailer Loads
- Cool containers with flooding quantities of water until well after fire is out.
- Do not get water inside containers.
- Withdraw immediately in case of rising sound from venting safety devices or discoloration of tank.
- ALWAYS stay away from tanks engulfed in fire.

SPILL OR LEAK
- Fully encapsulating, vapor protective clothing should be worn for spills and leaks with no fire.
- Do not touch damaged containers or spilled material unless wearing appropriate protective clothing.
- Stop leak if you can do it without risk.
- Use water spray to reduce vapors; do not put water directly on leak, spill area or inside container.
- Keep combustibles (wood, paper, oil, etc.) away from spilled material.
- **Small Spill** • Cover with DRY earth, DRY sand or other non-combustible material followed with plastic sheet to minimize spreading or contact with rain.
- Use clean non-sparking tools to collect material and place it into loosely covered plastic containers for later disposal.
- Prevent entry into waterways, sewers, basements or confined areas.

FIRST AID
- Move victim to fresh air. • Call 911 or emergency medical service.
- Give artificial respiration if victim is not breathing.
- **Do not use mouth-to-mouth method if victim ingested or inhaled the substance; give artificial respiration with the aid of a pocket mask equipped with a one-way valve or other proper respiratory medical device.**
- Administer oxygen if breathing is difficult.
- Remove and isolate contaminated clothing and shoes.
- In case of contact with substance, immediately flush skin or eyes with running water for at least 20 minutes.
- For minor skin contact, avoid spreading material on unaffected skin.
- Removal of solidified molten material from skin requires medical assistance.
- Keep victim warm and quiet.
- Effects of exposure (inhalation, ingestion or skin contact) to substance may be delayed.
- Ensure that medical personnel are aware of the material(s) involved and take precautions to protect themselves.

POTENTIAL HAZARDS

FIRE OR EXPLOSION
- Produce flammable gases on contact with water.
- May ignite on contact with water or moist air.
- Some react vigorously or explosively on contact with water.
- May be ignited by heat, sparks or flames.
- May re-ignite after fire is extinguished.
- Some are transported in highly flammable liquids.
- Runoff may create fire or explosion hazard.

HEALTH
- Inhalation or contact with vapors, substance or decomposition products may cause severe injury or death.
- May produce corrosive solutions on contact with water.
- Fire will produce irritating, corrosive and/or toxic gases.
- Runoff from fire control may cause pollution.

PUBLIC SAFETY

- **CALL Emergency Response Telephone Number on Shipping Paper first. If Shipping Paper not available or no answer, refer to appropriate telephone number listed on the inside back cover.**
- As an immediate precautionary measure, isolate spill or leak area in all directions for at least 50 meters (150 feet) for liquids and at least 25 meters (75 feet) for solids.
- Keep unauthorized personnel away.
- Stay upwind.
- Keep out of low areas.
- Ventilate the area before entry.

PROTECTIVE CLOTHING
- Wear positive pressure self-contained breathing apparatus (SCBA).
- Wear chemical protective clothing that is specifically recommended by the manufacturer. It may provide little or no thermal protection.
- Structural firefighters' protective clothing provides limited protection in fire situations ONLY; it is not effective in spill situations where direct contact with the substance is possible.

EVACUATION
Large Spill
- See Table 1 - Initial Isolation and Protective Action Distances for highlighted materials. For non-highlighted materials, increase, in the downwind direction, as necessary, the isolation distance shown under "PUBLIC SAFETY".

Fire
- If tank, rail car or tank truck is involved in a fire, ISOLATE for 800 meters (1/2 mile) in all directions; also, consider initial evacuation for 800 meters (1/2 mile) in all directions.

EMERGENCY RESPONSE

FIRE
- **DO NOT USE WATER OR FOAM.**

Small Fire
- Dry chemical, soda ash, lime or sand.

Large Fire
- DRY sand, dry chemical, soda ash or lime or withdraw from area and let fire burn.
- Move containers from fire area if you can do it without risk.

Fire Involving Metals or Powders (Aluminum, Lithium, Magnesium, etc.)
- Use dry chemical, DRY sand, sodium chloride powder, graphite powder or Met-L-X® powder; in addition, for Lithium you may use Lith-X® powder or copper powder. Also, see GUIDE 170.

Fire involving Tanks or Car/Trailer Loads
- Fight fire from maximum distance or use unmanned hose holders or monitor nozzles.
- Do not get water inside containers.
- Cool containers with flooding quantities of water until well after fire is out.
- Withdraw immediately in case of rising sound from venting safety devices or discoloration of tank.
- ALWAYS stay away from tanks engulfed in fire.

SPILL OR LEAK
- ELIMINATE all ignition sources (no smoking, flares, sparks or flames in immediate area).
- Do not touch or walk through spilled material.
- Stop leak if you can do it without risk.
- Use water spray to reduce vapors or divert vapor cloud drift. Avoid allowing water runoff to contact spilled material.
- **DO NOT GET WATER on spilled substance or inside containers.**

Small Spill • Cover with DRY earth, DRY sand or other non-combustible material followed with plastic sheet to minimize spreading or contact with rain.
- Dike for later disposal; do not apply water unless directed to do so.

Powder Spill • Cover powder spill with plastic sheet or tarp to minimize spreading and keep powder dry.
- **DO NOT CLEAN-UP OR DISPOSE OF, EXCEPT UNDER SUPERVISION OF A SPECIALIST.**

FIRST AID
- Move victim to fresh air.　• Call 911 or emergency medical service.
- Give artificial respiration if victim is not breathing.
- Administer oxygen if breathing is difficult.
- Remove and isolate contaminated clothing and shoes.
- In case of contact with substance, wipe from skin immediately; flush skin or eyes with running water for at least 20 minutes.
- Keep victim warm and quiet.
- Ensure that medical personnel are aware of the material(s) involved and take precautions to protect themselves.

POTENTIAL HAZARDS

FIRE OR EXPLOSION
- Produce flammable and toxic gases on contact with water.
- May ignite on contact with water or moist air.
- Some react vigorously or explosively on contact with water.
- May be ignited by heat, sparks or flames.
- May re-ignite after fire is extinguished.
- Some are transported in highly flammable liquids.
- Containers may explode when heated.
- Runoff may create fire or explosion hazard.

HEALTH
- Highly toxic: contact with water produces toxic gas, may be fatal if inhaled.
- Inhalation or contact with vapors, substance or decomposition products may cause severe injury or death.
- May produce corrosive solutions on contact with water.
- Fire will produce irritating, corrosive and/or toxic gases.
- Runoff from fire control may cause pollution.

PUBLIC SAFETY

- **CALL Emergency Response Telephone Number on Shipping Paper first. If Shipping Paper not available or no answer, refer to appropriate telephone number listed on the inside back cover.**
- As an immediate precautionary measure, isolate spill or leak area in all directions for at least 50 meters (150 feet) for liquids and at least 25 meters (75 feet) for solids.
- Keep unauthorized personnel away.
- Stay upwind.
- Keep out of low areas.
- Ventilate the area before entry.

PROTECTIVE CLOTHING
- Wear positive pressure self-contained breathing apparatus (SCBA).
- Wear chemical protective clothing that is specifically recommended by the manufacturer. It may provide little or no thermal protection.
- Structural firefighters' protective clothing provides limited protection in fire situations ONLY; it is not effective in spill situations where direct contact with the substance is possible.

EVACUATION
Large Spill
- See Table 1 - Initial Isolation and Protective Action Distances for highlighted materials. For non-highlighted materials, increase, in the downwind direction, as necessary, the isolation distance shown under "PUBLIC SAFETY".

Fire
- If tank, rail car or tank truck is involved in a fire, ISOLATE for 800 meters (1/2 mile) in all directions; also, consider initial evacuation for 800 meters (1/2 mile) in all directions.

EMERGENCY RESPONSE

FIRE
- **DO NOT USE WATER OR FOAM. (FOAM MAY BE USED FOR CHLOROSILANES, SEE BELOW)**

Small Fire
- Dry chemical, soda ash, lime or sand.

Large Fire
- DRY sand, dry chemical, soda ash or lime or withdraw from area and let fire burn.
- **FOR CHLOROSILANES, DO NOT USE WATER;** use AFFF alcohol-resistant medium expansion foam; **DO NOT USE** dry chemicals, soda ash or lime on chlorosilane fires (large or small) as they may release large quantities of hydrogen gas that may explode.
- Move containers from fire area if you can do it without risk.

Fire involving Tanks or Car/Trailer Loads
- Fight fire from maximum distance or use unmanned hose holders or monitor nozzles.
- Cool containers with flooding quantities of water until well after fire is out.
- Do not get water inside containers.
- Withdraw immediately in case of rising sound from venting safety devices or discoloration of tank.
- ALWAYS stay away from tanks engulfed in fire.

SPILL OR LEAK
- Fully encapsulating, vapor protective clothing should be worn for spills and leaks with no fire.
- ELIMINATE all ignition sources (no smoking, flares, sparks or flames in immediate area).
- Do not touch or walk through spilled material.
- Stop leak if you can do it without risk.
- **DO NOT GET WATER on spilled substance or inside containers.**
- Use water spray to reduce vapors or divert vapor cloud drift. Avoid allowing water runoff to contact spilled material.
- **FOR CHLOROSILANES,** use AFFF alcohol-resistant medium expansion foam to reduce vapors.

Small Spill • Cover with DRY earth, DRY sand or other non-combustible material followed with plastic sheet to minimize spreading or contact with rain.
- Dike for later disposal; do not apply water unless directed to do so.

Powder Spill • Cover powder spill with plastic sheet or tarp to minimize spreading and keep powder dry.
- **DO NOT CLEAN-UP OR DISPOSE OF, EXCEPT UNDER SUPERVISION OF A SPECIALIST.**

FIRST AID
- Move victim to fresh air. • Call 911 or emergency medical service.
- Give artificial respiration if victim is not breathing.
- **Do not use mouth-to-mouth method if victim ingested or inhaled the substance; give artificial respiration with the aid of a pocket mask equipped with a one-way valve or other proper respiratory medical device.**
- Administer oxygen if breathing is difficult.
- Remove and isolate contaminated clothing and shoes.
- In case of contact with substance, wipe from skin immediately; flush skin or eyes with running water for at least 20 minutes.
- Keep victim warm and quiet.
- Ensure that medical personnel are aware of the material(s) involved and take precautions to protect themselves.

POTENTIAL HAZARDS

FIRE OR EXPLOSION

- These substances will accelerate burning when involved in a fire.
- Some may decompose explosively when heated or involved in a fire.
- May explode from heat or contamination.
- Some will react explosively with hydrocarbons (fuels).
- May ignite combustibles (wood, paper, oil, clothing, etc.).
- Containers may explode when heated.
- Runoff may create fire or explosion hazard.

HEALTH

- Inhalation, ingestion or contact (skin, eyes) with vapors or substance may cause severe injury, burns or death.
- Fire may produce irritating, corrosive and/or toxic gases.
- Runoff from fire control or dilution water may cause pollution.

PUBLIC SAFETY

- **CALL Emergency Response Telephone Number on Shipping Paper first. If Shipping Paper not available or no answer, refer to appropriate telephone number listed on the inside back cover.**
- As an immediate precautionary measure, isolate spill or leak area in all directions for at least 50 meters (150 feet) for liquids and at least 25 meters (75 feet) for solids.
- Keep unauthorized personnel away.
- Stay upwind.
- Keep out of low areas.
- Ventilate closed spaces before entering.

PROTECTIVE CLOTHING

- Wear positive pressure self-contained breathing apparatus (SCBA).
- Wear chemical protective clothing that is specifically recommended by the manufacturer. It may provide little or no thermal protection.
- Structural firefighters' protective clothing will only provide limited protection.

EVACUATION

Large Spill

- Consider initial downwind evacuation for at least 100 meters (330 feet).

Fire

- If tank, rail car or tank truck is involved in a fire, ISOLATE for 800 meters (1/2 mile) in all directions; also, consider initial evacuation for 800 meters (1/2 mile) in all directions.

EMERGENCY RESPONSE

FIRE

Small Fire

- Use water. Do not use dry chemicals or foams. CO_2 or Halon® may provide limited control.

Large Fire

- Flood fire area with water from a distance.
- Do not move cargo or vehicle if cargo has been exposed to heat.
- Move containers from fire area if you can do it without risk.

Fire involving Tanks or Car/Trailer Loads

- Fight fire from maximum distance or use unmanned hose holders or monitor nozzles.
- Cool containers with flooding quantities of water until well after fire is out.
- ALWAYS stay away from tanks engulfed in fire.
- For massive fire, use unmanned hose holders or monitor nozzles; if this is impossible, withdraw from area and let fire burn.

SPILL OR LEAK

- Keep combustibles (wood, paper, oil, etc.) away from spilled material.
- Do not touch damaged containers or spilled material unless wearing appropriate protective clothing.
- Stop leak if you can do it without risk.
- Do not get water inside containers.

Small Dry Spill

- With clean shovel place material into clean, dry container and cover loosely; move containers from spill area.

Small Liquid Spill

- Use a non-combustible material like vermiculite or sand to soak up the product and place into a container for later disposal.

Large Spill

- Dike far ahead of liquid spill for later disposal.
- **Following product recovery, flush area with water.**

FIRST AID

- Move victim to fresh air. • Call 911 or emergency medical service.
- Give artificial respiration if victim is not breathing.
- Administer oxygen if breathing is difficult.
- Remove and isolate contaminated clothing and shoes.
- Contaminated clothing may be a fire risk when dry.
- In case of contact with substance, immediately flush skin or eyes with running water for at least 20 minutes.
- Keep victim warm and quiet.
- Ensure that medical personnel are aware of the material(s) involved and take precautions to protect themselves.

POTENTIAL HAZARDS

FIRE OR EXPLOSION
- These substances will accelerate burning when involved in a fire.
- May explode from heat or contamination.
- Some may burn rapidly.
- Some will react explosively with hydrocarbons (fuels).
- May ignite combustibles (wood, paper, oil, clothing, etc.).
- Containers may explode when heated.
- Runoff may create fire or explosion hazard.

HEALTH
- Toxic by ingestion.
- Inhalation of dust is toxic.
- Fire may produce irritating, corrosive and/or toxic gases.
- Contact with substance may cause severe burns to skin and eyes.
- Runoff from fire control or dilution water may cause pollution.

PUBLIC SAFETY

- **CALL Emergency Response Telephone Number on Shipping Paper first. If Shipping Paper not available or no answer, refer to appropriate telephone number listed on the inside back cover.**
- As an immediate precautionary measure, isolate spill or leak area in all directions for at least 50 meters (150 feet) for liquids and at least 25 meters (75 feet) for solids.
- Keep unauthorized personnel away.
- Stay upwind.
- Keep out of low areas.
- Ventilate closed spaces before entering.

PROTECTIVE CLOTHING
- Wear positive pressure self-contained breathing apparatus (SCBA).
- Wear chemical protective clothing that is specifically recommended by the manufacturer. It may provide little or no thermal protection.
- Structural firefighters' protective clothing will only provide limited protection.

EVACUATION
Large Spill
- Consider initial downwind evacuation for at least 100 meters (330 feet).
Fire
- If tank, rail car or tank truck is involved in a fire, ISOLATE for 800 meters (1/2 mile) in all directions; also, consider initial evacuation for 800 meters (1/2 mile) in all directions.

EMERGENCY RESPONSE

FIRE

Small Fire

- Use water. Do not use dry chemicals or foams. CO_2 or Halon® may provide limited control.

Large Fire

- Flood fire area with water from a distance.
- Do not move cargo or vehicle if cargo has been exposed to heat.
- Move containers from fire area if you can do it without risk.

Fire involving Tanks or Car/Trailer Loads

- Fight fire from maximum distance or use unmanned hose holders or monitor nozzles.
- Cool containers with flooding quantities of water until well after fire is out.
- ALWAYS stay away from tanks engulfed in fire.
- For massive fire, use unmanned hose holders or monitor nozzles; if this is impossible, withdraw from area and let fire burn.

SPILL OR LEAK

- Keep combustibles (wood, paper, oil, etc.) away from spilled material.
- Do not touch damaged containers or spilled material unless wearing appropriate protective clothing.
- Stop leak if you can do it without risk.

Small Dry Spill

- With clean shovel place material into clean, dry container and cover loosely; move containers from spill area.

Large Spill

- Dike far ahead of spill for later disposal.

FIRST AID

- Move victim to fresh air.   • Call 911 or emergency medical service.
- Give artificial respiration if victim is not breathing.
- Administer oxygen if breathing is difficult.
- Remove and isolate contaminated clothing and shoes.
- Contaminated clothing may be a fire risk when dry.
- In case of contact with substance, immediately flush skin or eyes with running water for at least 20 minutes.
- Keep victim warm and quiet.
- Ensure that medical personnel are aware of the material(s) involved and take precautions to protect themselves.

POTENTIAL HAZARDS

FIRE OR EXPLOSION

- These substances will accelerate burning when involved in a fire.
- May explode from heat or contamination.
- Some will react explosively with hydrocarbons (fuels).
- May ignite combustibles (wood, paper, oil, clothing, etc.).
- Containers may explode when heated.
- Runoff may create fire or explosion hazard.

HEALTH

- **TOXIC**; inhalation, ingestion or contact (skin, eyes) with vapors or substance may cause severe injury, burns or death.
- Fire may produce irritating, corrosive and/or toxic gases.
- Toxic/flammable fumes may accumulate in confined areas (basement, tanks, tank cars, etc.).
- Runoff from fire control or dilution water may cause pollution.

PUBLIC SAFETY

- **CALL Emergency Response Telephone Number on Shipping Paper first. If Shipping Paper not available or no answer, refer to appropriate telephone number listed on the inside back cover.**
- As an immediate precautionary measure, isolate spill or leak area for at least 50 meters (150 feet) in all directions.
- Keep unauthorized personnel away.
- Stay upwind.
- Keep out of low areas.
- Ventilate closed spaces before entering.

PROTECTIVE CLOTHING

- Wear positive pressure self-contained breathing apparatus (SCBA).
- Wear chemical protective clothing that is specifically recommended by the manufacturer. It may provide little or no thermal protection.
- Structural firefighters' protective clothing provides limited protection in fire situations ONLY; it is not effective in spill situations where direct contact with the substance is possible.

EVACUATION

Spill

- See Table 1 - Initial Isolation and Protective Action Distances for highlighted materials. For non-highlighted materials, increase, in the downwind direction, as necessary, the isolation distance shown under "PUBLIC SAFETY".

Fire

- If tank, rail car or tank truck is involved in a fire, ISOLATE for 800 meters (1/2 mile) in all directions; also, consider initial evacuation for 800 meters (1/2 mile) in all directions.

EMERGENCY RESPONSE

FIRE

Small Fire
- Use water. Do not use dry chemicals or foams. CO_2 or Halon® may provide limited control.

Large Fire
- Flood fire area with water from a distance.
- Do not move cargo or vehicle if cargo has been exposed to heat.
- Move containers from fire area if you can do it without risk.

Fire involving Tanks or Car/Trailer Loads
- Fight fire from maximum distance or use unmanned hose holders or monitor nozzles.
- Cool containers with flooding quantities of water until well after fire is out.
- ALWAYS stay away from tanks engulfed in fire.
- For massive fire, use unmanned hose holders or monitor nozzles; if this is impossible, withdraw from area and let fire burn.

SPILL OR LEAK

- Keep combustibles (wood, paper, oil, etc.) away from spilled material.
- Fully encapsulating, vapor protective clothing should be worn for spills and leaks with no fire.
- Do not touch damaged containers or spilled material unless wearing appropriate protective clothing.
- Stop leak if you can do it without risk.
- Use water spray to reduce vapors or divert vapor cloud drift.
- Do not get water inside containers.

Small Liquid Spill
- Use a non-combustible material like vermiculite or sand to soak up the product and place into a container for later disposal.

Large Spill
- Dike far ahead of liquid spill for later disposal.

FIRST AID

- Move victim to fresh air.   • Call 911 or emergency medical service.
- Give artificial respiration if victim is not breathing.
- **Do not use mouth-to-mouth method if victim ingested or inhaled the substance; give artificial respiration with the aid of a pocket mask equipped with a one-way valve or other proper respiratory medical device.**
- Administer oxygen if breathing is difficult.
- Remove and isolate contaminated clothing and shoes.
- Contaminated clothing may be a fire risk when dry.
- In case of contact with substance, immediately flush skin or eyes with running water for at least 20 minutes.
- Keep victim warm and quiet.
- Ensure that medical personnel are aware of the material(s) involved and take precautions to protect themselves.

POTENTIAL HAZARDS

FIRE OR EXPLOSION
- May explode from friction, heat or contamination.
- These substances will accelerate burning when involved in a fire.
- May ignite combustibles (wood, paper, oil, clothing, etc.).
- Some will react explosively with hydrocarbons (fuels).
- Containers may explode when heated.
- Runoff may create fire or explosion hazard.

HEALTH
- **TOXIC**; inhalation, ingestion or contact (skin, eyes) with vapors, dusts or substance may cause severe injury, burns or death.
- Fire may produce irritating and/or toxic gases.
- Toxic fumes or dust may accumulate in confined areas (basement, tanks, hopper/tank cars, etc.).
- Runoff from fire control or dilution water may cause pollution.

PUBLIC SAFETY

- **CALL Emergency Response Telephone Number on Shipping Paper first. If Shipping Paper not available or no answer, refer to appropriate telephone number listed on the inside back cover.**
- As an immediate precautionary measure, isolate spill or leak area in all directions for at least 50 meters (150 feet) for liquids and at least 25 meters (75 feet) for solids.
- Keep unauthorized personnel away.
- Stay upwind.
- Keep out of low areas.
- Ventilate closed spaces before entering.

PROTECTIVE CLOTHING
- Wear positive pressure self-contained breathing apparatus (SCBA).
- Wear chemical protective clothing that is specifically recommended by the manufacturer. It may provide little or no thermal protection.
- Structural firefighters' protective clothing provides limited protection in fire situations ONLY; it is not effective in spill situations where direct contact with the substance is possible.

EVACUATION
Spill
- See Table 1 - Initial Isolation and Protective Action Distances for highlighted materials. For non-highlighted materials, increase, in the downwind direction, as necessary, the isolation distance shown under "PUBLIC SAFETY".

Fire
- If tank, rail car or tank truck is involved in a fire, ISOLATE for 800 meters (1/2 mile) in all directions; also, consider initial evacuation for 800 meters (1/2 mile) in all directions.

EMERGENCY RESPONSE

FIRE

Small Fire
- Use water. Do not use dry chemicals or foams. CO_2 or Halon® may provide limited control.

Large Fire
- Flood fire area with water from a distance.
- Do not move cargo or vehicle if cargo has been exposed to heat.
- Move containers from fire area if you can do it without risk.
- Do not get water inside containers: a violent reaction may occur.

Fire involving Tanks or Car/Trailer Loads
- Cool containers with flooding quantities of water until well after fire is out.
- Dike fire-control water for later disposal.
- ALWAYS stay away from tanks engulfed in fire.
- For massive fire, use unmanned hose holders or monitor nozzles; if this is impossible, withdraw from area and let fire burn.

SPILL OR LEAK

- Keep combustibles (wood, paper, oil, etc.) away from spilled material.
- Do not touch damaged containers or spilled material unless wearing appropriate protective clothing.
- Use water spray to reduce vapors or divert vapor cloud drift.
- Prevent entry into waterways, sewers, basements or confined areas.

Small Spill
- Flush area with flooding quantities of water.

Large Spill
- **DO NOT CLEAN-UP OR DISPOSE OF, EXCEPT UNDER SUPERVISION OF A SPECIALIST.**

FIRST AID

- Move victim to fresh air.   • Call 911 or emergency medical service.
- Give artificial respiration if victim is not breathing.
- Administer oxygen if breathing is difficult.
- Remove and isolate contaminated clothing and shoes.
- Contaminated clothing may be a fire risk when dry.
- In case of contact with substance, immediately flush skin or eyes with running water for at least 20 minutes.
- Keep victim warm and quiet.
- Ensure that medical personnel are aware of the material(s) involved and take precautions to protect themselves.

POTENTIAL HAZARDS

FIRE OR EXPLOSION
- May ignite combustibles (wood, paper, oil, clothing, etc.).
- React vigorously and/or explosively with water.
- Produce toxic and/or corrosive substances on contact with water.
- Flammable/toxic gases may accumulate in tanks and hopper cars.
- Some may produce flammable hydrogen gas upon contact with metals.
- Containers may explode when heated.
- Runoff may create fire or explosion hazard.

HEALTH
- **TOXIC**; inhalation or contact with vapor, substance, or decomposition products may cause severe injury or death.
- Fire will produce irritating, corrosive and/or toxic gases.
- Runoff from fire control or dilution water may cause pollution.

PUBLIC SAFETY

- **CALL Emergency Response Telephone Number on Shipping Paper first. If Shipping Paper not available or no answer, refer to appropriate telephone number listed on the inside back cover.**
- As an immediate precautionary measure, isolate spill or leak area in all directions for at least 50 meters (150 feet) for liquids and at least 25 meters (75 feet) for solids.
- Keep unauthorized personnel away.
- Stay upwind.
- Keep out of low areas.
- Ventilate closed spaces before entering.

PROTECTIVE CLOTHING
- Wear positive pressure self-contained breathing apparatus (SCBA).
- Wear chemical protective clothing that is specifically recommended by the manufacturer. It may provide little or no thermal protection.
- Structural firefighters' protective clothing provides limited protection in fire situations ONLY; it is not effective in spill situations where direct contact with the substance is possible.

EVACUATION
Spill
- See Table 1 - Initial Isolation and Protective Action Distances for highlighted materials. For non-highlighted materials, increase, in the downwind direction, as necessary, the isolation distance shown under "PUBLIC SAFETY".

Fire
- If tank, rail car or tank truck is involved in a fire, ISOLATE for 800 meters (1/2 mile) in all directions; also, consider initial evacuation for 800 meters (1/2 mile) in all directions.

EMERGENCY RESPONSE

FIRE

- **DO NOT USE WATER OR FOAM.**

Small Fire

- Dry chemical, soda ash or lime.

Large Fire

- DRY sand, dry chemical, soda ash or lime or withdraw from area and let fire burn.
- Do not move cargo or vehicle if cargo has been exposed to heat.
- Move containers from fire area if you can do it without risk.

Fire involving Tanks or Car/Trailer Loads

- Fight fire from maximum distance or use unmanned hose holders or monitor nozzles.
- Cool containers with flooding quantities of water until well after fire is out.
- Withdraw immediately in case of rising sound from venting safety devices or discoloration of tank.
- ALWAYS stay away from tanks engulfed in fire.

SPILL OR LEAK

- ELIMINATE all ignition sources (no smoking, flares, sparks or flames in immediate area).
- Do not touch damaged containers or spilled material unless wearing appropriate protective clothing.
- Stop leak if you can do it without risk.
- Use water spray to reduce vapors or divert vapor cloud drift. Avoid allowing water runoff to contact spilled material.
- **DO NOT GET WATER on spilled substance or inside containers.**

Small Spill

- Cover with DRY earth, DRY sand or other non-combustible material followed with plastic sheet to minimize spreading or contact with rain.

Large Spill

- **DO NOT CLEAN-UP OR DISPOSE OF, EXCEPT UNDER SUPERVISION OF A SPECIALIST.**

FIRST AID

- Move victim to fresh air.   • Call 911 or emergency medical service.
- Give artificial respiration if victim is not breathing.
- **Do not use mouth-to-mouth method if victim ingested or inhaled the substance; give artificial respiration with the aid of a pocket mask equipped with a one-way valve or other proper respiratory medical device.**
- Administer oxygen if breathing is difficult.
- Remove and isolate contaminated clothing and shoes.
- Contaminated clothing may be a fire risk when dry.
- In case of contact with substance, immediately flush skin or eyes with running water for at least 20 minutes.
- Keep victim warm and quiet.   • Keep victim under observation.
- Effects of contact or inhalation may be delayed.
- Ensure that medical personnel are aware of the material(s) involved and take precautions to protect themselves.

POTENTIAL HAZARDS

FIRE OR EXPLOSION
- May explode from heat or contamination.
- May ignite combustibles (wood, paper, oil, clothing, etc.).
- May be ignited by heat, sparks or flames.
- May burn rapidly with flare-burning effect.
- Containers may explode when heated.
- Runoff may create fire or explosion hazard.

HEALTH
- Fire may produce irritating, corrosive and/or toxic gases.
- Ingestion or contact (skin, eyes) with substance may cause severe injury or burns.
- Runoff from fire control or dilution water may cause pollution.

PUBLIC SAFETY
- **CALL Emergency Response Telephone Number on Shipping Paper first. If Shipping Paper not available or no answer, refer to appropriate telephone number listed on the inside back cover.**
- As an immediate precautionary measure, isolate spill or leak area in all directions for at least 50 meters (150 feet) for liquids and at least 25 meters (75 feet) for solids.
- Keep unauthorized personnel away.
- Stay upwind.
- Keep out of low areas.

PROTECTIVE CLOTHING
- Wear positive pressure self-contained breathing apparatus (SCBA).
- Wear chemical protective clothing that is specifically recommended by the manufacturer. It may provide little or no thermal protection.
- Structural firefighters' protective clothing will only provide limited protection.

EVACUATION

Large Spill
- Consider initial evacuation for at least 250 meters (800 feet).

Fire
- If tank, rail car or tank truck is involved in a fire, ISOLATE for 800 meters (1/2 mile) in all directions; also, consider initial evacuation for 800 meters (1/2 mile) in all directions.

EMERGENCY RESPONSE

FIRE

Small Fire

- Water spray or fog is preferred; if water not available use dry chemical, CO_2 or regular foam.

Large Fire

- Flood fire area with water from a distance.
- Use water spray or fog; do not use straight streams.
- Do not move cargo or vehicle if cargo has been exposed to heat.
- Move containers from fire area if you can do it without risk.

Fire involving Tanks or Car/Trailer Loads

- Fight fire from maximum distance or use unmanned hose holders or monitor nozzles.
- Cool containers with flooding quantities of water until well after fire is out.
- ALWAYS stay away from tanks engulfed in fire.
- For massive fire, use unmanned hose holders or monitor nozzles; if this is impossible, withdraw from area and let fire burn.

SPILL OR LEAK

- ELIMINATE all ignition sources (no smoking, flares, sparks or flames in immediate area).
- Keep combustibles (wood, paper, oil, etc.) away from spilled material.
- Do not touch damaged containers or spilled material unless wearing appropriate protective clothing.
- Keep substance wet using water spray.
- Stop leak if you can do it without risk.

Small Spill

- Take up with inert, damp, non-combustible material using clean non-sparking tools and place into loosely covered plastic containers for later disposal.

Large Spill

- Wet down with water and dike for later disposal.
- Prevent entry into waterways, sewers, basements or confined areas.
- **DO NOT CLEAN-UP OR DISPOSE OF, EXCEPT UNDER SUPERVISION OF A SPECIALIST.**

FIRST AID

- Move victim to fresh air.   • Call 911 or emergency medical service.
- Give artificial respiration if victim is not breathing.
- Administer oxygen if breathing is difficult.
- Remove and isolate contaminated clothing and shoes.
- Contaminated clothing may be a fire risk when dry.
- Remove material from skin immediately.
- In case of contact with substance, immediately flush skin or eyes with running water for at least 20 minutes.
- Keep victim warm and quiet.
- Ensure that medical personnel are aware of the material(s) involved and take precautions to protect themselves.

POTENTIAL HAZARDS

FIRE OR EXPLOSION
- May explode from heat, shock, friction or contamination.
- May ignite combustibles (wood, paper, oil, clothing, etc.).
- May be ignited by heat, sparks or flames.
- May burn rapidly with flare-burning effect.
- Containers may explode when heated.
- Runoff may create fire or explosion hazard.

HEALTH
- Fire may produce irritating, corrosive and/or toxic gases.
- Ingestion or contact (skin, eyes) with substance may cause severe injury or burns.
- Runoff from fire control or dilution water may cause pollution.

PUBLIC SAFETY
- **CALL Emergency Response Telephone Number on Shipping Paper first. If Shipping Paper not available or no answer, refer to appropriate telephone number listed on the inside back cover.**
- As an immediate precautionary measure, isolate spill or leak area in all directions for at least 50 meters (150 feet) for liquids and at least 25 meters (75 feet) for solids.
- Keep unauthorized personnel away.
- Stay upwind.
- Keep out of low areas.

PROTECTIVE CLOTHING
- Wear positive pressure self-contained breathing apparatus (SCBA).
- Wear chemical protective clothing that is specifically recommended by the manufacturer. It may provide little or no thermal protection.
- Structural firefighters' protective clothing will only provide limited protection.

EVACUATION
Large Spill
- Consider initial evacuation for at least 250 meters (800 feet).

Fire
- If tank, rail car or tank truck is involved in a fire, ISOLATE for 800 meters (1/2 mile) in all directions; also, consider initial evacuation for 800 meters (1/2 mile) in all directions.

EMERGENCY RESPONSE

FIRE

Small Fire

- Water spray or fog is preferred; if water not available use dry chemical, CO_2 or regular foam.

Large Fire

- Flood fire area with water from a distance.
- Use water spray or fog; do not use straight streams.
- Do not move cargo or vehicle if cargo has been exposed to heat.
- Move containers from fire area if you can do it without risk.

Fire involving Tanks or Car/Trailer Loads

- Fight fire from maximum distance or use unmanned hose holders or monitor nozzles.
- Cool containers with flooding quantities of water until well after fire is out.
- ALWAYS stay away from tanks engulfed in fire.
- For massive fire, use unmanned hose holders or monitor nozzles; if this is impossible, withdraw from area and let fire burn.

SPILL OR LEAK

- ELIMINATE all ignition sources (no smoking, flares, sparks or flames in immediate area).
- Keep combustibles (wood, paper, oil, etc.) away from spilled material.
- Do not touch damaged containers or spilled material unless wearing appropriate protective clothing.
- Keep substance wet using water spray.
- Stop leak if you can do it without risk.

Small Spill

- Take up with inert, damp, non-combustible material using clean non-sparking tools and place into loosely covered plastic containers for later disposal.

Large Spill

- Wet down with water and dike for later disposal.
- Prevent entry into waterways, sewers, basements or confined areas.
- **DO NOT CLEAN-UP OR DISPOSE OF, EXCEPT UNDER SUPERVISION OF A SPECIALIST.**

FIRST AID

- Move victim to fresh air.   • Call 911 or emergency medical service.
- Give artificial respiration if victim is not breathing.
- Administer oxygen if breathing is difficult.
- Remove and isolate contaminated clothing and shoes.
- Contaminated clothing may be a fire risk when dry.
- Remove material from skin immediately.
- In case of contact with substance, immediately flush skin or eyes with running water for at least 20 minutes.
- Keep victim warm and quiet.
- Ensure that medical personnel are aware of the material(s) involved and take precautions to protect themselves.

POTENTIAL HAZARDS

FIRE OR EXPLOSION
- Lithium ion batteries contain flammable liquid electrolyte that may vent, ignite and produce sparks when subjected to high temperatures (> 150 ^{0}C (302 ^{0}F)), when damaged or abused (e.g., mechanical damage or electrical overcharging).
- May burn rapidly with flare-burning effect.
- May ignite other batteries in close proximity.

HEALTH
- Contact with battery electrolyte may be irritating to skin, eyes and mucous membranes.
- Fire will produce irritating, corrosive and/or toxic gases.
- Burning batteries may produce toxic hydrogen fluoride gas (see GUIDE 125).
- Fumes may cause dizziness or suffocation.

PUBLIC SAFETY

- **CALL Emergency Response Telephone Number on Shipping Paper first. If Shipping Paper not available or no answer, refer to appropriate telephone number listed on the inside back cover.**
- As an immediate precautionary measure, isolate spill or leak area for at least 25 meters (75 feet) in all directions.
- Keep unauthorized personnel away.
- Stay upwind.
- Keep out of low areas.
- Ventilate closed spaces before entering.

PROTECTIVE CLOTHING
- Wear positive pressure self-contained breathing apparatus (SCBA).
- Structural firefighters' protective clothing will only provide limited protection.

EVACUATION
Large Spill
- Consider initial downwind evacuation for at least 100 meters (330 feet).

Fire
- If rail car or trailer is involved in a fire, ISOLATE for 500 meters (1/3 mile) in all directions; also initiate evacuation including emergency responders for 500 meters (1/3 mile) in all directions.

EMERGENCY RESPONSE

FIRE
Small Fire
- Dry chemical, CO_2, water spray or regular foam.

Large Fire
- Water spray, fog or regular foam.
- Move containers from fire area if you can do it without risk.

SPILL OR LEAK
- ELIMINATE all ignition sources (no smoking, flares, sparks or flames in immediate area).
- Do not touch or walk through spilled material.
- Absorb with earth, sand or other non-combustible material.
- Leaking batteries and contaminated absorbent material should be placed in metal containers.

FIRST AID
- Move victim to fresh air.
- Call 911 or emergency medical service.
- Give artificial respiration if victim is not breathing.
- Administer oxygen if breathing is difficult.
- Remove and isolate contaminated clothing and shoes.
- In case of contact with substance, immediately flush skin or eyes with running water for at least 20 minutes.
- Ensure that medical personnel are aware of the material(s) involved and take precautions to protect themselves.

POTENTIAL HAZARDS

FIRE OR EXPLOSION
- May explode from heat, contamination or loss of temperature control.
- These materials are particularly sensitive to temperature rises. Above a given "Control Temperature" they decompose violently and catch fire.
- May ignite combustibles (wood, paper, oil, clothing, etc.).
- May ignite spontaneously if exposed to air.
- May be ignited by heat, sparks or flames.
- May burn rapidly with flare-burning effect.
- Containers may explode when heated.
- Runoff may create fire or explosion hazard.

HEALTH
- Fire may produce irritating, corrosive and/or toxic gases.
- Ingestion or contact (skin, eyes) with substance may cause severe injury or burns.
- Runoff from fire control or dilution water may cause pollution.

PUBLIC SAFETY

- **CALL Emergency Response Telephone Number on Shipping Paper first. If Shipping Paper not available or no answer, refer to appropriate telephone number listed on the inside back cover.**
- As an immediate precautionary measure, isolate spill or leak area in all directions for at least 50 meters (150 feet) for liquids and at least 25 meters (75 feet) for solids.
- Keep unauthorized personnel away.
- Stay upwind.
- Keep out of low areas.
- **DO NOT allow the substance to warm up. Obtain liquid nitrogen, dry ice or ice for cooling. If none can be obtained, evacuate the area immediately.**

PROTECTIVE CLOTHING
- Wear positive pressure self-contained breathing apparatus (SCBA).
- Wear chemical protective clothing that is specifically recommended by the manufacturer. It may provide little or no thermal protection.
- Structural firefighters' protective clothing will only provide limited protection.

EVACUATION
Large Spill
- Consider initial evacuation for at least 250 meters (800 feet).

Fire
- If tank, rail car or tank truck is involved in a fire, ISOLATE for 800 meters (1/2 mile) in all directions; also, consider initial evacuation for 800 meters (1/2 mile) in all directions.

EMERGENCY RESPONSE

FIRE

- The temperature of the substance must be maintained at or below the "Control Temperature" at all times.

Small Fire

- Water spray or fog is preferred; if water not available use dry chemical, CO_2 or regular foam.

Large Fire

- Flood fire area with water from a distance.
- Use water spray or fog; do not use straight streams.
- Do not move cargo or vehicle if cargo has been exposed to heat.
- Move containers from fire area if you can do it without risk.

Fire involving Tanks or Car/Trailer Loads

- Fight fire from maximum distance or use unmanned hose holders or monitor nozzles.
- Cool containers with flooding quantities of water until well after fire is out.
- **BEWARE OF POSSIBLE CONTAINER EXPLOSION.**
- ALWAYS stay away from tanks engulfed in fire.
- For massive fire, use unmanned hose holders or monitor nozzles; if this is impossible, withdraw from area and let fire burn.

SPILL OR LEAK

- ELIMINATE all ignition sources (no smoking, flares, sparks or flames in immediate area).
- Keep combustibles (wood, paper, oil, etc.) away from spilled material.
- Do not touch or walk through spilled material.
- Stop leak if you can do it without risk.

Small Spill

- Take up with inert, damp, non-combustible material using clean non-sparking tools and place into loosely covered plastic containers for later disposal.

Large Spill

- Dike far ahead of liquid spill for later disposal.
- Prevent entry into waterways, sewers, basements or confined areas.
- **DO NOT CLEAN-UP OR DISPOSE OF, EXCEPT UNDER SUPERVISION OF A SPECIALIST.**

FIRST AID

- Move victim to fresh air.   • Call 911 or emergency medical service.
- Give artificial respiration if victim is not breathing.
- Administer oxygen if breathing is difficult.
- Remove and isolate contaminated clothing and shoes.
- Contaminated clothing may be a fire risk when dry.
- Remove material from skin immediately.
- In case of contact with substance, immediately flush skin or eyes with running water for at least 20 minutes.
- Keep victim warm and quiet.
- Ensure that medical personnel are aware of the material(s) involved and take precautions to protect themselves.

POTENTIAL HAZARDS

FIRE OR EXPLOSION

- **Self-decomposition or self-ignition may be triggered by heat, chemical reaction, friction or impact.**
- May be ignited by heat, sparks or flames.
- Some may decompose explosively when heated or involved in a fire.
- May burn violently. Decomposition may be self-accelerating and produce large amounts of gases.
- Vapors or dust may form explosive mixtures with air.

HEALTH

- Inhalation or contact with vapors, substance or decomposition products may cause severe injury or death.
- May produce irritating, toxic and/or corrosive gases.
- Runoff from fire control may cause pollution.

PUBLIC SAFETY

- **CALL Emergency Response Telephone Number on Shipping Paper first. If Shipping Paper not available or no answer, refer to appropriate telephone number listed on the inside back cover.**
- As an immediate precautionary measure, isolate spill or leak area in all directions for at least 50 meters (150 feet) for liquids and at least 25 meters (75 feet) for solids.
- Keep unauthorized personnel away.
- Stay upwind.
- Keep out of low areas.

PROTECTIVE CLOTHING

- Wear positive pressure self-contained breathing apparatus (SCBA).
- Wear chemical protective clothing that is specifically recommended by the manufacturer. It may provide little or no thermal protection.
- Structural firefighters' protective clothing will only provide limited protection.

EVACUATION

Large Spill

- Consider initial downwind evacuation for at least 250 meters (800 feet).

Fire

- If tank, rail car or tank truck is involved in a fire, ISOLATE for 800 meters (1/2 mile) in all directions; also, consider initial evacuation for 800 meters (1/2 mile) in all directions.

EMERGENCY RESPONSE

FIRE

Small Fire

- Dry chemical, CO_2, water spray or regular foam.

Large Fire

- Flood fire area with water from a distance.
- Move containers from fire area if you can do it without risk.

Fire involving Tanks or Car/Trailer Loads

- **BEWARE OF POSSIBLE CONTAINER EXPLOSION.**
- Fight fire from maximum distance or use unmanned hose holders or monitor nozzles.
- Cool containers with flooding quantities of water until well after fire is out.
- Withdraw immediately in case of rising sound from venting safety devices or discoloration of tank.
- ALWAYS stay away from tanks engulfed in fire.

SPILL OR LEAK

- ELIMINATE all ignition sources (no smoking, flares, sparks or flames in immediate area).
- Do not touch or walk through spilled material.
- Stop leak if you can do it without risk.

Small Spill

- Take up with inert, damp, non-combustible material using clean non-sparking tools and place into loosely covered plastic containers for later disposal.
- Prevent entry into waterways, sewers, basements or confined areas.

FIRST AID

- Move victim to fresh air.   • Call 911 or emergency medical service.
- Give artificial respiration if victim is not breathing.
- Administer oxygen if breathing is difficult.
- Remove and isolate contaminated clothing and shoes.
- In case of contact with substance, immediately flush skin or eyes with running water for at least 20 minutes.
- Keep victim warm and quiet.
- Ensure that medical personnel are aware of the material(s) involved and take precautions to protect themselves.

POTENTIAL HAZARDS

FIRE OR EXPLOSION

- **Self-decomposition or self-ignition may be triggered by heat, chemical reaction, friction or impact.**
- Self-accelerating decomposition may occur if the specific control temperature is not maintained.
- These materials are particularly sensitive to temperature rises. Above a given "Control Temperature" they decompose violently and catch fire.
- May be ignited by heat, sparks or flames.
- Some may decompose explosively when heated or involved in a fire.
- May burn violently. Decomposition may be self-accelerating and produce large amounts of gases.
- Vapors or dust may form explosive mixtures with air.

HEALTH

- Inhalation or contact with vapors, substance or decomposition products may cause severe injury or death.
- May produce irritating, toxic and/or corrosive gases.
- Runoff from fire control may cause pollution.

PUBLIC SAFETY

- **CALL Emergency Response Telephone Number on Shipping Paper first. If Shipping Paper not available or no answer, refer to appropriate telephone number listed on the inside back cover.**
- As an immediate precautionary measure, isolate spill or leak area in all directions for at least 50 meters (150 feet) for liquids and at least 25 meters (75 feet) for solids.
- Keep unauthorized personnel away.
- Stay upwind.
- Keep out of low areas.
- **DO NOT allow the substance to warm up. Obtain liquid nitrogen, dry ice or ice for cooling. If none can be obtained, evacuate the area immediately.**

PROTECTIVE CLOTHING

- Wear positive pressure self-contained breathing apparatus (SCBA).
- Wear chemical protective clothing that is specifically recommended by the manufacturer. It may provide little or no thermal protection.
- Structural firefighters' protective clothing will only provide limited protection.

EVACUATION

Large Spill
- Consider initial downwind evacuation for at least 250 meters (800 feet).

Fire
- If tank, rail car or tank truck is involved in a fire, ISOLATE for 800 meters (1/2 mile) in all directions; also, consider initial evacuation for 800 meters (1/2 mile) in all directions.

EMERGENCY RESPONSE

FIRE

- **The temperature of the substance must be maintained at or below the "Control Temperature" at all times.**

Small Fire

- Dry chemical, CO_2, water spray or regular foam.

Large Fire

- Flood fire area with water from a distance.
- Move containers from fire area if you can do it without risk.

Fire involving Tanks or Car/Trailer Loads

- **BEWARE OF POSSIBLE CONTAINER EXPLOSION.**
- Fight fire from maximum distance or use unmanned hose holders or monitor nozzles.
- Cool containers with flooding quantities of water until well after fire is out.
- Withdraw immediately in case of rising sound from venting safety devices or discoloration of tank.
- ALWAYS stay away from tanks engulfed in fire.

SPILL OR LEAK

- ELIMINATE all ignition sources (no smoking, flares, sparks or flames in immediate area).
- Do not touch or walk through spilled material.
- Stop leak if you can do it without risk.

Small Spill

- Take up with inert, damp, non-combustible material using clean non-sparking tools and place into loosely covered plastic containers for later disposal.
- Prevent entry into waterways, sewers, basements or confined areas.
- **DO NOT CLEAN-UP OR DISPOSE OF, EXCEPT UNDER SUPERVISION OF A SPECIALIST.**

FIRST AID

- Move victim to fresh air.   • Call 911 or emergency medical service.
- Give artificial respiration if victim is not breathing.
- Administer oxygen if breathing is difficult.
- Remove and isolate contaminated clothing and shoes.
- In case of contact with substance, immediately flush skin or eyes with running water for at least 20 minutes.
- Keep victim warm and quiet.
- Ensure that medical personnel are aware of the material(s) involved and take precautions to protect themselves.

POTENTIAL HAZARDS

HEALTH
- **Highly toxic**, may be fatal if inhaled, swallowed or absorbed through skin.
- Avoid any skin contact.
- Effects of contact or inhalation may be delayed.
- Fire may produce irritating, corrosive and/or toxic gases.
- Runoff from fire control or dilution water may be corrosive and/or toxic and cause pollution.

FIRE OR EXPLOSION
- Non-combustible, substance itself does not burn but may decompose upon heating to produce corrosive and/or toxic fumes.
- Containers may explode when heated.
- Runoff may pollute waterways.

PUBLIC SAFETY
- **CALL Emergency Response Telephone Number on Shipping Paper first. If Shipping Paper not available or no answer, refer to appropriate telephone number listed on the inside back cover.**
- As an immediate precautionary measure, isolate spill or leak area in all directions for at least 50 meters (150 feet) for liquids and at least 25 meters (75 feet) for solids.
- Keep unauthorized personnel away.
- Stay upwind.
- Keep out of low areas.

PROTECTIVE CLOTHING
- Wear positive pressure self-contained breathing apparatus (SCBA).
- Wear chemical protective clothing that is specifically recommended by the manufacturer. It may provide little or no thermal protection.
- Structural firefighters' protective clothing provides limited protection in fire situations ONLY; it is not effective in spill situations where direct contact with the substance is possible.

EVACUATION
Spill
- See Table 1 - Initial Isolation and Protective Action Distances for highlighted materials. For non-highlighted materials, increase, in the downwind direction, as necessary, the isolation distance shown under "PUBLIC SAFETY".

Fire
- If tank, rail car or tank truck is involved in a fire, ISOLATE for 800 meters (1/2 mile) in all directions; also, consider initial evacuation for 800 meters (1/2 mile) in all directions.

EMERGENCY RESPONSE

FIRE

Small Fire

• Dry chemical, CO_2 or water spray.

Large Fire

• Water spray, fog or regular foam.
• Move containers from fire area if you can do it without risk.
• Dike fire-control water for later disposal; do not scatter the material.
• Use water spray or fog; do not use straight streams.

Fire involving Tanks or Car/Trailer Loads

• Fight fire from maximum distance or use unmanned hose holders or monitor nozzles.
• Do not get water inside containers.
• Cool containers with flooding quantities of water until well after fire is out.
• Withdraw immediately in case of rising sound from venting safety devices or discoloration of tank.
• ALWAYS stay away from tanks engulfed in fire.
• For massive fire, use unmanned hose holders or monitor nozzles; if this is impossible, withdraw from area and let fire burn.

SPILL OR LEAK

• Do not touch damaged containers or spilled material unless wearing appropriate protective clothing.
• Stop leak if you can do it without risk.
• Prevent entry into waterways, sewers, basements or confined areas.
• Cover with plastic sheet to prevent spreading.
• Absorb or cover with dry earth, sand or other non-combustible material and transfer to containers.
• DO NOT GET WATER INSIDE CONTAINERS.

FIRST AID

• Move victim to fresh air.   • Call 911 or emergency medical service.
• Give artificial respiration if victim is not breathing.
• **Do not use mouth-to-mouth method if victim ingested or inhaled the substance; give artificial respiration with the aid of a pocket mask equipped with a one-way valve or other proper respiratory medical device.**
• Administer oxygen if breathing is difficult.
• Remove and isolate contaminated clothing and shoes.
• In case of contact with substance, immediately flush skin or eyes with running water for at least 20 minutes.
• For minor skin contact, avoid spreading material on unaffected skin.
• Keep victim warm and quiet.
• Effects of exposure (inhalation, ingestion or skin contact) to substance may be delayed.
• Ensure that medical personnel are aware of the material(s) involved and take precautions to protect themselves.

POTENTIAL HAZARDS

HEALTH

- **Highly toxic**, may be fatal if inhaled, swallowed or absorbed through skin.
- Contact with molten substance may cause severe burns to skin and eyes.
- Avoid any skin contact.
- Effects of contact or inhalation may be delayed.
- Fire may produce irritating, corrosive and/or toxic gases.
- Runoff from fire control or dilution water may be corrosive and/or toxic and cause pollution.

FIRE OR EXPLOSION

- Combustible material: may burn but does not ignite readily.
- Containers may explode when heated.
- Runoff may pollute waterways.
- Substance may be transported in a molten form.

PUBLIC SAFETY

- **CALL Emergency Response Telephone Number on Shipping Paper first. If Shipping Paper not available or no answer, refer to appropriate telephone number listed on the inside back cover.**
- As an immediate precautionary measure, isolate spill or leak area in all directions for at least 50 meters (150 feet) for liquids and at least 25 meters (75 feet) for solids.
- Keep unauthorized personnel away.
- Stay upwind.
- Keep out of low areas.

PROTECTIVE CLOTHING

- Wear positive pressure self-contained breathing apparatus (SCBA).
- Wear chemical protective clothing that is specifically recommended by the manufacturer. It may provide little or no thermal protection.
- Structural firefighters' protective clothing provides limited protection in fire situations ONLY; it is not effective in spill situations where direct contact with the substance is possible.

EVACUATION

Spill

- See Table 1 - Initial Isolation and Protective Action Distances for highlighted materials. For non-highlighted materials, increase, in the downwind direction, as necessary, the isolation distance shown under "PUBLIC SAFETY".

Fire

- If tank, rail car or tank truck is involved in a fire, ISOLATE for 800 meters (1/2 mile) in all directions; also, consider initial evacuation for 800 meters (1/2 mile) in all directions.

EMERGENCY RESPONSE

FIRE

Small Fire

- Dry chemical, CO_2 or water spray.

Large Fire

- Water spray, fog or regular foam.
- Move containers from fire area if you can do it without risk.
- Dike fire-control water for later disposal; do not scatter the material.
- Use water spray or fog; do not use straight streams.

Fire involving Tanks or Car/Trailer Loads

- Fight fire from maximum distance or use unmanned hose holders or monitor nozzles.
- Do not get water inside containers.
- Cool containers with flooding quantities of water until well after fire is out.
- Withdraw immediately in case of rising sound from venting safety devices or discoloration of tank.
- ALWAYS stay away from tanks engulfed in fire.
- For massive fire, use unmanned hose holders or monitor nozzles; if this is impossible, withdraw from area and let fire burn.

SPILL OR LEAK

- ELIMINATE all ignition sources (no smoking, flares, sparks or flames in immediate area).
- Do not touch damaged containers or spilled material unless wearing appropriate protective clothing.
- Stop leak if you can do it without risk.
- Prevent entry into waterways, sewers, basements or confined areas.
- Cover with plastic sheet to prevent spreading.
- Absorb or cover with dry earth, sand or other non-combustible material and transfer to containers.
- DO NOT GET WATER INSIDE CONTAINERS.

FIRST AID

- Move victim to fresh air.   • Call 911 or emergency medical service.
- Give artificial respiration if victim is not breathing.
- **Do not use mouth-to-mouth method if victim ingested or inhaled the substance; give artificial respiration with the aid of a pocket mask equipped with a one-way valve or other proper respiratory medical device.**
- Administer oxygen if breathing is difficult.
- Remove and isolate contaminated clothing and shoes.
- In case of contact with substance, immediately flush skin or eyes with running water for at least 20 minutes.
- For minor skin contact, avoid spreading material on unaffected skin.
- Keep victim warm and quiet.
- Effects of exposure (inhalation, ingestion or skin contact) to substance may be delayed.
- Ensure that medical personnel are aware of the material(s) involved and take precautions to protect themselves.

POTENTIAL HAZARDS

HEALTH
- **TOXIC**; inhalation, ingestion or skin contact with material may cause severe injury or death.
- Contact with molten substance may cause severe burns to skin and eyes.
- Avoid any skin contact.
- Effects of contact or inhalation may be delayed.
- Fire may produce irritating, corrosive and/or toxic gases.
- Runoff from fire control or dilution water may be corrosive and/or toxic and cause pollution.

FIRE OR EXPLOSION
- Combustible material: may burn but does not ignite readily.
- When heated, vapors may form explosive mixtures with air: indoors, outdoors and sewers explosion hazards.
- Those substances designated with a **"P"** may polymerize explosively when heated or involved in a fire.
- Contact with metals may evolve flammable hydrogen gas.
- Containers may explode when heated.
- Runoff may pollute waterways.
- Substance may be transported in a molten form.

PUBLIC SAFETY
- **CALL Emergency Response Telephone Number on Shipping Paper first. If Shipping Paper not available or no answer, refer to appropriate telephone number listed on the inside back cover.**
- As an immediate precautionary measure, isolate spill or leak area in all directions for at least 50 meters (150 feet) for liquids and at least 25 meters (75 feet) for solids.
- Keep unauthorized personnel away.
- Stay upwind.   • Keep out of low areas.   • Ventilate enclosed areas.

PROTECTIVE CLOTHING
- Wear positive pressure self-contained breathing apparatus (SCBA).
- Wear chemical protective clothing that is specifically recommended by the manufacturer. It may provide little or no thermal protection.
- Structural firefighters' protective clothing provides limited protection in fire situations ONLY; it is not effective in spill situations where direct contact with the substance is possible.

EVACUATION
Spill
- See Table 1 - Initial Isolation and Protective Action Distances for highlighted materials. For non-highlighted materials, increase, in the downwind direction, as necessary, the isolation distance shown under "PUBLIC SAFETY".
Fire
- If tank, rail car or tank truck is involved in a fire, ISOLATE for 800 meters (1/2 mile) in all directions; also, consider initial evacuation for 800 meters (1/2 mile) in all directions.

EMERGENCY RESPONSE

FIRE

Small Fire
- Dry chemical, CO_2 or water spray.

Large Fire
- Dry chemical, CO_2, alcohol-resistant foam or water spray.
- Move containers from fire area if you can do it without risk.
- Dike fire-control water for later disposal; do not scatter the material.

Fire involving Tanks or Car/Trailer Loads
- Fight fire from maximum distance or use unmanned hose holders or monitor nozzles.
- Do not get water inside containers.
- Cool containers with flooding quantities of water until well after fire is out.
- Withdraw immediately in case of rising sound from venting safety devices or discoloration of tank.
- ALWAYS stay away from tanks engulfed in fire.

SPILL OR LEAK

- ELIMINATE all ignition sources (no smoking, flares, sparks or flames in immediate area).
- Do not touch damaged containers or spilled material unless wearing appropriate protective clothing.
- Stop leak if you can do it without risk.
- Prevent entry into waterways, sewers, basements or confined areas.
- Absorb or cover with dry earth, sand or other non-combustible material and transfer to containers.
- DO NOT GET WATER INSIDE CONTAINERS.

FIRST AID

- Move victim to fresh air.   • Call 911 or emergency medical service.
- Give artificial respiration if victim is not breathing.
- **Do not use mouth-to-mouth method if victim ingested or inhaled the substance; give artificial respiration with the aid of a pocket mask equipped with a one-way valve or other proper respiratory medical device.**
- Administer oxygen if breathing is difficult.
- Remove and isolate contaminated clothing and shoes.
- In case of contact with substance, immediately flush skin or eyes with running water for at least 20 minutes.
- For minor skin contact, avoid spreading material on unaffected skin.
- Keep victim warm and quiet.
- Effects of exposure (inhalation, ingestion or skin contact) to substance may be delayed.
- Ensure that medical personnel are aware of the material(s) involved and take precautions to protect themselves.

POTENTIAL HAZARDS

HEALTH
- **TOXIC**; inhalation, ingestion or skin contact with material may cause severe injury or death.
- Contact with molten substance may cause severe burns to skin and eyes.
- Avoid any skin contact.
- Effects of contact or inhalation may be delayed.
- Fire may produce irritating, corrosive and/or toxic gases.
- Runoff from fire control or dilution water may be corrosive and/or toxic and cause pollution.

FIRE OR EXPLOSION
- Non-combustible, substance itself does not burn but may decompose upon heating to produce corrosive and/or toxic fumes.
- Some are oxidizers and may ignite combustibles (wood, paper, oil, clothing, etc.).
- Contact with metals may evolve flammable hydrogen gas.
- Containers may explode when heated.

PUBLIC SAFETY
- **CALL Emergency Response Telephone Number on Shipping Paper first. If Shipping Paper not available or no answer, refer to appropriate telephone number listed on the inside back cover.**
- As an immediate precautionary measure, isolate spill or leak area in all directions for at least 50 meters (150 feet) for liquids and at least 25 meters (75 feet) for solids.
- Keep unauthorized personnel away.
- Stay upwind.
- Keep out of low areas.
- Ventilate enclosed areas.

PROTECTIVE CLOTHING
- Wear positive pressure self-contained breathing apparatus (SCBA).
- Wear chemical protective clothing that is specifically recommended by the manufacturer. It may provide little or no thermal protection.
- Structural firefighters' protective clothing provides limited protection in fire situations ONLY; it is not effective in spill situations where direct contact with the substance is possible.

EVACUATION
Spill
- See Table 1 - Initial Isolation and Protective Action Distances for highlighted materials. For non-highlighted materials, increase, in the downwind direction, as necessary, the isolation distance shown under "PUBLIC SAFETY".

Fire
- If tank, rail car or tank truck is involved in a fire, ISOLATE for 800 meters (1/2 mile) in all directions; also, consider initial evacuation for 800 meters (1/2 mile) in all directions.

EMERGENCY RESPONSE

FIRE

Small Fire

- Dry chemical, CO_2 or water spray.

Large Fire

- Dry chemical, CO_2, alcohol-resistant foam or water spray.
- Move containers from fire area if you can do it without risk.
- Dike fire-control water for later disposal; do not scatter the material.

Fire involving Tanks or Car/Trailer Loads

- Fight fire from maximum distance or use unmanned hose holders or monitor nozzles.
- Do not get water inside containers.
- Cool containers with flooding quantities of water until well after fire is out.
- Withdraw immediately in case of rising sound from venting safety devices or discoloration of tank.
- ALWAYS stay away from tanks engulfed in fire.

SPILL OR LEAK

- ELIMINATE all ignition sources (no smoking, flares, sparks or flames in immediate area).
- Do not touch damaged containers or spilled material unless wearing appropriate protective clothing.
- Stop leak if you can do it without risk.
- Prevent entry into waterways, sewers, basements or confined areas.
- Absorb or cover with dry earth, sand or other non-combustible material and transfer to containers.
- DO NOT GET WATER INSIDE CONTAINERS.

FIRST AID

- Move victim to fresh air.   • Call 911 or emergency medical service.
- Give artificial respiration if victim is not breathing.
- **Do not use mouth-to-mouth method if victim ingested or inhaled the substance; give artificial respiration with the aid of a pocket mask equipped with a one-way valve or other proper respiratory medical device.**
- Administer oxygen if breathing is difficult.
- Remove and isolate contaminated clothing and shoes.
- In case of contact with substance, immediately flush skin or eyes with running water for at least 20 minutes.
- For minor skin contact, avoid spreading material on unaffected skin.
- Keep victim warm and quiet.
- Effects of exposure (inhalation, ingestion or skin contact) to substance may be delayed.
- Ensure that medical personnel are aware of the material(s) involved and take precautions to protect themselves.

POTENTIAL HAZARDS

FIRE OR EXPLOSION

- **HIGHLY FLAMMABLE: Will be easily ignited by heat, sparks or flames.**
- Vapors form explosive mixtures with air: indoors, outdoors and sewers explosion hazards.
- Most vapors are heavier than air. They will spread along ground and collect in low or confined areas (sewers, basements, tanks).
- Vapors may travel to source of ignition and flash back.
- Those substances designated with a "**P**" may polymerize explosively when heated or involved in a fire.
- Substance will react with water (some violently) releasing flammable, toxic or corrosive gases and runoff.
- Contact with metals may evolve flammable hydrogen gas.
- Containers may explode when heated or if contaminated with water.

HEALTH

- **TOXIC;** inhalation, ingestion or contact (skin, eyes) with vapors, dusts or substance may cause severe injury, burns or death.
- **Bromoacetates and chloroacetates are extremely irritating/lachrymators.**
- Reaction with water or moist air will release toxic, corrosive or flammable gases.
- Reaction with water may generate much heat that will increase the concentration of fumes in the air.
- Fire will produce irritating, corrosive and/or toxic gases.
- Runoff from fire control or dilution water may be corrosive and/or toxic and cause pollution.

PUBLIC SAFETY

- **CALL Emergency Response Telephone Number on Shipping Paper first. If Shipping Paper not available or no answer, refer to appropriate telephone number listed on the inside back cover.**
- As an immediate precautionary measure, isolate spill or leak area in all directions for at least 50 meters (150 feet) for liquids and at least 25 meters (75 feet) for solids.
- Keep unauthorized personnel away.
- Stay upwind. • Keep out of low areas. • Ventilate enclosed areas.

PROTECTIVE CLOTHING

- Wear positive pressure self-contained breathing apparatus (SCBA).
- Wear chemical protective clothing that is specifically recommended by the manufacturer. It may provide little or no thermal protection.
- Structural firefighters' protective clothing provides limited protection in fire situations ONLY; it is not effective in spill situations where direct contact with the substance is possible.

EVACUATION

Spill

- See Table 1 - Initial Isolation and Protective Action Distances for highlighted materials. For non-highlighted materials, increase, in the downwind direction, as necessary, the isolation distance shown under "PUBLIC SAFETY".

Fire

- If tank, rail car or tank truck is involved in a fire, ISOLATE for 800 meters (1/2 mile) in all directions; also, consider initial evacuation for 800 meters (1/2 mile) in all directions.

EMERGENCY RESPONSE

FIRE

- Note: Most foams will react with the material and release corrosive/toxic gases.
- **CAUTION: For Acetyl chloride (UN1717), use CO_2 or dry chemical only.**
- **Small Fire** • CO_2, dry chemical, dry sand, alcohol-resistant foam.
- **Large Fire**
- Water spray, fog or alcohol-resistant foam.
- **FOR CHLOROSILANES, DO NOT USE WATER**; use AFFF alcohol-resistant medium expansion foam.
- Move containers from fire area if you can do it without risk.
- Use water spray or fog; do not use straight streams.
- **Fire involving Tanks or Car/Trailer Loads**
- Fight fire from maximum distance or use unmanned hose holders or monitor nozzles.
- Do not get water inside containers.
- Cool containers with flooding quantities of water until well after fire is out.
- Withdraw immediately in case of rising sound from venting safety devices or discoloration of tank.
- ALWAYS stay away from tanks engulfed in fire.

SPILL OR LEAK

- ELIMINATE all ignition sources (no smoking, flares, sparks or flames in immediate area).
- All equipment used when handling the product must be grounded.
- Do not touch damaged containers or spilled material unless wearing appropriate protective clothing.
- Stop leak if you can do it without risk.
- A vapor suppressing foam may be used to reduce vapors.
- **FOR CHLOROSILANES**, use AFFF alcohol-resistant medium expansion foam to reduce vapors.
- **DO NOT GET WATER on spilled substance or inside containers.**
- Use water spray to reduce vapors or divert vapor cloud drift. Avoid allowing water runoff to contact spilled material.
- Prevent entry into waterways, sewers, basements or confined areas.
- **Small Spill** • Cover with DRY earth, DRY sand or other non-combustible material followed with plastic sheet to minimize spreading or contact with rain.
- Use clean non-sparking tools to collect material and place it into loosely covered plastic containers for later disposal.

FIRST AID

- Move victim to fresh air. • Call 911 or emergency medical service.
- Give artificial respiration if victim is not breathing.
- **Do not use mouth-to-mouth method if victim ingested or inhaled the substance; give artificial respiration with the aid of a pocket mask equipped with a one-way valve or other proper respiratory medical device.**
- Administer oxygen if breathing is difficult.
- Remove and isolate contaminated clothing and shoes.
- In case of contact with substance, immediately flush skin or eyes with running water for at least 20 minutes.
- For minor skin contact, avoid spreading material on unaffected skin.
- Keep victim warm and quiet.
- Effects of exposure (inhalation, ingestion or skin contact) to substance may be delayed.
- Ensure that medical personnel are aware of the material(s) involved and take precautions to protect themselves.

POTENTIAL HAZARDS

FIRE OR EXPLOSION

- Combustible material: may burn but does not ignite readily.
- Substance will react with water (some violently) releasing flammable, toxic or corrosive gases and runoff.
- When heated, vapors may form explosive mixtures with air: indoors, outdoors and sewers explosion hazards.
- Most vapors are heavier than air. They will spread along ground and collect in low or confined areas (sewers, basements, tanks).
- Vapors may travel to source of ignition and flash back.
- Contact with metals may evolve flammable hydrogen gas.
- Containers may explode when heated or if contaminated with water.

HEALTH

- **TOXIC;** inhalation, ingestion or contact (skin, eyes) with vapors, dusts or substance may cause severe injury, burns or death.
- Contact with molten substance may cause severe burns to skin and eyes.
- Reaction with water or moist air will release toxic, corrosive or flammable gases.
- Reaction with water may generate much heat that will increase the concentration of fumes in the air.
- Fire will produce irritating, corrosive and/or toxic gases.
- Runoff from fire control or dilution water may be corrosive and/or toxic and cause pollution.

PUBLIC SAFETY

- **CALL Emergency Response Telephone Number on Shipping Paper first. If Shipping Paper not available or no answer, refer to appropriate telephone number listed on the inside back cover.**
- As an immediate precautionary measure, isolate spill or leak area in all directions for at least 50 meters (150 feet) for liquids and at least 25 meters (75 feet) for solids.
- Keep unauthorized personnel away.
- Stay upwind.   • Keep out of low areas.   • Ventilate enclosed areas.

PROTECTIVE CLOTHING

- Wear positive pressure self-contained breathing apparatus (SCBA).
- Wear chemical protective clothing that is specifically recommended by the manufacturer. It may provide little or no thermal protection.
- Structural firefighters' protective clothing provides limited protection in fire situations ONLY; it is not effective in spill situations where direct contact with the substance is possible.

EVACUATION

Spill

- See Table 1 - Initial Isolation and Protective Action Distances for highlighted materials. For non-highlighted materials, increase, in the downwind direction, as necessary, the isolation distance shown under "PUBLIC SAFETY".

Fire

- If tank, rail car or tank truck is involved in a fire, ISOLATE for 800 meters (1/2 mile) in all directions; also, consider initial evacuation for 800 meters (1/2 mile) in all directions.

EMERGENCY RESPONSE

FIRE
- Note: Most foams will react with the material and release corrosive/toxic gases.
- **Small Fire** • CO_2, dry chemical, dry sand, alcohol-resistant foam.
- **Large Fire**
- Water spray, fog or alcohol-resistant foam.
- **FOR CHLOROSILANES, DO NOT USE WATER**; use AFFF alcohol-resistant medium expansion foam.
- Move containers from fire area if you can do it without risk.
- Use water spray or fog; do not use straight streams.
- **Fire involving Tanks or Car/Trailer Loads**
- Fight fire from maximum distance or use unmanned hose holders or monitor nozzles.
- Do not get water inside containers.
- Cool containers with flooding quantities of water until well after fire is out.
- Withdraw immediately in case of rising sound from venting safety devices or discoloration of tank.
- ALWAYS stay away from tanks engulfed in fire.

SPILL OR LEAK
- ELIMINATE all ignition sources (no smoking, flares, sparks or flames in immediate area).
- All equipment used when handling the product must be grounded.
- Do not touch damaged containers or spilled material unless wearing appropriate protective clothing.
- Stop leak if you can do it without risk.
- A vapor suppressing foam may be used to reduce vapors.
- **FOR CHLOROSILANES**, use AFFF alcohol-resistant medium expansion foam to reduce vapors.
- **DO NOT GET WATER on spilled substance or inside containers.**
- Use water spray to reduce vapors or divert vapor cloud drift. Avoid allowing water runoff to contact spilled material.
- Prevent entry into waterways, sewers, basements or confined areas.
- **Small Spill** • Cover with DRY earth, DRY sand or other non-combustible material followed with plastic sheet to minimize spreading or contact with rain.
- Use clean non-sparking tools to collect material and place it into loosely covered plastic containers for later disposal.

FIRST AID
- Move victim to fresh air. • Call 911 or emergency medical service.
- Give artificial respiration if victim is not breathing.
- **Do not use mouth-to-mouth method if victim ingested or inhaled the substance; give artificial respiration with the aid of a pocket mask equipped with a one-way valve or other proper respiratory medical device.**
- Administer oxygen if breathing is difficult.
- Remove and isolate contaminated clothing and shoes.
- In case of contact with substance, immediately flush skin or eyes with running water for at least 20 minutes.
- For minor skin contact, avoid spreading material on unaffected skin.
- Keep victim warm and quiet.
- Effects of exposure (inhalation, ingestion or skin contact) to substance may be delayed.
- Ensure that medical personnel are aware of the material(s) involved and take precautions to protect themselves.

POTENTIAL HAZARDS

HEALTH

- **TOXIC**; inhalation, ingestion or contact (skin, eyes) with vapors, dusts or substance may cause severe injury, burns or death.
- Reaction with water or moist air will release toxic, corrosive or flammable gases.
- Reaction with water may generate much heat that will increase the concentration of fumes in the air.
- Fire will produce irritating, corrosive and/or toxic gases.
- Runoff from fire control or dilution water may be corrosive and/or toxic and cause pollution.

FIRE OR EXPLOSION

- Non-combustible, substance itself does not burn but may decompose upon heating to produce corrosive and/or toxic fumes.
- Vapors may accumulate in confined areas (basement, tanks, hopper/tank cars etc.).
- Substance will react with water (some violently), releasing corrosive and/or toxic gases and runoff.
- Contact with metals may evolve flammable hydrogen gas.
- Containers may explode when heated or if contaminated with water.

PUBLIC SAFETY

- **CALL Emergency Response Telephone Number on Shipping Paper first. If Shipping Paper not available or no answer, refer to appropriate telephone number listed on the inside back cover.**
- As an immediate precautionary measure, isolate spill or leak area in all directions for at least 50 meters (150 feet) for liquids and at least 25 meters (75 feet) for solids.
- Keep unauthorized personnel away.
- Stay upwind.
- Keep out of low areas.
- Ventilate enclosed areas.

PROTECTIVE CLOTHING

- Wear positive pressure self-contained breathing apparatus (SCBA).
- Wear chemical protective clothing that is specifically recommended by the manufacturer. It may provide little or no thermal protection.
- Structural firefighters' protective clothing provides limited protection in fire situations ONLY; it is not effective in spill situations where direct contact with the substance is possible.

EVACUATION

Spill

- See Table 1 - Initial Isolation and Protective Action Distances for highlighted materials. For non-highlighted materials, increase, in the downwind direction, as necessary, the isolation distance shown under "PUBLIC SAFETY".

Fire

- If tank, rail car or tank truck is involved in a fire, ISOLATE for 800 meters (1/2 mile) in all directions; also, consider initial evacuation for 800 meters (1/2 mile) in all directions.

EMERGENCY RESPONSE

FIRE
- Note: Most foams will react with the material and release corrosive/toxic gases.

Small Fire • CO_2 (except for Cyanides), dry chemical, dry sand, alcohol-resistant foam.

Large Fire
- Water spray, fog or alcohol-resistant foam.
- Move containers from fire area if you can do it without risk.
- Use water spray or fog; do not use straight streams.
- Dike fire-control water for later disposal; do not scatter the material.

Fire involving Tanks or Car/Trailer Loads
- Fight fire from maximum distance or use unmanned hose holders or monitor nozzles.
- Do not get water inside containers.
- Cool containers with flooding quantities of water until well after fire is out.
- Withdraw immediately in case of rising sound from venting safety devices or discoloration of tank.
- ALWAYS stay away from tanks engulfed in fire.

SPILL OR LEAK
- ELIMINATE all ignition sources (no smoking, flares, sparks or flames in immediate area).
- All equipment used when handling the product must be grounded.
- Do not touch damaged containers or spilled material unless wearing appropriate protective clothing.
- Stop leak if you can do it without risk.
- A vapor suppressing foam may be used to reduce vapors.
- DO NOT GET WATER INSIDE CONTAINERS.
- Use water spray to reduce vapors or divert vapor cloud drift. Avoid allowing water runoff to contact spilled material.
- Prevent entry into waterways, sewers, basements or confined areas.

Small Spill • Cover with DRY earth, DRY sand or other non-combustible material followed with plastic sheet to minimize spreading or contact with rain.
- Use clean non-sparking tools to collect material and place it into loosely covered plastic containers for later disposal.

FIRST AID
- Move victim to fresh air.   • Call 911 or emergency medical service.
- Give artificial respiration if victim is not breathing.
- **Do not use mouth-to-mouth method if victim ingested or inhaled the substance; give artificial respiration with the aid of a pocket mask equipped with a one-way valve or other proper respiratory medical device.**
- Administer oxygen if breathing is difficult.
- Remove and isolate contaminated clothing and shoes.
- In case of contact with substance, immediately flush skin or eyes with running water for at least 20 minutes.
- For minor skin contact, avoid spreading material on unaffected skin.
- Keep victim warm and quiet.
- Effects of exposure (inhalation, ingestion or skin contact) to substance may be delayed.
- Ensure that medical personnel are aware of the material(s) involved and take precautions to protect themselves.

POTENTIAL HAZARDS

HEALTH

• Inhalation or contact with substance may cause infection, disease or death.
• Runoff from fire control may cause pollution.
• **Note: Damaged packages containing solid CO_2 as a refrigerant may produce water or frost from condensation of air. Do not touch this liquid as it could be contaminated by the contents of the parcel.**

FIRE OR EXPLOSION

• Some of these materials may burn, but none ignite readily.
• Some may be transported in flammable liquids.

PUBLIC SAFETY

• **CALL Emergency Response Telephone Number on Shipping Paper first. If Shipping Paper not available or no answer, refer to appropriate telephone number listed on the inside back cover.**
• As an immediate precautionary measure, isolate spill or leak area for at least 25 meters (75 feet) in all directions.
• Keep unauthorized personnel away.
• Stay upwind.
• Obtain identity of substance involved.

PROTECTIVE CLOTHING

• Wear positive pressure self-contained breathing apparatus (SCBA).
• Structural firefighters' protective clothing will only provide limited protection.

EMERGENCY RESPONSE

FIRE

Small Fire

- Dry chemical, soda ash, lime or sand.

Large Fire

- Use extinguishing agent suitable for type of surrounding fire.
- Do not scatter spilled material with high pressure water streams.
- Move containers from fire area if you can do it without risk.

SPILL OR LEAK

- Do not touch or walk through spilled material.
- Do not touch damaged containers or spilled material unless wearing appropriate protective clothing.
- Absorb with earth, sand or other non-combustible material.
- Cover damaged package or spilled material with damp towel or rag and keep wet with liquid bleach or other disinfectant.
- **DO NOT CLEAN-UP OR DISPOSE OF, EXCEPT UNDER SUPERVISION OF A SPECIALIST.**

FIRST AID

- Move victim to a safe isolated area.

CAUTION: Victim may be a source of contamination.

- Call 911 or emergency medical service.
- Remove and isolate contaminated clothing and shoes.
- In case of contact with substance, immediately flush skin or eyes with running water for at least 20 minutes.
- Effects of exposure (inhalation, ingestion or skin contact) to substance may be delayed.
- **For further assistance, contact your local Poison Control Center.**
- Ensure that medical personnel are aware of the material(s) involved and take precautions to protect themselves.

POTENTIAL HAZARDS

HEALTH

- Inhalation of vapors or dust is extremely irritating.
- May cause burning of eyes and flow of tears.
- May cause coughing, difficult breathing and nausea.
- Brief exposure effects last only a few minutes.
- Exposure in an enclosed area may be very harmful.
- Fire will produce irritating, corrosive and/or toxic gases.
- Runoff from fire control or dilution water may cause pollution.

FIRE OR EXPLOSION

- Some of these materials may burn, but none ignite readily.
- Containers may explode when heated.

PUBLIC SAFETY

- **CALL Emergency Response Telephone Number on Shipping Paper first. If Shipping Paper not available or no answer, refer to appropriate telephone number listed on the inside back cover.**
- As an immediate precautionary measure, isolate spill or leak area in all directions for at least 50 meters (150 feet) for liquids and at least 25 meters (75 feet) for solids.
- Keep unauthorized personnel away.
- Stay upwind.
- Keep out of low areas.
- Ventilate closed spaces before entering.

PROTECTIVE CLOTHING

- Wear positive pressure self-contained breathing apparatus (SCBA).
- Wear chemical protective clothing that is specifically recommended by the manufacturer. It may provide little or no thermal protection.
- Structural firefighters' protective clothing provides limited protection in fire situations ONLY; it is not effective in spill situations where direct contact with the substance is possible.

EVACUATION

Large Spill

- See Table 1 - Initial Isolation and Protective Action Distances for highlighted materials. For non-highlighted materials, increase, in the downwind direction, as necessary, the isolation distance shown under "PUBLIC SAFETY".

Fire

- If tank, rail car or tank truck is involved in a fire, ISOLATE for 800 meters (1/2 mile) in all directions; also, consider initial evacuation for 800 meters (1/2 mile) in all directions.

EMERGENCY RESPONSE

FIRE
Small Fire
- Dry chemical, CO_2, water spray or regular foam.

Large Fire
- Water spray, fog or regular foam.
- Move containers from fire area if you can do it without risk.
- Dike fire-control water for later disposal; do not scatter the material.

Fire involving Tanks or Car/Trailer Loads
- Fight fire from maximum distance or use unmanned hose holders or monitor nozzles.
- Do not get water inside containers.
- Cool containers with flooding quantities of water until well after fire is out.
- Withdraw immediately in case of rising sound from venting safety devices or discoloration of tank.
- ALWAYS stay away from tanks engulfed in fire.
- For massive fire, use unmanned hose holders or monitor nozzles; if this is impossible, withdraw from area and let fire burn.

SPILL OR LEAK
- Do not touch or walk through spilled material.
- Stop leak if you can do it without risk.
- Fully encapsulating, vapor protective clothing should be worn for spills and leaks with no fire.

Small Spill
- Take up with sand or other non-combustible absorbent material and place into containers for later disposal.

Large Spill
- Dike far ahead of liquid spill for later disposal.
- Prevent entry into waterways, sewers, basements or confined areas.

FIRST AID
- Move victim to fresh air.   • Call 911 or emergency medical service.
- Give artificial respiration if victim is not breathing.
- **Do not use mouth-to-mouth method if victim ingested or inhaled the substance; give artificial respiration with the aid of a pocket mask equipped with a one-way valve or other proper respiratory medical device.**
- Administer oxygen if breathing is difficult.
- Remove and isolate contaminated clothing and shoes.
- In case of contact with substance, immediately flush skin or eyes with running water for at least 20 minutes.
- For minor skin contact, avoid spreading material on unaffected skin.
- Keep victim warm and quiet.
- Effects should disappear after individual has been exposed to fresh air for approximately 10 minutes.
- Ensure that medical personnel are aware of the material(s) involved and take precautions to protect themselves.

POTENTIAL HAZARDS

HEALTH
- Toxic by ingestion.
- Vapors may cause dizziness or suffocation.
- Exposure in an enclosed area may be very harmful.
- Contact may irritate or burn skin and eyes.
- Fire may produce irritating and/or toxic gases.
- Runoff from fire control or dilution water may cause pollution.

FIRE OR EXPLOSION
- Some of these materials may burn, but none ignite readily.
- Most vapors are heavier than air.
- Air/vapor mixtures may explode when ignited.
- Container may explode in heat of fire.

PUBLIC SAFETY

- **CALL Emergency Response Telephone Number on Shipping Paper first. If Shipping Paper not available or no answer, refer to appropriate telephone number listed on the inside back cover.**
- As an immediate precautionary measure, isolate spill or leak area for at least 50 meters (150 feet) in all directions.
- Keep unauthorized personnel away.
- Stay upwind.
- Many gases are heavier than air and will spread along ground and collect in low or confined areas (sewers, basements, tanks).
- Keep out of low areas.
- Ventilate closed spaces before entering.

PROTECTIVE CLOTHING
- Wear positive pressure self-contained breathing apparatus (SCBA).
- Wear chemical protective clothing that is specifically recommended by the manufacturer.
- Structural firefighters' protective clothing will only provide limited protection.

EVACUATION
Large Spill
- Consider initial downwind evacuation for at least 100 meters (330 feet).

Fire
- If tank, rail car or tank truck is involved in a fire, ISOLATE for 800 meters (1/2 mile) in all directions; also, consider initial evacuation for 800 meters (1/2 mile) in all directions.

EMERGENCY RESPONSE

FIRE

Small Fire

- Dry chemical, CO_2 or water spray.

Large Fire

- Dry chemical, CO_2, alcohol-resistant foam or water spray.
- Move containers from fire area if you can do it without risk.
- Dike fire-control water for later disposal; do not scatter the material.

Fire involving Tanks or Car/Trailer Loads

- Fight fire from maximum distance or use unmanned hose holders or monitor nozzles.
- Cool containers with flooding quantities of water until well after fire is out.
- Withdraw immediately in case of rising sound from venting safety devices or discoloration of tank.
- ALWAYS stay away from tanks engulfed in fire.

SPILL OR LEAK

- ELIMINATE all ignition sources (no smoking, flares, sparks or flames in immediate area).
- Stop leak if you can do it without risk.

Small Liquid Spill

- Take up with sand, earth or other non-combustible absorbent material.

Large Spill

- Dike far ahead of liquid spill for later disposal.
- Prevent entry into waterways, sewers, basements or confined areas.

FIRST AID

- Move victim to fresh air.   • Call 911 or emergency medical service.
- Give artificial respiration if victim is not breathing.
- Administer oxygen if breathing is difficult.
- Remove and isolate contaminated clothing and shoes.
- In case of contact with substance, immediately flush skin or eyes with running water for at least 20 minutes.
- For minor skin contact, avoid spreading material on unaffected skin.
- Wash skin with soap and water.
- Keep victim warm and quiet.
- Ensure that medical personnel are aware of the material(s) involved and take precautions to protect themselves.

POTENTIAL HAZARDS

HEALTH

- Radiation presents minimal risk to transport workers, emergency response personnel and the public during transportation accidents. Packaging durability increases as potential hazard of radioactive content increases.
- Very low levels of contained radioactive materials and low radiation levels outside packages result in low risks to people. Damaged packages may release measurable amounts of radioactive material, but the resulting risks are expected to be low.
- Some radioactive materials cannot be detected by commonly available instruments.
- Packages do not have RADIOACTIVE I, II, or III labels. Some may have EMPTY labels or may have the word "Radioactive" in the package marking.

FIRE OR EXPLOSION

- Some of these materials may burn, but most do not ignite readily.
- Many have cardboard outer packaging; content (physically large or small) can be of many different physical forms.
- Radioactivity does not change flammability or other properties of materials.

PUBLIC SAFETY

- **CALL Emergency Response Telephone Number on Shipping Paper first. If Shipping Paper not available or no answer, refer to appropriate telephone number listed on the inside back cover.**
- **Priorities for rescue, life-saving, first aid, fire control and other hazards are higher than the priority for measuring radiation levels.**
- Radiation Authority must be notified of accident conditions. Radiation Authority is usually responsible for decisions about radiological consequences and closure of emergencies.
- As an immediate precautionary measure, isolate spill or leak area for at least 25 meters (75 feet) in all directions.
- Stay upwind.
- Keep unauthorized personnel away.
- Detain or isolate uninjured persons or equipment suspected to be contaminated; delay decontamination and cleanup until instructions are received from Radiation Authority.

PROTECTIVE CLOTHING

- Positive pressure self-contained breathing apparatus (SCBA) and structural firefighters' protective clothing will provide adequate protection.

EVACUATION

Large Spill

- Consider initial downwind evacuation for at least 100 meters (330 feet).

Fire

- When a large quantity of this material is involved in a major fire, consider an initial evacuation distance of 300 meters (1000 feet) in all directions.

EMERGENCY RESPONSE

FIRE
- Presence of radioactive material will not influence the fire control processes and should not influence selection of techniques.
- Move containers from fire area if you can do it without risk.
- Do not move damaged packages; move undamaged packages out of fire zone.

Small Fire
- Dry chemical, CO_2, water spray or regular foam.

Large Fire
- Water spray, fog (flooding amounts).

SPILL OR LEAK
- Do not touch damaged packages or spilled material.
- Cover liquid spill with sand, earth or other non-combustible absorbent material.
- Cover powder spill with plastic sheet or tarp to minimize spreading.

FIRST AID
- Call 911 or emergency medical service.
- Medical problems take priority over radiological concerns.
- Use first aid treatment according to the nature of the injury.
- Do not delay care and transport of a seriously injured person.
- Give artificial respiration if victim is not breathing.
- Administer oxygen if breathing is difficult.
- In case of contact with substance, immediately flush skin or eyes with running water for at least 20 minutes.
- Injured persons contaminated by contact with released material are not a serious hazard to health care personnel, equipment or facilities.
- Ensure that medical personnel are aware of the material(s) involved, take precautions to protect themselves and prevent spread of contamination.

POTENTIAL HAZARDS

HEALTH

• Radiation presents minimal risk to transport workers, emergency response personnel and the public during transportation accidents. Packaging durability increases as potential hazard of radioactive content increases.
• Undamaged packages are safe. Contents of damaged packages may cause higher external radiation exposure, or both external and internal radiation exposure if contents are released.
• Low radiation hazard when material is inside container. If material is released from package or bulk container, hazard will vary from low to moderate. Level of hazard will depend on the type and amount of radioactivity, the kind of material it is in, and/or the surfaces it is on.
• Some material may be released from packages during accidents of moderate severity but risks to people are not great.
• Released radioactive materials or contaminated objects usually will be visible if packaging fails.
• Some exclusive use shipments of bulk and packaged materials will not have "RADIOACTIVE" labels. Placards, markings and shipping papers provide identification.
• Some packages may have a "RADIOACTIVE" label and a second hazard label. The second hazard is usually greater than the radiation hazard; so follow this GUIDE as well as the response GUIDE for the second hazard class label.
• Some radioactive materials cannot be detected by commonly available instruments.
• Runoff from control of cargo fire may cause low-level pollution.

FIRE OR EXPLOSION

• Some of these materials may burn, but most do not ignite readily.
• Uranium and Thorium metal cuttings may ignite spontaneously if exposed to air (see GUIDE 136).
• Nitrates are oxidizers and may ignite other combustibles (see GUIDE 141).

PUBLIC SAFETY

• **CALL Emergency Response Telephone Number on Shipping Paper first. If Shipping Paper not available or no answer, refer to appropriate telephone number listed on the inside back cover.**
• **Priorities for rescue, life-saving, first aid, fire control and other hazards are higher than the priority for measuring radiation levels.**
• Radiation Authority must be notified of accident conditions. Radiation Authority is usually responsible for decisions about radiological consequences and closure of emergencies.
• As an immediate precautionary measure, isolate spill or leak area for at least 25 meters (75 feet) in all directions.   • Stay upwind.   • Keep unauthorized personnel away.
• Detain or isolate uninjured persons or equipment suspected to be contaminated; delay decontamination and cleanup until instructions are received from Radiation Authority.

PROTECTIVE CLOTHING

• Positive pressure self-contained breathing apparatus (SCBA) and structural firefighters' protective clothing will provide adequate protection.

EVACUATION

Large Spill
• Consider initial downwind evacuation for at least 100 meters (330 feet).

Fire
• When a large quantity of this material is involved in a major fire, consider an initial evacuation distance of 300 meters (1000 feet) in all directions.

EMERGENCY RESPONSE

FIRE
- Presence of radioactive material will not influence the fire control processes and should not influence selection of techniques.
- Move containers from fire area if you can do it without risk.
- Do not move damaged packages; move undamaged packages out of fire zone.

Small Fire
- Dry chemical, CO_2, water spray or regular foam.

Large Fire
- Water spray, fog (flooding amounts).
- Dike fire-control water for later disposal.

SPILL OR LEAK
- Do not touch damaged packages or spilled material.
- Cover liquid spill with sand, earth or other non-combustible absorbent material.
- Dike to collect large liquid spills.
- Cover powder spill with plastic sheet or tarp to minimize spreading.

FIRST AID
- Call 911 or emergency medical service.
- Medical problems take priority over radiological concerns.
- Use first aid treatment according to the nature of the injury.
- Do not delay care and transport of a seriously injured person.
- Give artificial respiration if victim is not breathing.
- Administer oxygen if breathing is difficult.
- In case of contact with substance, wipe from skin immediately; flush skin or eyes with running water for at least 20 minutes.
- Injured persons contaminated by contact with released material are not a serious hazard to health care personnel, equipment or facilities.
- Ensure that medical personnel are aware of the material(s) involved, take precautions to protect themselves and prevent spread of contamination.

POTENTIAL HAZARDS

HEALTH

- Radiation presents minimal risk to transport workers, emergency response personnel and the public during transportation accidents. Packaging durability increases as potential hazard of radioactive content increases.
- Undamaged packages are safe. Contents of damaged packages may cause higher external radiation exposure, or both external and internal radiation exposure if contents are released.
- Type A packages (cartons, boxes, drums, articles, etc.) identified as "Type A" by marking on packages or by shipping papers contain non-life endangering amounts. Partial releases might be expected if "Type A" packages are damaged in moderately severe accidents.
- Type B packages, and the rarely occurring Type C packages, (large and small, usually metal) contain the most hazardous amounts. They can be identified by package markings or by shipping papers. Life threatening conditions may exist only if contents are released or package shielding fails. Because of design, evaluation and testing of packages, these conditions would be expected only for accidents of utmost severity.
- The rarely occurring "Special Arrangement" shipments may be of Type A, Type B or Type C packages. Package type will be marked on packages, and shipment details will be on shipping papers.
- Radioactive White-I labels indicate radiation levels outside single, isolated, undamaged packages are very low (less than 0.005 mSv/h (0.5 mrem/h)).
- Radioactive Yellow-II and Yellow-III labeled packages have higher radiation levels. The transport index (TI) on the label identifies the maximum radiation level in mrem/h one meter from a single, isolated, undamaged package.
- Some radioactive materials cannot be detected by commonly available instruments.
- Water from cargo fire control may cause pollution.

FIRE OR EXPLOSION

- Some of these materials may burn, but most do not ignite readily.
- Radioactivity does not change flammability or other properties of materials.
- Type B packages are designed and evaluated to withstand total engulfment in flames at temperatures of 800°C (1475°F) for a period of 30 minutes.

PUBLIC SAFETY

- **CALL Emergency Response Telephone Number on Shipping Paper first. If Shipping Paper not available or no answer, refer to appropriate telephone number listed on the inside back cover.**
- **Priorities for rescue, life-saving, first aid, fire control and other hazards are higher than the priority for measuring radiation levels.**
- Radiation Authority must be notified of accident conditions. Radiation Authority is usually responsible for decisions about radiological consequences and closure of emergencies.
- As an immediate precautionary measure, isolate spill or leak area for at least 25 meters (75 feet) in all directions. • Stay upwind. • Keep unauthorized personnel away.
- Detain or isolate uninjured persons or equipment suspected to be contaminated; delay decontamination and cleanup until instructions are received from Radiation Authority.

PROTECTIVE CLOTHING

- Positive pressure self-contained breathing apparatus (SCBA) and structural firefighters' protective clothing will provide adequate protection against internal radiation exposure, but not external radiation exposure.

EVACUATION

Large Spill
- Consider initial downwind evacuation for at least 100 meters (330 feet).

Fire
- When a large quantity of this material is involved in a major fire, consider an initial evacuation distance of 300 meters (1000 feet) in all directions.

EMERGENCY RESPONSE

FIRE
- Presence of radioactive material will not influence the fire control processes and should not influence selection of techniques.
- Move containers from fire area if you can do it without risk.
- Do not move damaged packages; move undamaged packages out of fire zone.

Small Fire
- Dry chemical, CO_2, water spray or regular foam.

Large Fire
- Water spray, fog (flooding amounts).
- Dike fire-control water for later disposal.

SPILL OR LEAK
- Do not touch damaged packages or spilled material.
- Damp surfaces on undamaged or slightly damaged packages are seldom an indication of packaging failure. Most packaging for liquid content have inner containers and/or inner absorbent materials.
- Cover liquid spill with sand, earth or other non-combustible absorbent material.

FIRST AID
- Call 911 or emergency medical service.
- Medical problems take priority over radiological concerns.
- Use first aid treatment according to the nature of the injury.
- Do not delay care and transport of a seriously injured person.
- Give artificial respiration if victim is not breathing.
- Administer oxygen if breathing is difficult.
- In case of contact with substance, immediately flush skin or eyes with running water for at least 20 minutes.
- Injured persons contaminated by contact with released material are not a serious hazard to health care personnel, equipment or facilities.
- Ensure that medical personnel are aware of the material(s) involved, take precautions to protect themselves and prevent spread of contamination.

POTENTIAL HAZARDS

HEALTH

- Radiation presents minimal risk to transport workers, emergency response personnel and the public during transportation accidents. Packaging durability increases as potential hazard of radioactive content increases.
- Undamaged packages are safe; contents of damaged packages may cause external radiation exposure, and much higher external exposure if contents (source capsules) are released.
- Contamination and internal radiation hazards are not expected, but not impossible.
- Type A packages (cartons, boxes, drums, articles, etc.) identified as "Type A" by marking on packages or by shipping papers contain non-life endangering amounts. Radioactive sources may be released if "Type A" packages are damaged in moderately severe accidents.
- Type B packages, and the rarely occurring Type C packages, (large and small, usually metal) contain the most hazardous amounts. They can be identified by package markings or by shipping papers. Life threatening conditions may exist only if contents are released or package shielding fails. Because of design, evaluation and testing of packages, these conditions would be expected only for accidents of utmost severity.
- Radioactive White-I labels indicate radiation levels outside single, isolated, undamaged packages are very low (less than 0.005 mSv/h (0.5 mrem/h)).
- Radioactive Yellow-II and Yellow-III labeled packages have higher radiation levels. The transport index (TI) on the label identifies the maximum radiation level in mrem/h one meter from a single, isolated, undamaged package.
- Radiation from the package contents, usually in durable metal capsules, can be detected by most radiation instruments.
- Water from cargo fire control is not expected to cause pollution.

FIRE OR EXPLOSION

- Packagings can burn completely without risk of content loss from sealed source capsule.
- Radioactivity does not change flammability or other properties of materials.
- Radioactive source capsules and Type B packages are designed and evaluated to withstand total engulfment in flames at temperatures of 800°C (1475°F) for a period of 30 minutes.

PUBLIC SAFETY

- **CALL Emergency Response Telephone Number on Shipping Paper first. If Shipping Paper not available or no answer, refer to appropriate telephone number listed on the inside back cover.**
- **Priorities for rescue, life-saving, first aid, fire control and other hazards are higher than the priority for measuring radiation levels.**
- Radiation Authority must be notified of accident conditions. Radiation Authority is usually responsible for decisions about radiological consequences and closure of emergencies.
- As an immediate precautionary measure, isolate spill or leak area for at least 25 meters (75 feet) in all directions.
- Stay upwind. • Keep unauthorized personnel away.
- Delay final cleanup until instructions or advice is received from Radiation Authority.

PROTECTIVE CLOTHING

- Positive pressure self-contained breathing apparatus (SCBA) and structural firefighters' protective clothing will provide adequate protection against internal radiation exposure, but not external radiation exposure.

EVACUATION

Large Spill
- Consider initial downwind evacuation for at least 100 meters (330 feet).

Fire
- When a large quantity of this material is involved in a major fire, consider an initial evacuation distance of 300 meters (1000 feet) in all directions.

EMERGENCY RESPONSE

FIRE
- Presence of radioactive material will not influence the fire control processes and should not influence selection of techniques.
- Move containers from fire area if you can do it without risk.
- Do not move damaged packages; move undamaged packages out of fire zone.

Small Fire
- Dry chemical, CO_2, water spray or regular foam.

Large Fire
- Water spray, fog (flooding amounts).

SPILL OR LEAK
- Do not touch damaged packages or spilled material.
- Damp surfaces on undamaged or slightly damaged packages are seldom an indication of packaging failure. Contents are seldom liquid. Content is usually a metal capsule, easily seen if released from package.
- If source capsule is identified as being out of package, **DO NOT TOUCH**. Stay away and await advice from Radiation Authority.

FIRST AID
- Call 911 or emergency medical service.
- Medical problems take priority over radiological concerns.
- Use first aid treatment according to the nature of the injury.
- Do not delay care and transport of a seriously injured person.
- Persons exposed to special form sources are not likely to be contaminated with radioactive material.
- Give artificial respiration if victim is not breathing.
- Administer oxygen if breathing is difficult.
- Injured persons contaminated by contact with released material are not a serious hazard to health care personnel, equipment or facilities.
- Ensure that medical personnel are aware of the material(s) involved, take precautions to protect themselves and prevent spread of contamination.

POTENTIAL HAZARDS

HEALTH

- Radiation presents minimal risk to transport workers, emergency response personnel and the public during transportation accidents. Packaging durability increases as potential radiation and criticality hazards of the content increase.
- Undamaged packages are safe. Contents of damaged packages may cause higher external radiation exposure, or both external and internal radiation exposure if contents are released.
- Type AF or IF packages, identified by package markings, do not contain life-threatening amounts of material. External radiation levels are low and packages are designed, evaluated and tested to control releases and to prevent a fission chain reaction under severe transport conditions.
- Type B(U)F, B(M)F and CF packages (identified by markings on packages or shipping papers) contain potentially life endangering amounts. Because of design, evaluation and testing of packages, fission chain reactions are prevented and releases are not expected to be life endangering for all accidents except those of utmost severity.
- The rarely occurring "Special Arrangement" shipments may be of Type AF, BF or CF packages. Package type will be marked on packages, and shipment details will be on shipping papers.
- The transport index (TI) shown on labels or a shipping paper might not indicate the radiation level at one meter from a single, isolated, undamaged package; instead, it might relate to controls needed during transport because of the fissile properties of the materials. Alternatively, the fissile nature of the contents may be indicated by a criticality safety index (CSI) on a special FISSILE label or on the shipping paper.
- Some radioactive materials cannot be detected by commonly available instruments.
- Water from cargo fire control is not expected to cause pollution.

FIRE OR EXPLOSION

- These materials are seldom flammable. Packages are designed to withstand fires without damage to contents.
- Radioactivity does not change flammability or other properties of materials.
- Type AF, IF, B(U)F, B(M)F and CF packages are designed and evaluated to withstand total engulfment in flames at temperatures of 800°C (1475°F) for a period of 30 minutes.

PUBLIC SAFETY

- **CALL Emergency Response Telephone Number on Shipping Paper first. If Shipping Paper not available or no answer, refer to appropriate telephone number listed on the inside back cover.**
- **Priorities for rescue, life-saving, first aid, fire control and other hazards are higher than the priority for measuring radiation levels.**
- Radiation Authority must be notified of accident conditions. Radiation Authority is usually responsible for decisions about radiological consequences and closure of emergencies.
- As an immediate precautionary measure, isolate spill or leak area for at least 25 meters (75 feet) in all directions. • Stay upwind. • Keep unauthorized personnel away.
- Detain or isolate uninjured persons or equipment suspected to be contaminated; delay decontamination and cleanup until instructions are received from Radiation Authority.

PROTECTIVE CLOTHING

- Positive pressure self-contained breathing apparatus (SCBA) and structural firefighters' protective clothing will provide adequate protection against internal radiation exposure, but not external radiation exposure.

EVACUATION

Large Spill
- Consider initial downwind evacuation for at least 100 meters (330 feet).

Fire
- When a large quantity of this material is involved in a major fire, consider an initial evacuation distance of 300 meters (1000 feet) in all directions.

EMERGENCY RESPONSE

FIRE
- Presence of radioactive material will not influence the fire control processes and should not influence selection of techniques.
- Move containers from fire area if you can do it without risk.
- Do not move damaged packages; move undamaged packages out of fire zone.

Small Fire
- Dry chemical, CO_2, water spray or regular foam.

Large Fire
- Water spray, fog (flooding amounts).

SPILL OR LEAK
- Do not touch damaged packages or spilled material.
- Damp surfaces on undamaged or slightly damaged packages are seldom an indication of packaging failure. Most packaging for liquid content have inner containers and/or inner absorbent materials.

Liquid Spill
- Package contents are seldom liquid. If any radioactive contamination resulting from a liquid release is present, it probably will be low-level.

FIRST AID
- Call 911 or emergency medical service.
- Medical problems take priority over radiological concerns.
- Use first aid treatment according to the nature of the injury.
- Do not delay care and transport of a seriously injured person.
- Give artificial respiration if victim is not breathing.
- Administer oxygen if breathing is difficult.
- In case of contact with substance, immediately flush skin or eyes with running water for at least 20 minutes.
- Injured persons contaminated by contact with released material are not a serious hazard to health care personnel, equipment or facilities.
- Ensure that medical personnel are aware of the material(s) involved, take precautions to protect themselves and prevent spread of contamination.

POTENTIAL HAZARDS

HEALTH

- Radiation presents minimal risk to transport workers, emergency response personnel and the public during transportation accidents. Packaging durability increases as potential radiation and criticality hazards of the content increase.
- Chemical hazard greatly exceeds radiation hazard.
- Substance reacts with water and water vapor in air to form toxic and corrosive hydrogen fluoride gas and an extremely irritating and corrosive, white-colored, water-soluble residue.
- If inhaled, may be fatal.
- Direct contact causes burns to skin, eyes, and respiratory tract.
- Low-level radioactive material; very low radiation hazard to people.
- Runoff from control of cargo fire may cause low-level pollution.

FIRE OR EXPLOSION

- Substance does not burn.   • The material may react violently with fuels.
- Containers in protective overpacks (horizontal cylindrical shape with short legs for tie-downs), are identified with "AF", "B(U)F" or "H(U)" on shipping papers or by markings on the overpacks. They are designed and evaluated to withstand severe conditions including total engulfment in flames at temperatures of 800°C (1475°F) for a period of 30 minutes.
- Bare filled cylinders, identified with UN2978 as part of the marking (may also be marked H(U) or H(M)), may rupture in heat of engulfing fire; bare empty (except for residue) cylinders will not rupture in fires.
- Radioactivity does not change flammability or other properties of materials.

PUBLIC SAFETY

- **CALL Emergency Response Telephone Number on Shipping Paper first. If Shipping Paper not available or no answer, refer to appropriate telephone number listed on the inside back cover.**
- **Priorities for rescue, life-saving, first aid, fire control and other hazards are higher than the priority for measuring radiation levels.**
- Radiation Authority must be notified of accident conditions. Radiation Authority is usually responsible for decisions about radiological consequences and closure of emergencies.
- As an immediate precautionary measure, isolate spill or leak area for at least 25 meters (75 feet) in all directions. • Stay upwind. • Keep unauthorized personnel away.
- Detain or isolate uninjured persons or equipment suspected to be contaminated; delay decontamination and cleanup until instructions are received from Radiation Authority.

PROTECTIVE CLOTHING

- Wear positive pressure self-contained breathing apparatus (SCBA).
- Wear chemical protective clothing that is specifically recommended by the manufacturer. It may provide little or no thermal protection.
- Structural firefighters' protective clothing provides limited protection in fire situations ONLY; it is not effective in spill situations where direct contact with the substance is possible.

EVACUATION

Large Spill
- See Table 1 - Initial Isolation and Protective Action Distances.

Fire
- When a large quantity of this material is involved in a major fire, consider an initial evacuation distance of 300 meters (1000 feet) in all directions.

EMERGENCY RESPONSE

FIRE
- DO NOT USE WATER OR FOAM ON MATERIAL ITSELF.
- Move containers from fire area if you can do it without risk.

Small Fire
- Dry chemical or CO_2.

Large Fire
- Water spray, fog or regular foam.
- Cool containers with flooding quantities of water until well after fire is out.
- If this is impossible, withdraw from area and let fire burn.
- ALWAYS stay away from tanks engulfed in fire.

SPILL OR LEAK
- Do not touch damaged packages or spilled material.
- Without fire or smoke, leak will be evident by visible and irritating vapors and residue forming at the point of release.
- Use fine water spray to reduce vapors; do not put water directly on point of material release from container.
- Residue buildup may self-seal small leaks.
- Dike far ahead of spill to collect runoff water.

FIRST AID
- Call 911 or emergency medical service.
- Medical problems take priority over radiological concerns.
- Use first aid treatment according to the nature of the injury.
- Do not delay care and transport of a seriously injured person.
- Give artificial respiration if victim is not breathing.
- Administer oxygen if breathing is difficult.
- In case of contact with substance, immediately flush skin or eyes with running water for at least 20 minutes.
- Effects of exposure (inhalation, ingestion or skin contact) to substance may be delayed.
- Injured persons contaminated by contact with released material are not a serious hazard to health care personnel, equipment or facilities.
- Ensure that medical personnel are aware of the material(s) involved, take precautions to protect themselves and prevent spread of contamination.

POTENTIAL HAZARDS

HEALTH
- **TOXIC; may be fatal if inhaled.**
- Vapors are extremely irritating.
- Contact with gas or liquefied gas will cause burns, severe injury and/or frostbite.
- Vapors from liquefied gas are initially heavier than air and spread along ground.
- Runoff from fire control may cause pollution.

FIRE OR EXPLOSION
- Substance does not burn but will support combustion.
- This is a strong oxidizer and will react vigorously or explosively with many materials including fuels.
- May ignite combustibles (wood, paper, oil, clothing, etc.).
- Vapor explosion and poison hazard indoors, outdoors or in sewers.
- Containers may explode when heated.
- Ruptured cylinders may rocket.

PUBLIC SAFETY

- **CALL Emergency Response Telephone Number on Shipping Paper first. If Shipping Paper not available or no answer, refer to appropriate telephone number listed on the inside back cover.**
- As an immediate precautionary measure, isolate spill or leak area for at least 100 meters (330 feet) in all directions.
- Keep unauthorized personnel away.
- Stay upwind.
- Many gases are heavier than air and will spread along ground and collect in low or confined areas (sewers, basements, tanks).
- Keep out of low areas.
- Ventilate closed spaces before entering.

PROTECTIVE CLOTHING
- Wear positive pressure self-contained breathing apparatus (SCBA).
- Wear chemical protective clothing that is specifically recommended by the manufacturer. It may provide little or no thermal protection.
- Structural firefighters' protective clothing provides limited protection in fire situations ONLY; it is not effective in spill situations where direct contact with the substance is possible.
- Always wear thermal protective clothing when handling refrigerated/cryogenic liquids.

EVACUATION
Spill
- See Table 1 - Initial Isolation and Protective Action Distances.

Fire
- If tank, rail car or tank truck is involved in a fire, ISOLATE for 1600 meters (1 mile) in all directions; also, consider initial evacuation for 1600 meters (1 mile) in all directions.

EMERGENCY RESPONSE

FIRE

Small Fire
- Dry chemical, soda ash, lime or sand.

Large Fire
- Water spray, fog (flooding amounts).
- Do not get water inside containers.
- Move containers from fire area if you can do it without risk.

Fire involving Tanks
- Fight fire from maximum distance or use unmanned hose holders or monitor nozzles.
- Cool containers with flooding quantities of water until well after fire is out.
- Do not direct water at source of leak or safety devices; icing may occur.
- Withdraw immediately in case of rising sound from venting safety devices or discoloration of tank.
- ALWAYS stay away from tanks engulfed in fire.
- For massive fire, use unmanned hose holders or monitor nozzles; if this is impossible, withdraw from area and let fire burn.

SPILL OR LEAK

- Do not touch or walk through spilled material.
- If you have not donned special protective clothing approved for this material, do not expose yourself to any risk of this material touching you.
- **Do not direct water at spill or source of leak.**
- A fine water spray remotely directed to the edge of the spill pool can be used to direct and maintain a hot flare fire that will burn the spilled material in a controlled manner.
- Keep combustibles (wood, paper, oil, etc.) away from spilled material.
- Stop leak if you can do it without risk.
- Use water spray to reduce vapors or divert vapor cloud drift. Avoid allowing water runoff to contact spilled material.
- If possible, turn leaking containers so that gas escapes rather than liquid.
- Prevent entry into waterways, sewers, basements or confined areas.
- Isolate area until gas has dispersed.
- Ventilate the area.

FIRST AID

- Move victim to fresh air.   • Call 911 or emergency medical service.
- Give artificial respiration if victim is not breathing.
- Administer oxygen if breathing is difficult.
- Clothing frozen to the skin should be thawed before being removed.
- Remove and isolate contaminated clothing and shoes.
- In case of contact with substance, immediately flush skin or eyes with running water for at least 20 minutes.
- Keep victim warm and quiet.   • Keep victim under observation.
- Effects of contact or inhalation may be delayed.
- Ensure that medical personnel are aware of the material(s) involved and take precautions to protect themselves.

POTENTIAL HAZARDS

HEALTH
- **TOXIC; Extremely Hazardous.**
- Inhalation extremely dangerous; may be fatal.
- Contact with gas or liquefied gas may cause burns, severe injury and/or frostbite.
- Odorless, will not be detected by sense of smell.

FIRE OR EXPLOSION
- **EXTREMELY FLAMMABLE.**
- May be ignited by heat, sparks or flames.
- Flame may be invisible.
- Containers may explode when heated.
- Vapor explosion and poison hazard indoors, outdoors or in sewers.
- Vapors from liquefied gas are initially heavier than air and spread along ground.
- Vapors may travel to source of ignition and flash back.
- Runoff may create fire or explosion hazard.

PUBLIC SAFETY

- **CALL Emergency Response Telephone Number on Shipping Paper first. If Shipping Paper not available or no answer, refer to appropriate telephone number listed on the inside back cover.**
- As an immediate precautionary measure, isolate spill or leak area for at least 100 meters (330 feet) in all directions.
- Keep unauthorized personnel away.
- Stay upwind.
- Many gases are heavier than air and will spread along ground and collect in low or confined areas (sewers, basements, tanks).
- Keep out of low areas.
- Ventilate closed spaces before entering.

PROTECTIVE CLOTHING
- Wear positive pressure self-contained breathing apparatus (SCBA).
- Wear chemical protective clothing that is specifically recommended by the manufacturer. It may provide little or no thermal protection.
- Structural firefighters' protective clothing provides limited protection in fire situations ONLY; it is not effective in spill situations where direct contact with the substance is possible.
- Always wear thermal protective clothing when handling refrigerated/cryogenic liquids.

EVACUATION
Spill
- See Table 1 - Initial Isolation and Protective Action Distances.

Fire
- If tank, rail car or tank truck is involved in a fire, ISOLATE for 800 meters (1/2 mile) in all directions; also, consider initial evacuation for 800 meters (1/2 mile) in all directions.

EMERGENCY RESPONSE

FIRE
- **DO NOT EXTINGUISH A LEAKING GAS FIRE UNLESS LEAK CAN BE STOPPED.**

Small Fire
- Dry chemical, CO_2 or water spray.

Large Fire
- Water spray, fog or regular foam.
- Move containers from fire area if you can do it without risk.

Fire involving Tanks
- Fight fire from maximum distance or use unmanned hose holders or monitor nozzles.
- Cool containers with flooding quantities of water until well after fire is out.
- Do not direct water at source of leak or safety devices; icing may occur.
- Withdraw immediately in case of rising sound from venting safety devices or discoloration of tank.
- ALWAYS stay away from tanks engulfed in fire.

SPILL OR LEAK
- ELIMINATE all ignition sources (no smoking, flares, sparks or flames in immediate area).
- All equipment used when handling the product must be grounded.
- Fully encapsulating, vapor protective clothing should be worn for spills and leaks with no fire.
- Do not touch or walk through spilled material.
- Stop leak if you can do it without risk.
- Use water spray to reduce vapors or divert vapor cloud drift. Avoid allowing water runoff to contact spilled material.
- Do not direct water at spill or source of leak.
- If possible, turn leaking containers so that gas escapes rather than liquid.
- Prevent entry into waterways, sewers, basements or confined areas.
- Isolate area until gas has dispersed.

FIRST AID
- Move victim to fresh air. • Call 911 or emergency medical service.
- Give artificial respiration if victim is not breathing.
- Administer oxygen if breathing is difficult.
- Remove and isolate contaminated clothing and shoes.
- In case of contact with substance, immediately flush skin or eyes with running water for at least 20 minutes.
- In case of contact with liquefied gas, thaw frosted parts with lukewarm water.
- Keep victim warm and quiet. • Keep victim under observation.
- Effects of contact or inhalation may be delayed.
- Ensure that medical personnel are aware of the material(s) involved and take precautions to protect themselves.

POTENTIAL HAZARDS

FIRE OR EXPLOSION

- Substance is transported in molten form at a temperature above 705°C (1300°F).
- Violent reaction with water; contact may cause an explosion or may produce a flammable gas.
- Will ignite combustible materials (wood, paper, oil, debris, etc.).
- Contact with nitrates or other oxidizers may cause an explosion.
- Contact with containers or other materials, including cold, wet or dirty tools, may cause an explosion.
- Contact with concrete will cause spalling and small pops.

HEALTH

- Contact causes severe burns to skin and eyes.
- Fire may produce irritating and/or toxic gases.

PUBLIC SAFETY

- **CALL Emergency Response Telephone Number on Shipping Paper first. If Shipping Paper not available or no answer, refer to appropriate telephone number listed on the inside back cover.**
- As an immediate precautionary measure, isolate spill or leak area for at least 50 meters (150 feet) in all directions.
- Keep unauthorized personnel away.
- Ventilate closed spaces before entering.

PROTECTIVE CLOTHING

- Wear positive pressure self-contained breathing apparatus (SCBA).
- Wear flame retardant structural firefighters' protective clothing, including faceshield, helmet and gloves, this will provide limited thermal protection.

EMERGENCY RESPONSE

FIRE
- **Do Not Use Water, except in life threatening situations and then only in a fine spray.**
- **Do not use halogenated extinguishing agents or foam.**
- Move combustibles out of path of advancing pool if you can do so without risk.
- Extinguish fires started by molten material by using appropriate method for the burning material; keep water, halogenated extinguishing agents and foam away from the molten material.

SPILL OR LEAK
- Do not touch or walk through spilled material.
- Do not attempt to stop leak, due to danger of explosion.
- Keep combustibles (wood, paper, oil, etc.) away from spilled material.
- Substance is very fluid, spreads quickly, and may splash. Do not try to stop it with shovels or other objects.
- Dike far ahead of spill; use dry sand to contain the flow of material.
- Where possible allow molten material to solidify naturally.
- Avoid contact even after material solidifies. Molten, heated and cold aluminum look alike; do not touch unless you know it is cold.
- Clean up under the supervision of an expert after material has solidified.

FIRST AID
- Move victim to fresh air.   • Call 911 or emergency medical service.
- Give artificial respiration if victim is not breathing.
- Administer oxygen if breathing is difficult.
- For severe burns, immediate medical attention is required.
- Removal of solidified molten material from skin requires medical assistance.
- Remove and isolate contaminated clothing and shoes.
- In case of contact with substance, immediately flush skin or eyes with running water for at least 20 minutes.
- Keep victim warm and quiet.

POTENTIAL HAZARDS

FIRE OR EXPLOSION

- May react violently or explosively on contact with water.
- Some are transported in flammable liquids.
- May be ignited by friction, heat, sparks or flames.
- Some of these materials will burn with intense heat.
- Dusts or fumes may form explosive mixtures in air.
- Containers may explode when heated.
- May re-ignite after fire is extinguished.

HEALTH

- Oxides from metallic fires are a severe health hazard.
- Inhalation or contact with substance or decomposition products may cause severe injury or death.
- Fire may produce irritating, corrosive and/or toxic gases.
- Runoff from fire control or dilution water may cause pollution.

PUBLIC SAFETY

- **CALL Emergency Response Telephone Number on Shipping Paper first. If Shipping Paper not available or no answer, refer to appropriate telephone number listed on the inside back cover.**
- As an immediate precautionary measure, isolate spill or leak area in all directions for at least 50 meters (150 feet) for liquids and at least 25 meters (75 feet) for solids.
- Stay upwind.
- Keep unauthorized personnel away.

PROTECTIVE CLOTHING

- Wear positive pressure self-contained breathing apparatus (SCBA).
- Structural firefighters' protective clothing will only provide limited protection.

EVACUATION

Large Spill
- Consider initial downwind evacuation for at least 50 meters (160 feet).

Fire
- If tank, rail car or tank truck is involved in a fire, ISOLATE for 800 meters (1/2 mile) in all directions; also, consider initial evacuation for 800 meters (1/2 mile) in all directions.

EMERGENCY RESPONSE

FIRE

- **DO NOT USE WATER, FOAM OR CO$_2$.**
- Dousing metallic fires with water will generate hydrogen gas, an extremely dangerous explosion hazard, particularly if fire is in a confined environment (i.e., building, cargo hold, etc.).
- Use DRY sand, graphite powder, dry sodium chloride based extinguishers, G-1® or Met-L-X® powder.
- Confining and smothering metal fires is preferable rather than applying water.
- Move containers from fire area if you can do it without risk.

Fire involving Tanks or Car/Trailer Loads

- If impossible to extinguish, protect surroundings and allow fire to burn itself out.

SPILL OR LEAK

- ELIMINATE all ignition sources (no smoking, flares, sparks or flames in immediate area).
- Do not touch or walk through spilled material.
- Stop leak if you can do it without risk.
- Prevent entry into waterways, sewers, basements or confined areas.

FIRST AID

- Move victim to fresh air. • Call 911 or emergency medical service.
- Give artificial respiration if victim is not breathing.
- Administer oxygen if breathing is difficult.
- Remove and isolate contaminated clothing and shoes.
- In case of contact with substance, immediately flush skin or eyes with running water for at least 20 minutes.
- Keep victim warm and quiet.
- Ensure that medical personnel are aware of the material(s) involved and take precautions to protect themselves.

POTENTIAL HAZARDS

FIRE OR EXPLOSION
- Some may burn but none ignite readily.
- Containers may explode when heated.
- Some may be transported hot.

HEALTH
- Inhalation of material may be harmful.
- Contact may cause burns to skin and eyes.
- Inhalation of Asbestos dust may have a damaging effect on the lungs.
- Fire may produce irritating, corrosive and/or toxic gases.
- Some liquids produce vapors that may cause dizziness or suffocation.
- Runoff from fire control may cause pollution.

PUBLIC SAFETY

- **CALL Emergency Response Telephone Number on Shipping Paper first. If Shipping Paper not available or no answer, refer to appropriate telephone number listed on the inside back cover.**
- As an immediate precautionary measure, isolate spill or leak area in all directions for at least 50 meters (150 feet) for liquids and at least 25 meters (75 feet) for solids.
- Keep unauthorized personnel away.
- Stay upwind.

PROTECTIVE CLOTHING
- Wear positive pressure self-contained breathing apparatus (SCBA).
- Structural firefighters' protective clothing will only provide limited protection.

EVACUATION
Spill
- See Table 1 - Initial Isolation and Protective Action Distances for highlighted materials. For non-highlighted materials, increase, in the downwind direction, as necessary, the isolation distance shown under "PUBLIC SAFETY".

Fire
- If tank, rail car or tank truck is involved in a fire, ISOLATE for 800 meters (1/2 mile) in all directions; also, consider initial evacuation for 800 meters (1/2 mile) in all directions.

EMERGENCY RESPONSE

FIRE

Small Fire

- Dry chemical, CO_2, water spray or regular foam.

Large Fire

- Water spray, fog or regular foam.
- Do not scatter spilled material with high pressure water streams.
- Move containers from fire area if you can do it without risk.
- Dike fire-control water for later disposal.

Fire involving Tanks

- Cool containers with flooding quantities of water until well after fire is out.
- Withdraw immediately in case of rising sound from venting safety devices or discoloration of tank.
- ALWAYS stay away from tanks engulfed in fire.

SPILL OR LEAK

- Do not touch or walk through spilled material.
- Stop leak if you can do it without risk.
- Prevent dust cloud.
- Avoid inhalation of asbestos dust.

Small Dry Spill

- With clean shovel place material into clean, dry container and cover loosely; move containers from spill area.

Small Spill

- Take up with sand or other non-combustible absorbent material and place into containers for later disposal.

Large Spill

- Dike far ahead of liquid spill for later disposal.
- Cover powder spill with plastic sheet or tarp to minimize spreading.
- Prevent entry into waterways, sewers, basements or confined areas.

FIRST AID

- Move victim to fresh air.   • Call 911 or emergency medical service.
- Give artificial respiration if victim is not breathing.
- Administer oxygen if breathing is difficult.
- Remove and isolate contaminated clothing and shoes.
- In case of contact with substance, immediately flush skin or eyes with running water for at least 20 minutes.
- Ensure that medical personnel are aware of the material(s) involved and take precautions to protect themselves.

POTENTIAL HAZARDS

HEALTH
- Inhalation of vapors or contact with substance will result in contamination and potential harmful effects.
- Fire will produce irritating, corrosive and/or toxic gases.

FIRE OR EXPLOSION
- Non-combustible, substance itself does not burn but may react upon heating to produce corrosive and/or toxic fumes.
- Runoff may pollute waterways.

PUBLIC SAFETY
- **CALL Emergency Response Telephone Number on Shipping Paper first. If Shipping Paper not available or no answer, refer to appropriate telephone number listed on the inside back cover.**
- As an immediate precautionary measure, isolate spill or leak area for at least 50 meters (150 feet) in all directions.
- Stay upwind.
- Keep unauthorized personnel away.

PROTECTIVE CLOTHING
- Wear positive pressure self-contained breathing apparatus (SCBA).
- Structural firefighters' protective clothing will only provide limited protection.

EVACUATION
Large Spill
- Consider initial downwind evacuation for at least 100 meters (330 feet).

Fire
- When any large container is involved in a fire, consider initial evacuation for 500 meters (1/3 mile) in all directions.

EMERGENCY RESPONSE

FIRE
- Use extinguishing agent suitable for type of surrounding fire.
- **Do not direct water at the heated metal.**

SPILL OR LEAK
- Do not touch or walk through spilled material.
- Do not touch damaged containers or spilled material unless wearing appropriate protective clothing.
- Stop leak if you can do it without risk.
- Prevent entry into waterways, sewers, basements or confined areas.
- Do not use steel or aluminum tools or equipment.
- Cover with earth, sand or other non-combustible material followed with plastic sheet to minimize spreading or contact with rain.
- For mercury, use a mercury spill kit.
- Mercury spill areas may be subsequently treated with calcium sulphide/calcium sulfide or with sodium thiosulphate/sodium thiosulfate wash to neutralize any residual mercury.

FIRST AID
- Move victim to fresh air.   • Call 911 or emergency medical service.
- Give artificial respiration if victim is not breathing.
- Administer oxygen if breathing is difficult.
- Remove and isolate contaminated clothing and shoes.
- In case of contact with substance, immediately flush skin or eyes with running water for at least 20 minutes.
- Keep victim warm and quiet.
- Ensure that medical personnel are aware of the material(s) involved and take precautions to protect themselves.

NOTES

INTRODUCTION TO TABLE 1 - INITIAL ISOLATION
AND PROTECTIVE ACTION DISTANCES

Table 1 - Initial Isolation and Protective Action Distances suggests distances useful to protect people from vapors resulting from spills involving dangerous goods that are considered toxic by inhalation (TIH), including certain chemical warfare agents, or which produce toxic gases upon contact with water. Table 1 provides first responders with initial guidance until technically qualified emergency response personnel are available. **Distances show areas likely to be affected during the first 30 minutes after materials are spilled and could increase with time.**

The **Initial Isolation Zone** defines an area SURROUNDING the incident in which persons may be exposed to dangerous (upwind) and life threatening (downwind) concentrations of material. The **Protective Action Zone** defines an area DOWNWIND from the incident in which persons may become incapacitated and unable to take protective action and/or incur serious or irreversible health effects. Table 1 provides specific guidance for small and large spills occurring day or night.

Adjusting distances for a specific incident involves many interdependent variables and should be made only by personnel technically qualified to make such adjustments. For this reason, no precise guidance can be provided in this document to aid in adjusting the table distances; however, general guidance follows.

Factors That May Change the Protective Action Distances

The GUIDE for a material (orange-bordered pages) clearly indicates under the section EVACUATION – Fire, the evacuation distance required to protect against fragmentation hazard of a large container. If the material becomes involved in a **FIRE**, the toxic hazard may become less important than the fire or explosion hazard.

If more than one tank car, cargo tank, portable tank, or large cylinder involved in the incident is leaking, LARGE SPILL distances may need to be increased.

For a material with a protective action distance of 11.0+ km (7.0+ miles), the actual distance can be larger in certain atmospheric conditions. If the dangerous goods vapor plume is channeled in a valley or between many tall buildings, distances may be larger than shown in Table 1 due to less mixing of the plume with the atmosphere. Daytime spills in regions with known strong inversions or snow cover, or occurring near sunset, may require an increase of the protective action distance because airborne contaminants mix and disperse more slowly and may travel much farther downwind. In such cases, the nighttime protective action distance may be more appropriate. In addition, protective action distances may be larger for liquid spills when either the material or outdoor temperature exceeds 30°C (86°F).

Materials which react with water to produce large amounts of toxic gases are included in Table 1 - Initial Isolation and Protective Action Distances. Note that some water-reactive materials (WRM) which are also TIH (e.g., Bromine trifluoride (1746), Thionyl chloride (1836), etc.) produce additional TIH materials when spilled in water. For these materials, two entries are provided in Table 1 - Initial Isolation and Protective Action Distances (i.e., for spills on land and for spills in water). If it is not clear whether the spill is on land or in water, or in cases where the spill occurs both on land and in water, choose the larger Protective Action Distance. Following Table 1, Table 2 – Materials which produce large amounts of Toxic Inhalation Hazard gases (TIH) when spilled in water lists the toxic gases that are produced when these water-reactive materials (WRM) are spilled in water.

When a water-reactive TIH producing material is spilled into a river or stream, the source of the toxic gas may move with the current and stretch from the spill point downstream for a substantial distance.

Initial isolation and protective action distances in this guidebook are derived from historical data on transportation incidents and the use of statistical models. For worst case scenarios involving the instantaneous release of the entire contents of a package (e.g., as a result of terrorism, sabotage or catastrophic accident) the distances may increase substantially. For such events, doubling of the initial isolation and protective action distances is appropriate in absence of other information.

PROTECTIVE ACTION DECISION FACTORS TO CONSIDER

The choice of protective actions for a given situation depends on a number of factors. For some cases, evacuation may be the best option; in others, sheltering in-place may be the best course. Sometimes, these two actions may be used in combination. In any emergency, officials need to quickly give the public instructions. The public will need continuing information and instructions while being evacuated or sheltered in-place.

Proper evaluation of the factors listed below will determine the effectiveness of evacuation or in-place protection. The importance of these factors can vary with emergency conditions. In specific emergencies, other factors may need to be identified and considered as well. This list indicates what kind of information may be needed to make the initial decision.

The Dangerous Goods

- Degree of health hazard
- Chemical and physical properties
- Amount involved
- Containment/control of release
- Rate of vapor movement

The Population Threatened

- Location
- Number of people
- Time available to evacuate or shelter in-place
- Ability to control evacuation or shelter in-place
- Building types and availability
- Special institutions or populations, e.g., nursing homes, hospitals, prisons

Weather Conditions

- Effect on vapor and cloud movement
- Potential for change
- Effect on evacuation or protection in-place

PROTECTIVE ACTIONS

Protective Actions are those steps taken to preserve the health and safety of emergency responders and the public during an incident involving releases of dangerous goods. Table 1 - Initial Isolation and Protective Action Distances (green-bordered pages) predicts the size of downwind areas which could be affected by a cloud of toxic gas. People in this area should be evacuated and/or sheltered in-place inside buildings.

Isolate Hazard Area and Deny Entry means keep everybody away from the area if they are not directly involved in emergency response operations. Unprotected emergency responders should not be allowed to enter the isolation zone. This "isolation" task is done first to establish control over the area of operations. This is the first step for any protective actions that may follow. See Table 1 - Isolation and Protective Action Distances (green-bordered pages) for more detailed information on specific materials.

Evacuate means move all people from a threatened area to a safer place. To perform an evacuation, there must be enough time for people to be warned, to get ready, and to leave an area. If there is enough time, evacuation is the best protective action. Begin evacuating people nearby and those outdoors in direct view of the scene. When additional help arrives, expand the area to be evacuated downwind and crosswind to at least the extent recommended in this guidebook. Even after people move to the distances recommended, they may not be completely safe from harm. They should not be permitted to congregate at such distances. Send evacuees to a definite place, by a specific route, far enough away so they will not have to be moved again if the wind shifts.

Shelter In-Place means people should seek shelter inside a building and remain inside until the danger passes. **Sheltering in-place is used when evacuating the public would cause greater risk than staying where they are, or when an evacuation cannot be performed.** Direct the people inside to **close all doors and windows** and to **shut off all ventilating, heating and cooling systems.** In-place protection may not be the best option if (a) the vapors are flammable; (b) if it will take a long time for the gas to clear the area; or (c) if buildings cannot be closed tightly. Vehicles can offer some protection for a short period if the windows are closed and the ventilating systems are shut off. Vehicles are not as effective as buildings for in-place protection.

It is vital to maintain communications with competent persons inside the building so that they are advised about changing conditions. **Persons protected-in-place should be warned to stay far from windows** because of the danger from glass and projected metal fragments in a fire and/or explosion.

Every dangerous goods incident is different. Each will have special problems and concerns. Action to protect the public must be selected carefully. These pages can help with **initial** decisions on how to protect the public. Officials must continue to gather information and monitor the situation until the threat is removed.

BACKGROUND ON TABLE 1 - INITIAL ISOLATION
AND PROTECTIVE ACTION DISTANCES

Initial Isolation and Protective Action Distances in this guidebook were determined for small and large spills occurring during day or night. The overall analysis was statistical in nature and utilized state-of-the-art emission rate and dispersion models; statistical release data from the U.S. DOT HMIS (Hazardous Materials Incident Reporting System) database; meteorological observations from over 120 locations in United States, Canada and Mexico; and the most current toxicological exposure guidelines.

For each chemical, thousands of hypothetical releases were modeled to account for the statistical variation in both release amount and atmospheric conditions. Based on this statistical sample, the 90% percentile Protective Action Distance for each chemical and category was selected to appear in the Table. A brief description of the analysis is provided below. A detailed report outlining the methodology and data used in the generation of the Initial Isolation and Protective Action Distances may be obtained from the U.S. Department of Transportation, Pipeline and Hazardous Materials Safety Administration.

Release amounts and emission rates into the atmosphere were statistically modeled based on (1) data from the U.S. DOT HMIS database; (2) container types and sizes authorized for transport as specified in 49 CFR §172.101 and Part 173; (3) physical properties of the individual materials, and (4) atmospheric data from a historical database. The emission model calculated the release of vapor due to evaporation of pools on the ground, direct release of vapors from the container, or a combination of both, as would occur for liquefied gases which can flash to form both a vapor/aerosol mixture and an evaporating pool. In addition, the emission model also calculated the emission of toxic vapor by-products generated from spilling water-reactive materials in water. Spills that involve releases of approximately 200 liters (300 kg for solids)or less are considered Small Spills, while spills that involve quantities greater than 200 liters (300 kg for solids) are considered Large Spills. An exception to this is certain chemical warfare agents where Small Spills include releases up to 2 kg, and Large Spills include releases up to 25 kg. These agents are BZ, CX, GA, GB, GD, GF, HD, HL, HN1, HN2, HN3, L and VX.

Downwind dispersion of the vapor was estimated for each case modeled. Atmospheric parameters affecting the dispersion, and the emission rate, were selected in a statistical fashion from a database containing hourly meteorological data from 120 cities in the United States, Canada and Mexico. The dispersion calculation accounted for the time dependent emission rate from the source as well as the density of the vapor plume (i.e., heavy gas effects). Since atmospheric mixing is less effective at dispersing vapor plumes during nighttime, day and night were separated in the analysis. In Table 1, "Day" refers to time periods after sunrise and before sunset, while "Night" includes all hours between sunset and sunrise.

Toxicological short-term exposure guidelines for the materials were applied to determine the downwind distance to which persons may become incapacitated and unable to take protective action or may incur serious health effects. When available, toxicological exposure guidelines were chosen from AEGL-2 or ERPG-2 emergency response guidelines, with AEGL-2 values being the first choice. For materials that do not have AEGL-2 or ERPG-2 values, emergency response guidelines estimated from lethal concentration limits derived from animal studies were used, as recommended by an independent panel of toxicological experts from industry and academia.

HOW TO USE TABLE 1 - INITIAL ISOLATION AND PROTECTIVE ACTION DISTANCES

(1) The responder should already have:

- Identified the material by its ID Number and Name; (if an ID Number cannot be found, use the Name of Material index in the blue-bordered pages to locate that number.)
- Found the three-digit guide for that material in order to consult the emergency actions recommended jointly with this table;
- **Noted the wind direction.**

(2) Look in Table 1 (the green-bordered pages) for the ID Number and Name of the Material involved in the incident. Some ID Numbers have more than one shipping name listed—look for the specific name of the material. (If the shipping name is not known and Table 1 lists more than one name for the same ID Number, use the entry with the largest protective action distances.)

(3) Determine if the incident involves a SMALL or LARGE spill and if DAY or NIGHT. Generally, a SMALL SPILL is one which involves a single, small package (e.g., a drum containing up to approximately 200 liters), a small cylinder, or a small leak from a large package. A LARGE SPILL is one which involves a spill from a large package, or multiple spills from many small packages. DAY is any time after sunrise and before sunset. NIGHT is any time between sunset and sunrise.

(4) Look up the INITIAL ISOLATION DISTANCE. Direct all persons to move, in a crosswind direction, away from the spill to the distance specified—in meters and feet.

(5) Look up the initial PROTECTIVE ACTION DISTANCE shown in Table 1. For a given material, spill size, and whether day or night, Table 1 gives the downwind distance—in kilometers and miles— for which protective actions should be considered. For practical purposes, the Protective Action Zone (i.e., the area in which people are at risk of harmful exposure) is a square, whose length and width are the same as the downwind distance shown in Table 1.

(6) Initiate Protective Actions to the extent possible, beginning with those closest to the spill site and working away from the site in the downwind direction. When a water-reactive TIH producing material is spilled into a river or stream, the source of the toxic gas may move with the current or stretch from the spill point downstream for a substantial distance.

The shape of the area in which protective actions should be taken (the Protective Action Zone) is shown in this figure. The spill is located at the center of the small circle. The larger circle represents the INITIAL ISOLATION zone around the spill.

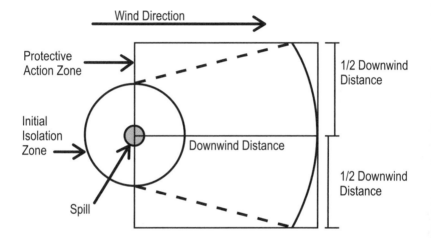

NOTE 1: See "Introduction To Table 1 - Initial Isolation And Protective Action Distances" for factors which may increase or decrease Protective Action Distances.

NOTE 2: See Table 2 – Water-Reactive Materials which Produce Toxic Gases for the list of gases produced when these materials are spilled in water.

Call the emergency response telephone number listed on the shipping paper, or the appropriate response agency as soon as possible for additional information on the material, safety precautions, and mitigation procedures.

TABLE 1 - INITIAL ISOLATION AND PROTECTIVE ACTION DISTANCES

ID No.	NAME OF MATERIAL	SMALL SPILLS (From a small package or small leak from a large package)				LARGE SPILLS (From a large package or from many small packages)				
		First ISOLATE in all Directions		Then PROTECT persons Downwind during-		First ISOLATE in all Directions		Then PROTECT persons Downwind during-		
		Meters	(Feet)	DAY Kilometers (Miles)	NIGHT Kilometers (Miles)	Meters	(Feet)	DAY Kilometers (Miles)	NIGHT Kilometers (Miles)	
1005 1005	Ammonia, anhydrous Anhydrous ammonia	30 m	(100 ft)	0.1 km (0.1 mi)	0.2 km (0.1 mi)	150 m	(500 ft)	0.8 km (0.5 mi)	2.3 km (1.4 mi)	
1008 1008	Boron trifluoride Boron trifluoride, compressed	30 m	(100 ft)	0.1 km (0.1 mi)	0.6 km (0.4 mi)	300 m	(1000 ft)	1.9 km (1.2 mi)	4.8 km (3.0 mi)	
1016 1016	Carbon monoxide Carbon monoxide, compressed	30 m	(100 ft)	0.1 km (0.1 mi)	0.1 km (0.1 mi)	150 m	(500 ft)	0.7 km (0.5 mi)	2.7 km (1.7 mi)	
1017	Chlorine	60 m	(200 ft)	0.4 km (0.3 mi)	1.6 km (1.0 mi)	600 m	(2000 ft)	3.5 km (2.2 mi)	8.0 km (5.0 mi)	
1023 1023	Coal gas Coal gas, compressed	30 m	(100 ft)	0.1 km (0.1 mi)	0.1 km (0.1 mi)	60 m	(200 ft)	0.3 km (0.2 mi)	0.4 km (0.3 mi)	
1026 1026	Cyanogen Cyanogen gas	30 m	(100 ft)	0.2 km (0.1 mi)	0.9 km (0.5 mi)	150 m	(500 ft)	1.0 km (0.7 mi)	3.5 km (2.2 mi)	
1040 1040	Ethylene oxide Ethylene oxide with Nitrogen	30 m	(100 ft)	0.1 km (0.1 mi)	0.2 km (0.1 mi)	150 m	(500 ft)	0.8 km (0.5 mi)	2.5 km (1.6 mi)	
1045 1045	Fluorine Fluorine, compressed	30 m	(100 ft)	0.1 km (0.1 mi)	0.3 km (0.2 mi)	150 m	(500 ft)	0.8 km (0.5 mi)	3.1 km (1.9 mi)	
1048	Hydrogen bromide, anhydrous	30 m	(100 ft)	0.1 km (0.1 mi)	0.4 km (0.3 mi)	300 m	(1000 ft)	1.5 km (1.0 mi)	4.5 km (2.8 mi)	
1050	Hydrogen chloride, anhydrous	30 m	(100 ft)	0.1 km (0.1 mi)	0.4 km (0.2 mi)	60 m	(200 ft)	0.3 km (0.2 mi)	1.4 km (0.9 mi)	
1051	AC (when used as a weapon)	100 m	(300 ft)	0.3 km (0.2 mi)	1.1 km (0.7 mi)	1000 m	(3000 ft)	3.8 km (2.4 mi)	7.2 km (4.5 mi)	
1051	Hydrocyanic acid, aqueous solutions, with more than 20% Hydrogen cyanide	60 m	(200 ft)	0.2 km (0.1 mi)	0.6 km (0.4 mi)	400 m	(1250 ft)	1.6 km (1.0 mi)	4.1 km (2.5 mi)	
1051 1051	Hydrogen cyanide, anhydrous, stabilized Hydrogen cyanide, stabilized									
1052	Hydrogen fluoride, anhydrous	30 m	(100 ft)	0.1 km (0.1 mi)	0.5 km (0.3 mi)	300 m	(1000 ft)	1.7 km (1.1 mi)	3.6 km (2.2 mi)	

ID No.	Name of Material	SMALL SPILLS First ISOLATE in all Directions	Then PROTECT persons Downwind during DAY	Then PROTECT persons Downwind during NIGHT	LARGE SPILLS First ISOLATE in all Directions	Then PROTECT persons Downwind during DAY	Then PROTECT persons Downwind during NIGHT
1053 1053	Hydrogen sulfide Hydrogen sulphide	30 m (100 ft)	0.1 km (0.1 mi)	0.4 km (0.3 mi)	300 m (1000 ft)	2.0 km (1.3 mi)	6.2 km (3.9 mi)
1062	Methyl bromide	30 m (100 ft)	0.1 km (0.1 mi)	0.2 km (0.1 mi)	150 m (500 ft)	0.7 km (0.4 mi)	2.2 km (1.4 mi)
1064	Methyl mercaptan	30 m (100 ft)	0.1 km (0.1 mi)	0.3 km (0.2 mi)	200 m (600 ft)	1.3 km (0.8 mi)	4.1 km (2.6 mi)
1067 1067	Dinitrogen tetroxide Nitrogen dioxide	30 m (100 ft)	0.1 km (0.1 mi)	0.4 km (0.2 mi)	400 m (1250 ft)	1.1 km (0.7 mi)	3.0 km (1.9 mi)
1069	Nitrosyl chloride	30 m (100 ft)	0.2 km (0.2 mi)	1.1 km (0.7 mi)	800 m (2500 ft)	4.2 km (2.6 mi)	11.0+ km (7.0+ mi)
1071 1071	Oil gas Oil gas, compressed	30 m (100 ft)	0.1 km (0.1 mi)	0.1 km (0.1 mi)	60 m (200 ft)	0.3 km (0.2 mi)	0.4 km (0.3 mi)
1076	CG (when used as a weapon)	200 m (600 ft)	1.1 km (0.7 mi)	4.0 km (2.5 mi)	1000 m (3000 ft)	7.5 km (4.7 mi)	11.0+ km (7.0+ mi)
1076	Diphosgene	30 m (100 ft)	0.2 km (0.1 mi)	0.2 km (0.1 mi)	30 m (100 ft)	0.4 km (0.2 mi)	0.5 km (0.3 mi)
1076	DP (when used as a weapon)	30 m (100 ft)	0.2 km (0.2 mi)	0.7 km (0.5 mi)	200 m (600 ft)	1.1 km (0.7 mi)	2.6 km (1.6 mi)
1076	Phosgene	100 m (300 ft)	0.7 km (0.4 mi)	2.6 km (1.6 mi)	500 m (1500 ft)	3.3 km (2.0 mi)	9.7 km (6.1 mi)
1079 1079	Sulfur dioxide Sulphur dioxide	60 m (200 ft)	0.3 km (0.2 mi)	1.2 km (0.7 mi)	400 m (1250 ft)	2.1 km (1.3 mi)	5.7 km (3.6 mi)
1082	Trifluorochloroethylene, stabilized	30 m (100 ft)	0.1 km (0.1 mi)	0.2 km (0.1 mi)	60 m (200 ft)	0.4 km (0.3 mi)	1.0 km (0.6 mi)
1092	Acrolein, stabilized	100 m (300 ft)	1.1 km (0.7 mi)	3.3 km (2.0 mi)	1000 m (3000 ft)	11.0+ km (7.0+ mi)	11.0+ km (7.0+ mi)
1098	Allyl alcohol	30 m (100 ft)	0.1 km (0.1 mi)	0.2 km (0.1 mi)	60 m (200 ft)	0.6 km (0.4 mi)	1.1 km (0.7 mi)
1135	Ethylene chlorohydrin	30 m (100 ft)	0.2 km (0.1 mi)	0.3 km (0.2 mi)	60 m (200 ft)	0.7 km (0.5 mi)	1.2 km (0.7 mi)
1143 1143	Crotonaldehyde Crotonaldehyde, stabilized	30 m (100 ft)	0.1 km (0.1 mi)	0.1 km (0.1 mi)	60 m (200 ft)	0.4 km (0.3 mi)	0.7 km (0.5 mi)
1162	Dimethyldichlorosilane (when spilled in water)	30 m (100 ft)	0.1 km (0.1 mi)	0.3 km (0.2 mi)	60 m (200 ft)	0.6 km (0.4 mi)	2.0 km (1.3 mi)
1163 1163	1,1-Dimethylhydrazine Dimethylhydrazine, unsymmetrical	30 m (100 ft)	0.2 km (0.1 mi)	0.5 km (0.4 mi)	100 m (300 ft)	1.3 km (0.8 mi)	2.4 km (1.5 mi)
1182	Ethyl chloroformate	30 m (100 ft)	0.1 km (0.1 mi)	0.2 km (0.1 mi)	60 m (200 ft)	0.4 km (0.3 mi)	0.7 km (0.4 mi)

TABLE 1 - INITIAL ISOLATION AND PROTECTIVE ACTION DISTANCES

ID No.	NAME OF MATERIAL	SMALL SPILLS (From a small package or small leak from a large package)					LARGE SPILLS (From a large package or from many small packages)				
		First ISOLATE in all Directions		Then PROTECT persons Downwind during-			First ISOLATE in all Directions		Then PROTECT persons Downwind during-		
				DAY		NIGHT			DAY		NIGHT	
		Meters	(Feet)	Kilometers (Miles)		Kilometers (Miles)	Meters	(Feet)	Kilometers (Miles)		Kilometers (Miles)	
1183	Ethyldichlorosilane (when spilled in water)	30 m	(100 ft)	0.1 km	(0.1 mi)	0.3 km	(0.2 mi)	60 m	(200 ft)	0.7 km	(0.4 mi)	2.2 km	(1.4 mi)
1185	Ethyleneimine, stabilized	30 m	(100 ft)	0.2 km	(0.1 mi)	0.5 km	(0.3 mi)	100 m	(300 ft)	1.1 km	(0.7 mi)	2.2 km	(1.4 mi)
1196	Ethyltrichlorosilane (when spilled in water)	30 m	(100 ft)	0.1 km	(0.1 mi)	0.3 km	(0.2 mi)	300 m	(1000 ft)	0.8 km	(0.5 mi)	2.7 km	(1.7 mi)
1238	Methyl chloroformate	30 m	(100 ft)	0.2 km	(0.2 mi)	0.6 km	(0.4 mi)	150 m	(500 ft)	1.2 km	(0.8 mi)	2.5 km	(1.6 mi)
1239	Methyl chloromethyl ether	30 m	(100 ft)	0.3 km	(0.2 mi)	1.1 km	(0.7 mi)	200 m	(600 ft)	2.5 km	(1.5 mi)	5.1 km	(3.2 mi)
1242	Methyldichlorosilane (when spilled in water)	30 m	(100 ft)	0.1 km	(0.1 mi)	0.3 km	(0.2 mi)	60 m	(200 ft)	0.8 km	(0.5 mi)	2.5 km	(1.6 mi)
1244	Methylhydrazine	30 m	(100 ft)	0.3 km	(0.2 mi)	0.7 km	(0.4 mi)	150 m	(500 ft)	1.5 km	(1.0 mi)	2.5 km	(1.5 mi)
1250	Methyltrichlorosilane (when spilled in water)	30 m	(100 ft)	0.1 km	(0.1 mi)	0.2 km	(0.2 mi)	60 m	(200 ft)	0.6 km	(0.4 mi)	2.0 km	(1.3 mi)
1251	Methyl vinyl ketone, stabilized	150 m	(500 ft)	1.6 km	(1.0 mi)	3.6 km	(2.3 mi)	1000 m	(3000 ft)	11.0+ km	(7.0+ mi)	11.0+ km	7.0+ mi)
1259	Nickel carbonyl	150 m	(500 ft)	1.4 km	(0.9 mi)	4.9 km	(3.1 mi)	1000 m	(3000 ft)	11.0+ km	(7.0+ mi)	11.0+ km	(7.0+ mi)
1295	Trichlorosilane (when spilled in water)	30 m	(100 ft)	0.1 km	(0.1 mi)	0.3 km	(0.2 mi)	60 m	(200 ft)	0.7 km	(0.5 mi)	2.3 km	(1.4 mi)
1298	Trimethylchlorosilane (when spilled in water)	30 m	(100 ft)	0.1 km	(0.1 mi)	0.1 km	(0.1 mi)	30 m	(100 ft)	0.4 km	(0.3 mi)	1.2 km	(0.7 mi)
1305	Vinyltrichlorosilane (when spilled in water)	30 m	(100 ft)	0.1 km	(0.1 mi)	0.2 km	(0.2 mi)	60 m	(200 ft)	0.6 km	(0.4 mi)	2.0 km	(1.3 mi)
1305	Vinyltrichlorosilane, stabilized (when spilled in water)											

ID No.	Name of Material	SMALL SPILLS (From a small package or small leak from a large package)			LARGE SPILLS (From a large package or from many small packages)		
		First ISOLATE in all Directions	Then PROTECT persons Downwind during DAY	Then PROTECT persons Downwind during NIGHT	First ISOLATE in all Directions	Then PROTECT persons Downwind during DAY	Then PROTECT persons Downwind during NIGHT
1340	Phosphorus pentasulfide, free from yellow and white Phosphorus **(when spilled in water)**	30 m (100 ft)	0.1 km (0.1 mi)	0.2 km (0.1 mi)	60 m (200 ft)	0.4 km (0.2 mi)	1.5 km (0.9 mi)
1340	Phosphorus pentasulphide, free from yellow and white Phosphorus **(when spilled in water)**						
1360	Calcium phosphide **(when spilled in water)**	60 m (200 ft)	0.4 km (0.2 mi)	1.5 km (0.9 mi)	500 m (1500 ft)	4.4 km (2.8 mi)	11.0+ km (7.0+ mi)
1380	Pentaborane	60 m (200 ft)	0.7 km (0.4 mi)	2.3 km (1.4 mi)	400 m (1250 ft)	4.6 km (2.9 mi)	8.9 km (5.5 mi)
1384	Sodium dithionite **(when spilled in water)**	30 m (100 ft)	0.1 km (0.1 mi)	0.2 km (0.1 mi)	30 m (100 ft)	0.3 km (0.2 mi)	1.2 km (0.7 mi)
1384	Sodium hydrosulfite **(when spilled in water)**						
1384	Sodium hydrosulphite **(when spilled in water)**						
1397	Aluminum phosphide **(when spilled in water)**	60 m (200 ft)	0.5 km (0.3 mi)	1.9 km (1.2 mi)	600 m (2000 ft)	5.7 km (3.6 mi)	11.0+ km (7.0+ mi)
1412	Lithium amide **(when spilled in water)**	30 m (100 ft)	0.1 km (0.1 mi)	0.1 km (0.1 mi)	30 m (100 ft)	0.3 km (0.2 mi)	1.0 km (0.6 mi)
1419	Magnesium aluminum phosphide **(when spilled in water)**	60 m (200 ft)	0.4 km (0.3 mi)	1.7 km (1.1 mi)	600 m (2000 ft)	5.3 km (3.3 mi)	11.0+ km (7.0+ mi)
1432	Sodium phosphide **(when spilled in water)**	30 m (100 ft)	0.3 km (0.2 mi)	1.2 km (0.8 mi)	400 m (1250 ft)	3.5 km (2.2 mi)	10.6 km (6.6 mi)
1510	Tetranitromethane	30 m (100 ft)	0.2 km (0.2 mi)	0.4 km (0.2 mi)	60 m (200 ft)	0.6 km (0.4 mi)	1.0 km (0.6 mi)
1541	Acetone cyanohydrin, stabilized **(when spilled in water)**	30 m (100 ft)	0.1 km (0.1 mi)	0.1 km (0.1 mi)	100 m (300 ft)	0.3 km (0.2 mi)	1.0 km (0.7 mi)
1556	MD **(when used as a weapon)**	30 m (100 ft)	0.2 km (0.1 mi)	0.5 km (0.4 mi)	150 m (500 ft)	0.7 km (0.4 mi)	2.2 km (1.4 mi)
1556	Methyldichloroarsine	30 m (100 ft)	0.2 km (0.1 mi)	0.2 km (0.2 mi)	60 m (200 ft)	0.5 km (0.3 mi)	0.8 km (0.5 mi)
1556	PD **(when used as a weapon)**	30 m (100 ft)	0.1 km (0.1 mi)	0.1 km (0.1 mi)	30 m (100 ft)	0.2 km (0.1 mi)	0.2 km (0.1 mi)

TABLE 1 - INITIAL ISOLATION AND PROTECTIVE ACTION DISTANCES

ID No.	NAME OF MATERIAL	SMALL SPILLS (From a small package or small leak from a large package)			LARGE SPILLS (From a large package or from many small packages)			
		First ISOLATE in all Directions	Then PROTECT persons Downwind during-		First ISOLATE in all Directions	Then PROTECT persons Downwind during-		
			DAY	NIGHT		DAY	NIGHT	
		Meters (Feet)	Kilometers (Miles)	Kilometers (Miles)	Meters (Feet)	Kilometers (Miles)	Kilometers (Miles)	
1560 1560	Arsenic chloride Arsenic trichloride	30 m (100 ft)	0.2 km (0.1 mi)	0.3 km (0.2 mi)	100 m (300 ft)	1.1 km (0.7 mi)	1.8 km (1.1 mi)	
1569	Bromoacetone	30 m (100 ft)	0.2 km (0.2 mi)	0.8 km (0.5 mi)	100 m (300 ft)	1.1 km (0.7 mi)	2.3 km (1.5 mi)	
1580	Chloropicrin	30 m (100 ft)	0.4 km (0.3 mi)	1.0 km (0.6 mi)	150 m (500 ft)	1.9 km (1.2 mi)	3.3 km (2.1 mi)	
1581 1581	Chloropicrin and Methyl bromide mixture Methyl bromide and Chloropicrin mixture	30 m (100 ft)	0.1 km (0.1 mi)	0.6 km (0.4 mi)	300 m (1000 ft)	2.1 km (1.3 mi)	5.9 km (3.7 mi)	
1582 1582	Chloropicrin and Methyl chloride mixture Methyl chloride and Chloropicrin mixture	30 m (100 ft)	0.1 km (0.1 mi)	0.4 km (0.3 mi)	60 m (200 ft)	0.4 km (0.2 mi)	1.7 km (1.1 mi)	
1583	Chloropicrin mixture, n.o.s.	30 m (100 ft)	0.4 km (0.3 mi)	1.0 km (0.6 mi)	150 m (500 ft)	1.9 km (1.2 mi)	3.3 km (2.1 mi)	
1589	CK (when used as a weapon)	60 m (200 ft)	0.4 km (0.3 mi)	1.5 km (1.0 mi)	600 m (2000 ft)	4.1 km (2.5 mi)	8.0 km (5.0 mi)	
1589	Cyanogen chloride, stabilized	100 m (300 ft)	0.4 km (0.3 mi)	1.5 km (0.9 mi)	400 m (1250 ft)	3.1 km (2.0 mi)	6.8 km (4.3 mi)	
1595 1595	Dimethyl sulfate Dimethyl sulphate	30 m (100 ft)	0.1 km (0.1 mi)	0.2 km (0.1 mi)	60 m (200 ft)	0.5 km (0.3 mi)	0.7 km (0.5 mi)	
1605	Ethylene dibromide	30 m (100 ft)	0.1 km (0.1 mi)	0.1 km (0.1 mi)	30 m (100 ft)	0.3 km (0.2 mi)	0.5 km (0.3 mi)	
1612	Hexaethyl tetraphosphate and compressed gas mixture	100 m (300 ft)	0.8 km (0.5 mi)	2.7 km (1.7 mi)	400 m (1250 ft)	3.5 km (2.2 mi)	8.1 km (5.1 mi)	
1613 1613	Hydrocyanic acid, aqueous solution, with not more than 20% Hydrogen cyanide Hydrogen cyanide, aqueous solution, with not more than 20% Hydrogen cyanide	30 m (100 ft)	0.1 km (0.1 mi)	0.1 km (0.1 mi)	100 m (300 ft)	0.5 km (0.3 mi)	1.1 km (0.7 mi)	

ID No.	Name of Material	Small Spills First ISOLATE (all directions)	Small Spills Then PROTECT Day	Small Spills Then PROTECT Night	Large Spills First ISOLATE (all directions)	Large Spills Then PROTECT Day	Large Spills Then PROTECT Night
1614	Hydrogen cyanide, stabilized (absorbed)	60 m (200 ft)	0.2 km (0.1 mi)	0.6 km (0.4 mi)	150 m (500 ft)	0.6 km (0.4 mi)	1.7 km (1.1 mi)
1647 / 1647	Ethylene dibromide and Methyl bromide mixture, liquid / Methyl bromide and Ethylene dibromide mixture, liquid	30 m (100 ft)	0.1 km (0.1 mi)	0.2 km (0.1 mi)	150 m (500 ft)	0.7 km (0.4 mi)	2.2 km (1.4 mi)
1660 / 1660	Nitric oxide / Nitric oxide, compressed	30 m (100 ft)	0.1 km (0.1 mi)	0.6 km (0.4 mi)	100 m (300 ft)	0.6 km (0.4 mi)	2.2 km (1.4 mi)
1670	Perchloromethyl mercaptan	30 m (100 ft)	0.2 km (0.2 mi)	0.4 km (0.2 mi)	100 m (300 ft)	0.8 km (0.5 mi)	1.4 km (0.9 mi)
1680	Potassium cyanide (when spilled in water)	30 m (100 ft)	0.1 km (0.1 mi)	0.2 km (0.1 mi)	100 m (300 ft)	0.3 km (0.2 mi)	1.2 km (0.8 mi)
1680	Potassium cyanide, solid (when spilled in water)	30 m (100 ft)					
1689	Sodium cyanide (when spilled in water)	30 m (100 ft)	0.1 km (0.1 mi)	0.2 km (0.1 mi)	100 m (300 ft)	0.4 km (0.3 mi)	1.4 km (0.9 mi)
1689	Sodium cyanide, solid (when spilled in water)	30 m (100 ft)					
1694	CA (when used as a weapon)	30 m (100 ft)	0.1 km (0.1 mi)	0.4 km (0.3 mi)	100 m (300 ft)	0.6 km (0.4 mi)	2.7 km (1.7 mi)
1695	Chloroacetone, stabilized	30 m (100 ft)	0.2 km (0.1 mi)	0.3 km (0.2 mi)	60 m (200 ft)	0.6 km (0.4 mi)	1.1 km (0.7 mi)
1697	CN (when used as a weapon)	30 m (100 ft)	0.1 km (0.1 mi)	0.2 km (0.1 mi)	60 m (200 ft)	0.3 km (0.2 mi)	1.4 km (0.9 mi)
1698 / 1698	Adamsite (when used as a weapon) / DM (when used as a weapon)	30 m (100 ft)	0.1 km (0.1 mi)	0.3 km (0.2 mi)	60 m (200 ft)	0.3 km (0.2 mi)	1.4 km (0.9 mi)
1699	DA (when used as a weapon)	30 m (100 ft)	0.1 km (0.1 mi)	0.6 km (0.4 mi)	200 m (600 ft)	1.0 km (0.6 mi)	3.8 km (2.4 mi)
1716	Acetyl bromide (when spilled in water)	30 m (100 ft)	0.1 km (0.1 mi)	0.3 km (0.2 mi)	60 m (200 ft)	0.6 km (0.4 mi)	1.7 km (1.1 mi)
1717	Acetyl chloride (when spilled in water)	30 m (100 ft)	0.1 km (0.1 mi)	0.3 km (0.2 mi)	100 m (300 ft)	0.9 km (0.6 mi)	2.8 km (1.8 mi)

TABLE 1 - INITIAL ISOLATION AND PROTECTIVE ACTION DISTANCES

ID No.	NAME OF MATERIAL	SMALL SPILLS (From a small package or small leak from a large package)				LARGE SPILLS (From a large package or from many small packages)			
		First ISOLATE in all Directions		Then PROTECT persons Downwind during-		First ISOLATE in all Directions		Then PROTECT persons Downwind during-	
				DAY	NIGHT			DAY	NIGHT
		Meters	(Feet)	Kilometers (Miles)	Kilometers (Miles)	Meters	(Feet)	Kilometers (Miles)	Kilometers (Miles)
1722 1722	Allyl chlorocarbonate Allyl chloroformate	100 m	(300 ft)	1.2 km (0.8 mi)	2.8 km (1.8 mi)	600 m	(2000 ft)	7.8 km (4.9 mi)	11.0+ km (7.0+ mi)
1724	Allyltrichlorosilane, stabilized (when spilled in water)	30 m	(100 ft)	0.1 km (0.1 mi)	0.2 km (0.2 mi)	60 m	(200 ft)	0.6 km (0.4 mi)	1.9 km (1.2 mi)
1725	Aluminum bromide, anhydrous (when spilled in water)	30 m	(100 ft)	0.1 km (0.1 mi)	0.3 km (0.2 mi)	30 m	(100 ft)	0.4 km (0.2 mi)	1.2 km (0.8 mi)
1726	Aluminum chloride, anhydrous (when spilled in water)	30 m	(100 ft)	0.1 km (0.1 mi)	0.3 km (0.2 mi)	60 m	(200 ft)	0.6 km (0.4 mi)	2.1 km (1.3 mi)
1728	Amyltrichlorosilane (when spilled in water)	30 m	(100 ft)	0.1 km (0.1 mi)	0.2 km (0.2 mi)	60 m	(200 ft)	0.6 km (0.4 mi)	1.9 km (1.2 mi)
1732	Antimony pentafluoride (when spilled in water)	30 m	(100 ft)	0.1 km (0.1 mi)	0.5 km (0.3 mi)	150 m	(500 ft)	1.2 km (0.8 mi)	4.0 km (2.5 mi)
1741	Boron trichloride (when spilled on land)	30 m	(100 ft)	0.1 km (0.1 mi)	0.3 km (0.2 mi)	100 m	(300 ft)	0.6 km (0.4 mi)	1.5 km (1.0 mi)
1741	Boron trichloride (when spilled in water)	30 m	(100 ft)	0.1 km (0.1 mi)	0.5 km (0.3 mi)	100 m	(300 ft)	1.3 km (0.8 mi)	3.9 km (2.4 mi)
1744 1744 1744	Bromine Bromine, solution Bromine, solution (Inhalation Hazard Zone A)	60 m	(200 ft)	0.6 km (0.4 mi)	1.8 km (1.1 mi)	300 m	(1000 ft)	3.1 km (1.9 mi)	6.6 km (4.1 mi)
1744	Bromine, solution (Inhalation Hazard Zone B)	30 m	(100 ft)	0.5 km (0.3 mi)	1.1 km (0.7 mi)	150 m	(500 ft)	1.9 km (1.2 mi)	3.4 km (2.1 mi)
1745	Bromine pentafluoride (when spilled on land)	30 m	(100 ft)	0.2 km (0.2 mi)	0.9 km (0.6 mi)	150 m	(500 ft)	1.5 km (0.9 mi)	3.2 km (2.0 mi)
1745	Bromine pentafluoride (when spilled in water)	30 m	(100 ft)	0.1 km (0.1 mi)	0.5 km (0.4 mi)	150 m	(500 ft)	1.3 km (0.8 mi)	4.2 km (2.6 mi)

ID No.	NAME OF MATERIAL	SMALL SPILLS			LARGE SPILLS		
		First ISOLATE in all Directions	Then PROTECT persons Downwind during DAY	NIGHT	First ISOLATE in all Directions	Then PROTECT persons Downwind during DAY	NIGHT
1746	Bromine trifluoride **(when spilled on land)**	30 m (100 ft)	0.1 km (0.1 mi)	0.1 km (0.1 mi)	30 m (100 ft)	0.3 km (0.2 mi)	0.5 km (0.3 mi)
1746	Bromine trifluoride **(when spilled in water)**	30 m (100 ft)	0.1 km (0.1 mi)	0.5 km (0.3 mi)	100 m (300 ft)	1.1 km (0.7 mi)	3.9 km (2.4 mi)
1747	Butyltrichlorosilane **(when spilled in water)**	30 m (100 ft)	0.1 km (0.1 mi)	0.1 km (0.1 mi)	30 m (100 ft)	0.4 km (0.2 mi)	1.2 km (0.7 mi)
1749	Chlorine trifluoride	60 m (200 ft)	0.4 km (0.3 mi)	1.8 km (1.1 mi)	400 m (1250 ft)	2.7 km (1.7 mi)	7.2 km (4.5 mi)
1752	Chloroacetyl chloride **(when spilled on land)**	30 m (100 ft)	0.3 km (0.2 mi)	0.7 km (0.4 mi)	150 m (500 ft)	1.4 km (0.9 mi)	2.3 km (1.5 mi)
1752	Chloroacetyl chloride **(when spilled in water)**	30 m (100 ft)	0.1 km (0.1 mi)	0.1 km (0.1 mi)	30 m (100 ft)	0.3 km (0.2 mi)	0.9 km (0.5 mi)
1753	Chlorophenyltrichlorosilane **(when spilled in water)**	30 m (100 ft)	0.1 km (0.1 mi)	0.1 km (0.1 mi)	30 m (100 ft)	0.3 km (0.2 mi)	1.0 km (0.7 mi)
1754	Chlorosulfonic acid **(when spilled on land)**	30 m (100 ft)	0.1 km (0.1 mi)	0.1 km (0.1 mi)	30 m (100 ft)	0.3 km (0.2 mi)	0.4 km (0.3 mi)
1754	Chlorosulfonic acid **(when spilled in water)**	30 m (100 ft)	0.1 km (0.1 mi)	0.5 km (0.3 mi)	60 m (200 ft)	1.0 km (0.6 mi)	2.9 km (1.8 mi)
1754	Chlorosulfonic acid and Sulfur trioxide mixture **(when spilled on land)**	60 m (200 ft)	0.4 km (0.2 mi)	1.0 km (0.6 mi)	300 m (1000 ft)	2.9 km (1.8 mi)	5.7 km (3.6 mi)
1754	Chlorosulfonic acid and Sulfur trioxide mixture **(when spilled in water)**	30 m (100 ft)	0.1 km (0.1 mi)	0.5 km (0.3 mi)	60 m (200 ft)	1.0 km (0.6 mi)	2.9 km (1.8 mi)
1754	Chlorosulphonic acid **(when spilled on land)**	30 m (100 ft)	0.1 km (0.1 mi)	0.1 km (0.1 mi)	30 m (100 ft)	0.3 km (0.2 mi)	0.4 km (0.3 mi)
1754	Chlorosulphonic acid **(when spilled in water)**	30 m (100 ft)	0.1 km (0.1 mi)	0.5 km (0.3 mi)	60 m (200 ft)	1.0 km (0.6 mi)	2.9 km (1.8 mi)
1754	Chlorosulphonic acid and Sulphur trioxide mixture **(when spilled on land)**	60 m (200 ft)	0.4 km (0.2 mi)	1.0 km (0.6 mi)	300 m (1000 ft)	2.9 km (1.8 mi)	5.7 km (3.6 mi)

TABLE 1 - INITIAL ISOLATION AND PROTECTIVE ACTION DISTANCES

ID No.	NAME OF MATERIAL	SMALL SPILLS (From a small package or small leak from a large package)				LARGE SPILLS (From a large package or from many small packages)			
		First ISOLATE in all Directions	Then PROTECT persons Downwind during-			First ISOLATE in all Directions	Then PROTECT persons Downwind during-		
				DAY	NIGHT			DAY	NIGHT
		Meters (Feet)		Kilometers (Miles)	Kilometers (Miles)	Meters (Feet)		Kilometers (Miles)	Kilometers (Miles)
1754	Chlorosulphonic acid and Sulphur trioxide mixture (when spilled in water)	30 m	(100 ft)	0.1 km (0.1 mi)	0.5 km (0.3 mi)	60 m	(200 ft)	1.0 km (0.6 mi)	2.9 km (1.8 mi)
1754	Sulfur trioxide and Chlorosulfonic acid mixture (when spilled on land)	60 m	(200 ft)	0.4 km (0.2 mi)	1.0 km (0.6 mi)	300 m	(1000 ft)	2.9 km (1.8 mi)	5.7 km (3.6 mi)
1754	Sulfur trioxide and Chlorosulfonic acid mixture (when spilled in water)	30 m	(100 ft)	0.1 km (0.1 mi)	0.5 km (0.3 mi)	60 m	(200 ft)	1.0 km (0.6 mi)	2.9 km (1.8 mi)
1754	Sulphur trioxide and Chlorosulphonic acid mixture (when spilled on land)	60 m	(200 ft)	0.4 km (0.2 mi)	1.0 km (0.6 mi)	300 m	(1000 ft)	2.9 km (1.8 mi)	5.7 km (3.6 mi)
1754	Sulphur trioxide and Chlorosulphonic acid mixture (when spilled in water)	30 m	(100 ft)	0.1 km (0.1 mi)	0.5 km (0.3 mi)	60 m	(200 ft)	1.0 km (0.6 mi)	2.9 km (1.8 mi)
1758	Chromium oxychloride (when spilled in water)	30 m	(100 ft)	0.1 km (0.1 mi)	0.1 km (0.1 mi)	30 m	(100 ft)	0.2 km (0.2 mi)	0.8 km (0.5 mi)
1762	Cyclohexenyltrichlorosilane (when spilled in water)	30 m	(100 ft)	0.1 km (0.1 mi)	0.2 km (0.1 mi)	30 m	(100 ft)	0.4 km (0.3 mi)	1.4 km (0.9 mi)
1763	Cyclohexyltrichlorosilane (when spilled in water)	30 m	(100 ft)	0.1 km (0.1 mi)	0.2 km (0.1 mi)	30 m	(100 ft)	0.4 km (0.3 mi)	1.4 km (0.9 mi)
1765	Dichloroacetyl chloride (when spilled in water)	30 m	(100 ft)	0.1 km (0.1 mi)	0.1 km (0.1 mi)	30 m	(100 ft)	0.3 km (0.2 mi)	1.0 km (0.6 mi)
1766	Dichlorophenyltrichlorosilane (when spilled in water)	30 m	(100 ft)	0.1 km (0.1 mi)	0.2 km (0.2 mi)	60 m	(200 ft)	0.7 km (0.4 mi)	2.2 km (1.4 mi)
1767	Diethyldichlorosilane (when spilled in water)	30 m	(100 ft)	0.1 km (0.1 mi)	0.1 km (0.1 mi)	30 m	(100 ft)	0.4 km (0.2 mi)	1.1 km (0.7 mi)
1769	Diphenyldichlorosilane (when spilled in water)	30 m	(100 ft)	0.1 km (0.1 mi)	0.1 km (0.1 mi)	30 m	(100 ft)	0.2 km (0.2 mi)	0.6 km (0.4 mi)

ID No.	Name of Material	SMALL SPILLS First ISOLATE in all Directions	SMALL SPILLS Then PROTECT persons Downwind during DAY	SMALL SPILLS Then PROTECT persons Downwind during NIGHT	LARGE SPILLS First ISOLATE in all Directions	LARGE SPILLS Then PROTECT persons Downwind during DAY	LARGE SPILLS Then PROTECT persons Downwind during NIGHT
1771	Dodecyltrichlorosilane (when spilled in water)	30 m (100 ft)	0.1 km (0.1 mi)	0.2 km (0.1 mi)	60 m (200 ft)	0.5 km (0.3 mi)	1.4 km (0.9 mi)
1777 1777	Fluorosulfonic acid (when spilled in water) Fluorosulphonic acid (when spilled in water)	30 m (100 ft)	0.1 km (0.1 mi)	0.1 km (0.1 mi)	30 m (100 ft)	0.2 km (0.2 mi)	0.8 km (0.5 mi)
1781	Hexadecyltrichlorosilane (when spilled in water)	30 m (100 ft)	0.1 km (0.1 mi)	0.1 km (0.1 mi)	30 m (100 ft)	0.2 km (0.2 mi)	0.7 km (0.4 mi)
1784	Hexyltrichlorosilane (when spilled in water)	30 m (100 ft)	0.1 km (0.1 mi)	0.2 km (0.1 mi)	60 m (200 ft)	0.5 km (0.3 mi)	1.5 km (0.9 mi)
1799	Nonyltrichlorosilane (when spilled in water)	30 m (100 ft)	0.1 km (0.1 mi)	0.2 km (0.1 mi)	60 m (200 ft)	0.5 km (0.3 mi)	1.6 km (1.0 mi)
1800	Octadecyltrichlorosilane (when spilled in water)	30 m (100 ft)	0.1 km (0.1 mi)	0.2 km (0.1 mi)	30 m (100 ft)	0.4 km (0.3 mi)	1.4 km (0.9 mi)
1801	Octyltrichlorosilane (when spilled in water)	30 m (100 ft)	0.1 km (0.1 mi)	0.2 km (0.1 mi)	60 m (200 ft)	0.5 km (0.3 mi)	1.6 km (1.0 mi)
1804	Phenyltrichlorosilane (when spilled in water)	30 m (100 ft)	0.1 km (0.1 mi)	0.2 km (0.1 mi)	60 m (200 ft)	0.5 km (0.3 mi)	1.6 km (1.0 mi)
1806	Phosphorus pentachloride (when spilled in water)	30 m (100 ft)	0.1 km (0.1 mi)	0.2 km (0.2 mi)	30 m (100 ft)	0.4 km (0.3 mi)	1.6 km (1.0 mi)
1808	Phosphorus tribromide (when spilled in water)	30 m (100 ft)	0.1 km (0.1 mi)	0.3 km (0.2 mi)	60 m (200 ft)	0.6 km (0.4 mi)	2.0 km (1.2 mi)
1809	Phosphorus trichloride (when spilled on land)	30 m (100 ft)	0.2 km (0.2 mi)	0.7 km (0.4 mi)	150 m (500 ft)	1.5 km (0.9 mi)	3.0 km (1.9 mi)
1809	Phosphorus trichloride (when spilled in water)	30 m (100 ft)	0.1 km (0.1 mi)	0.4 km (0.2 mi)	60 m (200 ft)	0.8 km (0.5 mi)	2.8 km (1.7 mi)
1810	Phosphorus oxychloride (when spilled on land)	30 m (100 ft)	0.3 km (0.2 mi)	0.5 km (0.4 mi)	100 m (300 ft)	1.1 km (0.7 mi)	2.0 km (1.3 mi)
1810	Phosphorus oxychloride (when spilled in water)	30 m (100 ft)	0.1 km (0.1 mi)	0.3 km (0.2 mi)	60 m (200 ft)	0.7 km (0.5 mi)	2.3 km (1.4 mi)

TABLE 1 - INITIAL ISOLATION AND PROTECTIVE ACTION DISTANCES

		SMALL SPILLS (From a small package or small leak from a large package)						LARGE SPILLS (From a large package or from many small packages)					
		First ISOLATE in all Directions		Then PROTECT persons Downwind during-				First ISOLATE in all Directions		Then PROTECT persons Downwind during-			
				DAY		NIGHT				DAY		NIGHT	
ID No.	NAME OF MATERIAL	Meters	(Feet)	Kilometers (Miles)		Kilometers (Miles)		Meters	(Feet)	Kilometers (Miles)		Kilometers (Miles)	
1815	Propionyl chloride (when spilled in water)	30 m	(100 ft)	0.1 km	(0.1 mi)	0.1 km	(0.1 mi)	30 m	(100 ft)	0.3 km	(0.2 mi)	0.8 km	(0.5 mi)
1816	Propyltrichlorosilane (when spilled in water)	30 m	(100 ft)	0.1 km	(0.1 mi)	0.2 km	(0.2 mi)	60 m	(200 ft)	0.6 km	(0.4 mi)	2.0 km	(1.3 mi)
1818	Silicon tetrachloride (when spilled in water)	30 m	(100 ft)	0.1 km	(0.1 mi)	0.3 km	(0.2 mi)	100 m	(300 ft)	0.9 km	(0.6 mi)	2.9 km	(1.8 mi)
1828	Sulfur chlorides (when spilled on land)	30 m	(100 ft)	0.1 km	(0.1 mi)	0.2 km	(0.1 mi)	60 m	(200 ft)	0.7 km	(0.5 mi)	1.2 km	(0.8 mi)
1828	Sulfur chlorides (when spilled in water)	30 m	(100 ft)	0.1 km	(0.1 mi)	0.2 km	(0.1 mi)	30 m	(100 ft)	0.4 km	(0.2 mi)	1.2 km	(0.8 mi)
1828	Sulphur chlorides (when spilled on land)	30 m	(100 ft)	0.1 km	(0.1 mi)	0.2 km	(0.1 mi)	60 m	(200 ft)	0.7 km	(0.5 mi)	1.2 km	(0.8 mi)
1828	Sulphur chlorides (when spilled in water)	30 m	(100 ft)	0.1 km	(0.1 mi)	0.2 km	(0.1 mi)	30 m	(100 ft)	0.4 km	(0.2 mi)	1.2 km	(0.8 mi)
1829 1829 1829 1829 1829 1829	Sulfur trioxide, inhibited Sulfur trioxide, stabilized Sulfur trioxide, uninhibited Sulphur trioxide, inhibited Sulphur trioxide, stabilized Sulphur trioxide, uninhibited	60 m	(200 ft)	0.4 km	(0.2 mi)	1.0 km	(0.6 mi)	300 m	(1000 ft)	2.9 km	(1.8 mi)	5.7 km	(3.6 mi)
1831 1831 1831 1831	Sulfuric acid, fuming Sulfuric acid, fuming, with not less than 30% free Sulfur trioxide Sulphuric acid, fuming Sulphuric acid, fuming, with not less than 30% free Sulphur trioxide	60 m	(200 ft)	0.4 km	(0.2 mi)	1.0 km	(0.6 mi)	300 m	(1000 ft)	2.9 km	(1.8 mi)	5.7 km	(3.6 mi)

ID No.	Name of Material						
1834	Sulfuryl chloride (when spilled on land)	30 m (100 ft)	0.2 km (0.1 mi)	0.5 km (0.4 mi)	100 m (300 ft)	1.0 km (0.6 mi)	2.1 km (1.3 mi)
1834	Sulfuryl chloride (when spilled in water)	30 m (100 ft)	0.1 km (0.1 mi)	0.2 km (0.1 mi)	60 m (200 ft)	0.5 km (0.3 mi)	1.8 km (1.2 mi)
1834	Sulphuryl chloride (when spilled on land)	30 m (100 ft)	0.2 km (0.1 mi)	0.5 km (0.4 mi)	100 m (300 ft)	1.0 km (0.6 mi)	2.1 km (1.3 mi)
1834	Sulphuryl chloride (when spilled in water)	30 m (100 ft)	0.1 km (0.1 mi)	0.2 km (0.1 mi)	60 m (200 ft)	0.5 km (0.3 mi)	1.8 km (1.2 mi)
1836	Thionyl chloride (when spilled on land)	30 m (100 ft)	0.3 km (0.2 mi)	0.7 km (0.5 mi)	100 m (300 ft)	0.9 km (0.6 mi)	1.9 km (1.2 mi)
1836	Thionyl chloride (when spilled in water)	30 m (100 ft)	0.3 km (0.2 mi)	1.4 km (0.9 mi)	300 m (1000 ft)	3.3 km (2.1 mi)	7.5 km (4.7 mi)
1838	Titanium tetrachloride (when spilled on land)	30 m (100 ft)	0.1 km (0.1 mi)	0.2 km (0.1 mi)	60 m (200 ft)	0.5 km (0.3 mi)	0.8 km (0.5 mi)
1838	Titanium tetrachloride (when spilled in water)	30 m (100 ft)	0.1 km (0.1 mi)	0.2 km (0.1 mi)	60 m (200 ft)	0.6 km (0.4 mi)	1.9 km (1.2 mi)
1859	Silicon tetrafluoride Silicon tetrafluoride, compressed	30 m (100 ft)	0.1 km (0.1 mi)	0.5 km (0.3 mi)	100 m (300 ft)	0.5 km (0.3 mi)	1.9 km (1.2 mi)
1892	ED (when used as a weapon)	30 m (100 ft)	0.1 km (0.1 mi)	0.3 km (0.2 mi)	150 m (500 ft)	0.8 km (0.5 mi)	1.9 km (1.2 mi)
1892	Ethyldichloroarsine	30 m (100 ft)	0.2 km (0.1 mi)	0.3 km (0.2 mi)	60 m (200 ft)	0.6 km (0.4 mi)	0.9 km (0.6 mi)
1898	Acetyl iodide (when spilled in water)	30 m (100 ft)	0.1 km (0.1 mi)	0.3 km (0.2 mi)	60 m (200 ft)	0.5 km (0.3 mi)	1.4 km (0.9 mi)
1911	Diborane Diborane, compressed	60 m (200 ft)	0.3 km (0.2 mi)	1.2 km (0.8 mi)	300 m (1000 ft)	1.7 km (1.1 mi)	4.3 km (2.7 mi)
1923	Calcium dithionite (when spilled in water) Calcium hydrosulfite (when spilled in water) Calcium hydrosulphite (when spilled in water)	30 m (100 ft)	0.1 km (0.1 mi)	0.2 km (0.2 mi)	30 m (100 ft)	0.3 km (0.2 mi)	1.2 km (0.8 mi)

TABLE 1 - INITIAL ISOLATION AND PROTECTIVE ACTION DISTANCES

ID No.	NAME OF MATERIAL	SMALL SPILLS (From a small package or small leak from a large package)			LARGE SPILLS (From a large package or from many small packages)			
		First ISOLATE in all Directions	Then PROTECT persons Downwind during-		First ISOLATE in all Directions	Then PROTECT persons Downwind during-		
			DAY	NIGHT		DAY		NIGHT
		Meters (Feet)	Kilometers (Miles)	Kilometers (Miles)	Meters (Feet)	Kilometers (Miles)		Kilometers (Miles)
1929	Potassium dithionite (when spilled in water)	30 m (100 ft)	0.1 km (0.1 mi)	0.2 km (0.1 mi)	30 m (100 ft)	0.3 km (0.2 mi)		1.1 km (0.7 mi)
1929	Potassium hydrosulfite (when spilled in water)							
1929	Potassium hydrosulphite (when spilled in water)							
1931	Zinc dithionite (when spilled in water)	30 m (100 ft)	0.1 km (0.1 mi)	0.2 km (0.1 mi)	30 m (100 ft)	0.3 km (0.2 mi)		1.1 km (0.7 mi)
1931	Zinc hydrosulfite (when spilled in water)							
1931	Zinc hydrosulphite (when spilled in water)							
1953	Compressed gas, flammable, poisonous, n.o.s. (Inhalation Hazard Zone A)	100 m (300 ft)	0.6 km (0.4 mi)	2.5 km (1.5 mi)	800 m (2500 ft)	4.4 km (2.7 mi)		8.9 km (5.6 mi)
1953	Compressed gas, flammable, poisonous, n.o.s. (Inhalation Hazard Zone B)	30 m (100 ft)	0.2 km (0.1 mi)	0.8 km (0.5 mi)	400 m (1250 ft)	1.9 km (1.2 mi)		4.8 km (3.0 mi)
1953	Compressed gas, flammable, poisonous, n.o.s. (Inhalation Hazard Zone C)	30 m (100 ft)	0.1 km (0.1 mi)	0.3 km (0.2 mi)	300 m (1000 ft)	1.3 km (0.8 mi)		4.1 km (2.6 mi)
1953	Compressed gas, flammable, poisonous, n.o.s. (Inhalation Hazard Zone D)	30 m (100 ft)	0.1 km (0.1 mi)	0.2 km (0.1 mi)	150 m (500 ft)	0.7 km (0.5 mi)		2.7 km (1.7 mi)
1953	Compressed gas, flammable, toxic, n.o.s. (Inhalation Hazard Zone A)	100 m (300 ft)	0.6 km (0.4 mi)	2.5 km (1.5 mi)	800 m (2500 ft)	4.4 km (2.7 mi)		8.9 km (5.6 mi)

ID No.	Name of Material	First ISOLATE in all Directions	Then PROTECT persons Downwind during DAY	Then PROTECT persons Downwind during NIGHT	First ISOLATE in all Directions	Then PROTECT persons Downwind during DAY	Then PROTECT persons Downwind during NIGHT
1953	Compressed gas, flammable, toxic, n.o.s. (Inhalation Hazard Zone B)	30 m (100 ft)	0.2 km (0.1 mi)	0.8 km (0.5 mi)	400 m (1250 ft)	1.9 km (1.2 mi)	4.8 km (3.0 mi)
1953	Compressed gas, flammable, toxic, n.o.s. (Inhalation Hazard Zone C)	30 m (100 ft)	0.1 km (0.1 mi)	0.3 km (0.2 mi)	300 m (1000 ft)	1.3 km (0.8 mi)	4.1 km (2.6 mi)
1953	Compressed gas, flammable, toxic, n.o.s. (Inhalation Hazard Zone D)	30 m (100 ft)	0.1 km (0.1 mi)	0.2 km (0.1 mi)	150 m (500 ft)	0.7 km (0.5 mi)	2.7 km (1.7 mi)
1953	Compressed gas, poisonous, flammable, n.o.s.	100 m (300 ft)	0.6 km (0.4 mi)	2.5 km (1.5 mi)	800 m (2500 ft)	4.4 km (2.7 mi)	8.9 km (5.6 mi)
1953	Compressed gas, poisonous, flammable, n.o.s. (Inhalation Hazard Zone A)						
1953	Compressed gas, poisonous, flammable, n.o.s. (Inhalation Hazard Zone B)	30 m (100 ft)	0.2 km (0.1 mi)	0.8 km (0.5 mi)	400 m (1250 ft)	1.9 km (1.2 mi)	4.8 km (3.0 mi)
1953	Compressed gas, poisonous, flammable, n.o.s. (Inhalation Hazard Zone C)	30 m (100 ft)	0.1 km (0.1 mi)	0.3 km (0.2 mi)	300 m (1000 ft)	1.3 km (0.8 mi)	4.1 km (2.6 mi)
1953	Compressed gas, poisonous, flammable, n.o.s. (Inhalation Hazard Zone D)	30 m (100 ft)	0.1 km (0.1 mi)	0.2 km (0.1 mi)	150 m (500 ft)	0.7 km (0.5 mi)	2.7 km (1.7 mi)
1953	Compressed gas, toxic, flammable, n.o.s.	100 m (300 ft)	0.6 km (0.4 mi)	2.5 km (1.5 mi)	800 m (2500 ft)	4.4 km (2.7 mi)	8.9 km (5.6 mi)
1953	Compressed gas, toxic, flammable, n.o.s. (Inhalation Hazard Zone A)						
1953	Compressed gas, toxic, flammable, n.o.s. (Inhalation Hazard Zone B)	30 m (100 ft)	0.2 km (0.1 mi)	0.8 km (0.5 mi)	400 m (1250 ft)	1.9 km (1.2 mi)	4.8 km (3.0 mi)

TABLE 1 - INITIAL ISOLATION AND PROTECTIVE ACTION DISTANCES

ID No.	NAME OF MATERIAL	SMALL SPILLS (From a small package or small leak from a large package)			LARGE SPILLS (From a large package or from many small packages)			
		First ISOLATE in all Directions	Then PROTECT persons Downwind during-		First ISOLATE in all Directions	Then PROTECT persons Downwind during-		
			DAY	NIGHT		DAY		NIGHT
		Meters (Feet)	Kilometers (Miles)	Kilometers (Miles)	Meters (Feet)	Kilometers (Miles)		Kilometers (Miles)
1953	Compressed gas, toxic, flammable, n.o.s. (Inhalation Hazard Zone C)	30 m (100 ft)	0.1 km (0.1 mi)	0.3 km (0.2 mi)	300 m (1000 ft)	1.3 km (0.8 mi)		4.1 km (2.6 mi)
1953	Compressed gas, toxic, flammable, n.o.s. (Inhalation Hazard Zone D)	30 m (100 ft)	0.1 km (0.1 mi)	0.2 km (0.1 mi)	150 m (500 ft)	0.7 km (0.5 mi)		2.7 km (1.7 mi)
1955 1955	Compressed gas, poisonous, n.o.s. Compressed gas, poisonous, n.o.s. (Inhalation Hazard Zone A)	100 m (300 ft)	0.5 km (0.3 mi)	2.1 km (1.3 mi)	800 m (2500 ft)	4.4 km (2.7 mi)		8.9 km (5.6 mi)
1955	Compressed gas, poisonous, n.o.s. (Inhalation Hazard Zone B)	30 m (100 ft)	0.2 km (0.1 mi)	0.8 km (0.5 mi)	400 m (1250 ft)	1.9 km (1.2 mi)		4.8 km (3.0 mi)
1955	Compressed gas, poisonous, n.o.s. (Inhalation Hazard Zone C)	30 m (100 ft)	0.1 km (0.1 mi)	0.4 km (0.2 mi)	200 m (600 ft)	1.0 km (0.6 mi)		3.2 km (2.0 mi)
1955	Compressed gas, poisonous, n.o.s. (Inhalation Hazard Zone D)	30 m (100 ft)	0.1 km (0.1 mi)	0.2 km (0.1 mi)	150 m (500 ft)	0.7 km (0.5 mi)		2.7 km (1.7 mi)
1955 1955	Compressed gas, toxic, n.o.s. Compressed gas, toxic, n.o.s. (Inhalation Hazard Zone A)	100 m (300 ft)	0.5 km (0.3 mi)	2.1 km (1.3 mi)	800 m (2500 ft)	4.4 km (2.7 mi)		8.9 km (5.6 mi)
1955	Compressed gas, toxic, n.o.s. (Inhalation Hazard Zone B)	30 m (100 ft)	0.2 km (0.1 mi)	0.8 km (0.5 mi)	400 m (1250 ft)	1.9 km (1.2 mi)		4.8 km (3.0 mi)
1955	Compressed gas, toxic, n.o.s. (Inhalation Hazard Zone C)	30 m (100 ft)	0.1 km (0.1 mi)	0.4 km (0.2 mi)	200 m (600 ft)	1.0 km (0.6 mi)		3.2 km (2.0 mi)
1955	Compressed gas, toxic, n.o.s. (Inhalation Hazard Zone D)	30 m (100 ft)	0.1 km (0.1 mi)	0.2 km (0.1 mi)	150 m (500 ft)	0.7 km (0.5 mi)		2.7 km (1.7 mi)

ID No.	Name of Material	SMALL SPILLS First ISOLATE in all Directions	SMALL SPILLS Then PROTECT persons Downwind during DAY	SMALL SPILLS Then PROTECT persons Downwind during NIGHT	LARGE SPILLS First ISOLATE in all Directions	LARGE SPILLS Then PROTECT persons Downwind during DAY	LARGE SPILLS Then PROTECT persons Downwind during NIGHT
1955	Organic phosphate compound mixed with compressed gas	100 m (300 ft)	1.0 km (0.7 mi)	3.4 km (2.1 mi)	500 m (1500 ft)	4.4 km (2.7 mi)	9.6 km (6.0 mi)
1955	Organic phosphate mixed with compressed gas						
1955	Organic phosphorus compound mixed with compressed gas						
1967	Insecticide gas, poisonous, n.o.s.	100 m (300 ft)	1.0 km (0.7 mi)	3.4 km (2.1 mi)	500 m (1500 ft)	4.4 km (2.7 mi)	9.6 km (6.0 mi)
1967	Insecticide gas, toxic, n.o.s.						
1967	Parathion and compressed gas mixture						
1975	Dinitrogen tetroxide and Nitric oxide mixture	30 m (100 ft)	0.1 km (0.1 mi)	0.6 km (0.4 mi)	100 m (300 ft)	0.6 km (0.4 mi)	2.2 km (1.4 mi)
1975	Nitric oxide and Dinitrogen tetroxide mixture						
1975	Nitric oxide and Nitrogen dioxide mixture						
1975	Nitric oxide and Nitrogen tetroxide mixture						
1975	Nitrogen dioxide and Nitric oxide mixture						
1975	Nitrogen tetroxide and Nitric oxide mixture						
1994	Iron pentacarbonyl	100 m (300 ft)	0.9 km (0.6 mi)	2.1 km (1.3 mi)	500 m (1500 ft)	5.5 km (3.5 mi)	8.9 km (5.5 mi)
2004	Magnesium diamide (when spilled in water)	30 m (100 ft)	0.1 km (0.1 mi)	0.4 km (0.2 mi)	60 m (200 ft)	0.6 km (0.4 mi)	2.3 km (1.5 mi)
2011	Magnesium phosphide (when spilled in water)	60 m (200 ft)	0.4 km (0.3 mi)	1.6 km (1.0 mi)	500 m (1500 ft)	4.8 km (3.0 mi)	11.0+ km (7.0+ mi)
2012	Potassium phosphide (when spilled in water)	30 m (100 ft)	0.3 km (0.2 mi)	1.2 km (0.7 mi)	400 m (1250 ft)	3.1 km (2.0 mi)	9.4 km (5.9 mi)
2013	Strontium phosphide (when spilled in water)	30 m (100 ft)	0.3 km (0.2 mi)	1.1 km (0.7 mi)	400 m (1250 ft)	3.0 km (1.9 mi)	9.4 km (5.9 mi)
2032	Nitric acid, fuming	30 m (100 ft)	0.1 km (0.1 mi)	0.3 km (0.2 mi)	150 m (500 ft)	0.6 km (0.4 mi)	1.1 km (0.7 mi)
2032	Nitric acid, red fuming						

TABLE 1 - INITIAL ISOLATION AND PROTECTIVE ACTION DISTANCES

ID No.	NAME OF MATERIAL	SMALL SPILLS (From a small package or small leak from a large package)						LARGE SPILLS (From a large package or from many small packages)					
		First ISOLATE in all Directions		Then PROTECT persons Downwind during-				First ISOLATE in all Directions		Then PROTECT persons Downwind during-			
		Meters	(Feet)	DAY Kilometers	(Miles)	NIGHT Kilometers	(Miles)	Meters	(Feet)	DAY Kilometers	(Miles)	NIGHT Kilometers	(Miles)
2186	Hydrogen chloride, refrigerated liquid	30 m	(100 ft)	0.1 km	(0.1 mi)	0.4 km	(0.2 mi)	500 m	(1500 ft)	2.8 km	(1.7 mi)	10.2 km	(6.3 mi)
2188	Arsine	200 m	(600 ft)	1.1 km	(0.7 mi)	4.0 km	(2.5 mi)	1000 m	(3000 ft)	7.0 km	(4.4 mi)	11.0+ km	(7.0+ mi)
2188	SA (when used as a weapon)	400 m	(1250 ft)	2.0 km	(1.3 mi)	5.5 km	(3.4 mi)	1000 m	(3000 ft)	9.2 km	(5.7 mi)	11.0+ km	(7.0+ mi)
2189	Dichlorosilane	30 m	(100 ft)	0.2 km	(0.1 mi)	1.0 km	(0.6 mi)	800 m	(2500 ft)	4.2 km	(2.6 mi)	10.3 km	(6.4 mi)
2190 2190	Oxygen difluoride Oxygen difluoride, compressed	800 m	(2500 ft)	5.3 km	(3.3 mi)	11.0+ km	(7.0+ mi)	1000 m	(3000 ft)	11.0+ km	(7.0+ mi)	11.0+ km	(7.0+ mi)
2191 2191	Sulfuryl fluoride Sulphuryl fluoride	30 m	(100 ft)	0.1 km	(0.1 mi)	0.5 km	(0.3 mi)	300 m	(1000 ft)	1.7 km	(1.1 mi)	4.9 km	(3.1 mi)
2192	Germane	30 m	(100 ft)	0.2 km	(0.1 mi)	0.8 km	(0.5 mi)	150 m	(500 ft)	0.9 km	(0.5 mi)	2.8 km	(1.8 mi)
2194	Selenium hexafluoride	60 m	(200 ft)	0.4 km	(0.3 mi)	1.9 km	(1.2 mi)	500 m	(1500 ft)	2.9 km	(1.8 mi)	6.4 km	(4.0 mi)
2195	Tellurium hexafluoride	200 m	(600 ft)	1.2 km	(0.8 mi)	4.3 km	(2.7 mi)	1000 m	(3000 ft)	9.4 km	(5.9 mi)	11.0+ km	(7.0+ mi)
2196	Tungsten hexafluoride	30 m	(100 ft)	0.2 km	(0.1 mi)	0.8 km	(0.5 mi)	150 m	(500 ft)	1.0 km	(0.6 mi)	2.9 km	(1.8 mi)
2197	Hydrogen iodide, anhydrous	30 m	(100 ft)	0.1 km	(0.1 mi)	0.4 km	(0.2 mi)	150 m	(500 ft)	1.0 km	(0.6 mi)	3.2 km	(2.0 mi)
2198 2198	Phosphorus pentafluoride Phosphorus pentafluoride, compressed	30 m	(100 ft)	0.2 km	(0.2 mi)	1.1 km	(0.7 mi)	200 m	(600 ft)	1.3 km	(0.8 mi)	3.8 km	(2.4 mi)
2199	Phosphine	100 m	(300 ft)	0.6 km	(0.4 mi)	2.5 km	(1.5 mi)	800 m	(2500 ft)	4.4 km	(2.7 mi)	8.9 km	(5.6 mi)
2202	Hydrogen selenide, anhydrous	200 m	(600 ft)	1.3 km	(0.8 mi)	4.6 km	(2.9 mi)	1000 m	(3000 ft)	8.7 km	(5.4 mi)	11.0+ km	(7.0+ mi)
2204 2204	Carbonyl sulfide Carbonyl sulphide	30 m	(100 ft)	0.2 km	(0.1 mi)	0.7 km	(0.4 mi)	500 m	(1500 ft)	3.3 km	(2.1 mi)	8.7 km	(5.4 mi)
2232 2232	Chloroacetaldehyde 2-Chloroethanal	30 m	(100 ft)	0.2 km	(0.1 mi)	0.4 km	(0.3 mi)	100 m	(300 ft)	0.9 km	(0.5 mi)	1.5 km	(0.9 mi)

ID No.	Name of Material	SMALL SPILLS First ISOLATE in all Directions	SMALL SPILLS Then PROTECT persons Downwind during DAY	SMALL SPILLS Then PROTECT persons Downwind during NIGHT	LARGE SPILLS First ISOLATE in all Directions	LARGE SPILLS Then PROTECT persons Downwind during DAY	LARGE SPILLS Then PROTECT persons Downwind during NIGHT
2308	Nitrosylsulfuric acic (when spilled in water)	30 m (100 ft)	0.1 km (0.1 mi)	0.4 km (0.3 mi)	300 m (1000 ft)	0.8 km (0.5 mi)	2.5 km (1.6 mi)
2308	Nitrosylsulfuric acic, liquid (when spilled in water)						
2308	Nitrosylsulfuric acic, solid (when spilled in water)						
2308	Nitrosylsulphuric acic (when spilled in water)						
2308	Nitrosylsulphuric acic, liquid (when spilled in water)						
2308	Nitrosylsulphuric acic, solid (when spilled in water)						
2334	Allylamine	30 m (100 ft)	0.2 km (0.1 mi)	0.6 km (0.4 mi)	150 m (500 ft)	1.7 km (1.1 mi)	3.0 km (1.9 mi)
2337	Phenyl mercaptan	30 m (100 ft)	0.1 km (0.1 mi)	0.1 km (0.1 mi)	30 m (100 ft)	0.3 km (0.2 mi)	0.5 km (0.3 mi)
2353	Butyryl chloride (when spilled in water)	30 m (100 ft)	0.1 km (0.1 mi)	0.1 km (0.1 mi)	30 m (100 ft)	0.3 km (0.2 mi)	1.0 km (0.6 mi)
2382 2382	1,2-Dimethylhydrazine Dimethylhydrazine, symmetrical	30 m (100 ft)	0.2 km (0.1 mi)	0.4 km (0.3 mi)	100 m (300 ft)	1.0 km (0.6 mi)	1.7 km (1.1 mi)
2395	Isobutyryl chloride (when spilled in water)	30 m (100 ft)	0.1 km (0.1 mi)	0.1 km (0.1 mi)	30 m (100 ft)	0.2 km (0.2 mi)	0.6 km (0.4 mi)
2407	Isopropyl chloroformate	30 m (100 ft)	0.2 km (0.1 mi)	0.3 km (0.2 mi)	60 m (200 ft)	0.7 km (0.5 mi)	1.4 km (0.9 mi)
2417 2417	Carbonyl fluoride Carbonyl fluoride, compressed	30 m (100 ft)	0.2 km (0.1 mi)	0.8 km (0.5 mi)	150 m (500 ft)	0.9 km (0.5 mi)	3.0 km (1.9 mi)
2418 2418	Sulfur tetrafluoride Sulphur tetrafluoride	100 m (300 ft)	0.6 km (0.4 mi)	2.6 km (1.6 mi)	800 m (2500 ft)	4.7 km (2.9 mi)	10.3 km (6.4 mi)
2420	Hexafluoroacetone	60 m (200 ft)	0.3 km (0.2 mi)	1.5 km (0.9 mi)	1000 m (3000 ft)	8.4 km (5.2 mi)	11.0+ km (7.0+ mi)
2421	Nitrogen trioxide	30 m (100 ft)	0.1 km (0.1 mi)	0.3 km (0.2 mi)	100 m (300 ft)	0.3 km (0.2 mi)	1.2 km (0.8 mi)
2434	Dibenzyldichlorosilane (when spilled in water)	30 m (100 ft)	0.1 km (0.1 mi)	0.1 km (0.1 mi)	30 m (100 ft)	0.2 km (0.1 mi)	0.6 km (0.4 mi)
2435	Ethylphenyldichlorosilane (when spilled in water)	30 m (100 ft)	0.1 km (0.1 mi)	0.1 km (0.1 mi)	30 m (100 ft)	0.4 km (0.2 mi)	1.1 km (0.7 mi)

TABLE 1 - INITIAL ISOLATION AND PROTECTIVE ACTION DISTANCES

ID No.	NAME OF MATERIAL	SMALL SPILLS (From a small package or small leak from a large package)						LARGE SPILLS (From a large package or from many small packages)					
		First ISOLATE in all Directions		Then PROTECT persons Downwind during-				First ISOLATE in all Directions		Then PROTECT persons Downwind during-			
				DAY		NIGHT				DAY		NIGHT	
		Meters	(Feet)	Kilometers	(Miles)	Kilometers	(Miles)	Meters	(Feet)	Kilometers	(Miles)	Kilometers	(Miles)
2437	Methylphenyldichlorosilane (when spilled in water)	30 m	(100 ft)	0.1 km	(0.1 mi)	0.1 km	(0.1 mi)	30 m	(100 ft)	0.2 km	(0.1 mi)	0.6 km	(0.4 mi)
2438	Trimethylacetyl chloride	30 m	(100 ft)	0.1 km	(0.1 mi)	0.3 km	(0.2 mi)	60 m	(200 ft)	0.6 km	(0.4 mi)	1.1 km	(0.7 mi)
2442	Trichloroacetyl chloride	30 m	(100 ft)	0.2 km	(0.1 mi)	0.3 km	(0.2 mi)	60 m	(200 ft)	0.7 km	(0.5 mi)	1.3 km	(0.8 mi)
2474	Thiophosgene	60 m	(200 ft)	0.7 km	(0.4 mi)	2.0 km	(1.3 mi)	300 m	(1000 ft)	3.1 km	(1.9 mi)	5.3 km	(3.3 mi)
2477	Methyl isothiocyanate	30 m	(100 ft)	0.1 km	(0.1 mi)	0.2 km	(0.1 mi)	60 m	(200 ft)	0.5 km	(0.3 mi)	0.8 km	(0.5 mi)
2480	Methyl isocyanate	150 m	(500 ft)	1.8 km	(1.1 mi)	5.3 km	(3.3 mi)	1000 m	(3000 ft)	11.0+ km	(7.0+ mi)	11.0+ km	(7.0+ mi)
2481	Ethyl isocyanate	150 m	(500 ft)	1.5 km	(1.0 mi)	3.8 km	(2.4 mi)	1000 m	(3000 ft)	11.0+ km	(7.0+ mi)	11.0+ km	(7.0+ mi)
2482	n-Propyl isocyanate	100 m	(300 ft)	1.2 km	(0.8 mi)	2.8 km	(1.7 mi)	800 m	(2500 ft)	9.6 km	(6.0 mi)	11.0+ km	(7.0+ mi)
2483	Isopropyl isocyanate	100 m	(300 ft)	1.3 km	(0.8 mi)	3.0 km	(1.9 mi)	1000 m	(3000 ft)	11.0+ km	(7.0+ mi)	11.0+ km	(7.0+ mi)
2484	tert-Butyl isocyanate	100 m	(300 ft)	1.1 km	(0.7 mi)	2.6 km	(1.6 mi)	800 m	(2500 ft)	9.3 km	(5.8 mi)	11.0+ km	(7.0+ mi)
2485	n-Butyl isocyanate	60 m	(200 ft)	0.8 km	(0.5 mi)	1.7 km	(1.1 mi)	400 m	(1250 ft)	4.8 km	(3.0 mi)	6.9 km	(4.3 mi)
2486	Isobutyl isocyanate	60 m	(200 ft)	0.8 km	(0.5 mi)	1.8 km	(1.1 mi)	400 m	(1250 ft)	4.8 km	(3.0 mi)	7.4 km	(4.6 mi)
2487	Phenyl isocyanate	30 m	(100 ft)	0.4 km	(0.3 mi)	0.6 km	(0.4 mi)	150 m	(500 ft)	1.6 km	(1.0 mi)	2.5 km	(1.6 mi)
2488	Cyclohexyl isocyanate	30 m	(100 ft)	0.3 km	(0.2 mi)	0.4 km	(0.2 mi)	100 m	(300 ft)	1.0 km	(0.6 mi)	1.4 km	(0.9 mi)
2495	Iodine pentafluoride (when spilled in water)	30 m	(100 ft)	0.1 km	(0.1 mi)	0.5 km	(0.4 mi)	150 m	(500 ft)	1.2 km	(0.8 mi)	4.2 km	(2.6 mi)
2521	Diketene, stabilized	30 m	(100 ft)	0.1 km	(0.1 mi)	0.1 km	(0.1 mi)	30 m	(100 ft)	0.3 km	(0.2 mi)	0.5 km	(0.3 mi)
2534	Methylchlorosilane	30 m	(100 ft)	0.2 km	(0.1 mi)	0.7 km	(0.4 mi)	300 m	(1000 ft)	1.6 km	(1.0 mi)	4.3 km	(2.7 mi)
2548	Chlorine pentafluoride	60 m	(200 ft)	0.3 km	(0.2 mi)	1.4 km	(0.9 mi)	400 m	(1250 ft)	2.3 km	(1.4 mi)	6.5 km	(4.1 mi)

ID No.	NAME OF MATERIAL	SMALL SPILLS First ISOLATE in all Directions	Then PROTECT persons Downwind during DAY	Then PROTECT persons Downwind during NIGHT	LARGE SPILLS First ISOLATE in all Directions	Then PROTECT persons Downwind during DAY	Then PROTECT persons Downwind during NIGHT
2600	Carbon monoxide and Hydrogen mixture	30 m (100 ft)	0.1 km (0.1 mi)	0.1 km (0.1 mi)	150 m (500 ft)	0.7 km (0.5 mi)	2.7 km (1.7 mi)
2600	Carbon monoxide and Hydrogen mixture, compressed						
2600	Hydrogen and Carbon monoxide mixture						
2600	Hydrogen and Carbon monoxide mixture, compressed						
2605	Methoxymethyl isocyanate	30 m (100 ft)	0.4 km (0.3 mi)	0.6 km (0.4 mi)	150 m (500 ft)	1.6 km (1.0 mi)	2.5 km (1.6 mi)
2606	Methyl orthosilicate	30 m (100 ft)	0.1 km (0.1 mi)	0.1 km (0.1 mi)	30 m (100 ft)	0.3 km (0.2 mi)	0.5 km (0.3 mi)
2644	Methyl iodide	30 m (100 ft)	0.1 km (0.1 mi)	0.2 km (0.1 mi)	100 m (300 ft)	0.3 km (0.2 mi)	0.8 km (0.5 mi)
2646	Hexachlorocyclopentadiene	30 m (100 ft)	0.1 km (0.1 mi)	0.1 km (0.1 mi)	30 m (100 ft)	0.4 km (0.3 mi)	0.5 km (0.3 mi)
2668	Chloroacetonitrile	30 m (100 ft)	0.1 km (0.1 mi)	0.1 km (0.1 mi)	30 m (100 ft)	0.3 km (0.2 mi)	0.5 km (0.3 mi)
2676	Stibine	60 m (200 ft)	0.4 km (0.2 mi)	1.7 km (1.1 mi)	500 m (1500 ft)	2.8 km (1.7 mi)	7.2 km (4.5 mi)
2691	Phosphorus pentabromide (when spilled in water)	30 m (100 ft)	0.1 km (0.1 mi)	0.4 km (0.2 mi)	30 m (100 ft)	0.4 km (0.3 mi)	1.5 km (1.0 mi)
2692	Boron tribromide (when spilled on land)	30 m (100 ft)	0.1 km (0.1 mi)	0.4 km (0.2 mi)	60 m (200 ft)	0.5 km (0.3 mi)	1.0 km (0.6 mi)
2692	Boron tribromide (when spilled in water)	30 m (100 ft)	0.1 km (0.1 mi)	0.6 km (0.4 mi)	100 m (300 ft)	1.0 km (0.6 mi)	3.0 km (1.9 mi)
2740	n-Propyl chloroformate	30 m (100 ft)	0.2 km (0.1 mi)	0.3 km (0.2 mi)	60 m (200 ft)	0.7 km (0.5 mi)	1.3 km (0.8 mi)
2742	sec-Butyl chloroformate	30 m (100 ft)	0.1 km (0.1 mi)	0.1 km (0.1 mi)	30 m (100 ft)	0.4 km (0.2 mi)	0.6 km (0.4 mi)
2742	Isobutyl chloroformate	30 m (100 ft)	0.1 km (0.1 mi)	0.1 km (0.1 mi)	30 m (100 ft)	0.3 km (0.2 mi)	0.5 km (0.3 mi)
2743	n-Butyl chloroformate	30 m (100 ft)	0.1 km (0.1 mi)	0.1 km (0.1 mi)	30 m (100 ft)	0.3 km (0.2 mi)	0.5 km (0.3 mi)
2806	Lithium nitride (when spilled in water)	30 m (100 ft)	0.1 km (0.1 mi)	0.4 km (0.2 mi)	60 m (200 ft)	0.6 km (0.4 mi)	2.2 km (1.4 mi)
2810	Buzz (when used as a weapon) BZ (when used as a weapon)	30 m (100 ft)	0.1 km (0.1 mi)	0.1 km (0.1 mi)	30 m (100 ft)	0.1 km (0.1 mi)	0.5 km (0.3 mi)

TABLE 1 - INITIAL ISOLATION AND PROTECTIVE ACTION DISTANCES

ID No.	NAME OF MATERIAL	SMALL SPILLS (From a small package or small leak from a large package) First ISOLATE in all Directions Meters (Feet)		Then PROTECT persons Downwind during- DAY Kilometers (Miles)		NIGHT Kilometers (Miles)		LARGE SPILLS (From a large package or from many small packages) First ISOLATE in all Directions Meters (Feet)		Then PROTECT persons Downwind during- DAY Kilometers (Miles)		NIGHT Kilometers (Miles)	
2810	CS (when used as a weapon)	30 m	(100 ft)	0.2 km	(0.1 mi)	0.7 km	(0.4 mi)	100 m	(300 ft)	0.5 km	(0.3 mi)	2.1 km	(1.3 mi)
2810	DC (when used as a weapon)	30 m	(100 ft)	0.1 km	(0.1 mi)	0.6 km	(0.4 mi)	100 m	(300 ft)	0.5 km	(0.3 mi)	2.0 km	(1.3 mi)
2810	GA (when used as a weapon)	30 m	(100 ft)	0.2 km	(0.1 mi)	0.2 km	(0.1 mi)	100 m	(300 ft)	0.6 km	(0.4 mi)	0.7 km	(0.4 mi)
2810	GB (when used as a weapon)	60 m	(200 ft)	0.4 km	(0.3 mi)	1.2 km	(0.8 mi)	800 m	(2500 ft)	2.3 km	(1.4 mi)	4.5 km	(2.8 mi)
2810	GD (when used as a weapon)	60 m	(200 ft)	0.4 km	(0.3 mi)	0.8 km	(0.5 mi)	400 m	(1250 ft)	1.7 km	(1.1 mi)	2.4 km	(1.5 mi)
2810	GF (when used as a weapon)	60 m	(200 ft)	0.2 km	(0.2 mi)	0.3 km	(0.2 mi)	150 m	(500 ft)	0.9 km	(0.6 mi)	1.1 km	(0.7 mi)
2810 2810	H (when used as a weapon) HD (when used as a weapon)	30 m	(100 ft)	0.1 km	(0.1 mi)	0.1 km	(0.1 mi)	60 m	(200 ft)	0.4 km	(0.2 mi)	0.4 km	(0.3 mi)
2810	HL (when used as a weapon)	30 m	(100 ft)	0.2 km	(0.1 mi)	0.3 km	(0.2 mi)	100 m	(300 ft)	0.5 km	(0.3 mi)	1.0 km	(0.7 mi)
2810	HN-1 (when used as a weapon)	30 m	(100 ft)	0.1 km	(0.1 mi)	0.1 km	(0.1 mi)	60 m	(200 ft)	0.4 km	(0.2 mi)	0.5 km	(0.4 mi)
2810	HN-2 (when used as a weapon)	30 m	(100 ft)	0.1 km	(0.1 mi)	0.1 km	(0.1 mi)	60 m	(200 ft)	0.3 km	(0.2 mi)	0.5 km	(0.3 mi)
2810	HN-3 (when used as a weapon)	30 m	(100 ft)	0.1 km	(0.1 mi)	0.1 km	(0.1 mi)	30 m	(100 ft)	0.1 km	(0.1 mi)	0.1 km	(0.1 mi)
2810 2810	L (Lewisite) (when used as a weapon) Lewisite (when used as a weapon)	30 m	(100 ft)	0.2 km	(0.1 mi)	0.3 km	(0.2 mi)	100 m	(300 ft)	0.5 km	(0.3 mi)	1.0 km	(0.7 mi)
2810	Mustard (when used as a weapon)	30 m	(100 ft)	0.1 km	(0.1 mi)	0.1 km	(0.1 mi)	60 m	(200 ft)	0.4 km	(0.2 mi)	0.4 km	(0.3 mi)
2810	Mustard Lewisite (when used as a weapon)	30 m	(100 ft)	0.2 km	(0.1 mi)	0.3 km	(0.2 mi)	100 m	(300 ft)	0.5 km	(0.3 mi)	1.0 km	(0.7 mi)
2810 2810	Poisonous liquid, n.o.s. Poisonous liquid, n.o.s. (Inhalation Hazard Zone A)	60 m	(200 ft)	0.8 km	(0.5 mi)	1.8 km	(1.1 mi)	300 m	(1000 ft)	2.9 km	(1.8 mi)	5.7 km	(3.6 mi)
2810	Poisonous liquid, n.o.s. (Inhalation Hazard Zone B)	30 m	(100 ft)	0.1 km	(0.1 mi)	0.2 km	(0.1 mi)	60 m	(200 ft)	0.5 km	(0.3 mi)	0.8 km	(0.5 mi)

ID No.	Name of Material	SMALL SPILLS			LARGE SPILLS		
		First ISOLATE in all Directions	Then PROTECT persons downwind during DAY	NIGHT	First ISOLATE in all Directions	Then PROTECT persons downwind during DAY	NIGHT
2810 2810	Poisonous liquid, organic, n.o.s. Poisonous liquid, organic, n.o.s. (Inhalation Hazard Zone A)	60 m (200 ft)	0.8 km (0.5 mi)	1.8 km (1.1 mi)	400 m (1250 ft)	4.8 km (3.0 mi)	7.4 km (4.6 mi)
2810	Poisonous liquid, organic, n.o.s. (Inhalation Hazard Zone B)	30 m (100 ft)	0.1 km (0.1 mi)	0.2 km (0.1 mi)	60 m (200 ft)	0.5 km (0.3 mi)	0.8 km (0.5 mi)
2810	Sarin (when used as a weapon)	60 m (200 ft)	0.4 km (0.3 mi)	1.2 km (0.8 mi)	800 m (2500 ft)	2.3 km (1.4 mi)	4.5 km (2.8 mi)
2810	Soman (when used as a weapon)	60 m (200 ft)	0.4 km (0.3 mi)	0.8 km (0.5 mi)	400 m (1250 ft)	1.7 km (1.1 mi)	2.4 km (1.5 mi)
2810	Tabun (when used as a weapon)	30 m (100 ft)	0.2 km (0.1 mi)	0.2 km (0.1 mi)	100 m (300 ft)	0.6 km (0.4 mi)	0.7 km (0.4 mi)
2810	Thickened GD (when used as a weapon)	60 m (200 ft)	0.4 km (0.3 mi)	0.8 km (0.5 mi)	400 m (1250 ft)	1.7 km (1.1 mi)	2.4 km (1.5 mi)
2810 2810	Toxic liquid, n.o.s. Toxic liquid, n.o.s. (Inhalation Hazard Zone A)	60 m (200 ft)	0.8 km (0.5 mi)	1.8 km (1.1 mi)	300 m (1000 ft)	2.9 km (1.8 mi)	5.7 km (3.6 mi)
2810	Toxic liquid, n.o.s. (Inhalation Hazard Zone B)	30 m (100 ft)	0.1 km (0.1 mi)	0.2 km (0.1 mi)	60 m (200 ft)	0.5 km (0.3 mi)	0.8 km (0.5 mi)
2810 2810	Toxic liquid, organic, n.o.s. Toxic liquid, organic, n.o.s. (Inhalation Hazard Zone A)	60 m (200 ft)	0.8 km (0.5 mi)	1.8 km (1.1 mi)	400 m (1250 ft)	4.8 km (3.0 mi)	7.4 km (4.6 mi)
2810	Toxic liquid, organic, n.o.s. (Inhalation Hazard Zone B)	30 m (100 ft)	0.1 km (0.1 mi)	0.2 km (0.1 mi)	60 m (200 ft)	0.5 km (0.3 mi)	0.8 km (0.5 mi)
2810	VX (when used as a weapon)	30 m (100 ft)	0.1 km (0.1 mi)	0.1 km (0.1 mi)	60 m (200 ft)	0.4 km (0.2 mi)	0.4 km (0.3 mi)
2811	CX (when used as a weapon)	30 m (100 ft)	0.1 km (0.1 mi)	0.7 km (0.4 mi)	100 m (300 ft)	0.5 km (0.3 mi)	2.3 km (1.4 mi)
2826	Ethyl chlorothioformate	30 m (100 ft)	0.1 km (0.1 mi)	0.2 km (0.1 mi)	60 m (200 ft)	0.5 km (0.3 mi)	0.7 km (0.5 mi)
2845	Ethyl phosphonous dichloride, anhydrous	30 m (100 ft)	0.3 km (0.2 mi)	0.8 km (0.5 mi)	150 m (500 ft)	1.6 km (1.0 mi)	2.9 km (1.8 mi)
2845	Methyl phosphonous dichloride	30 m (100 ft)	0.4 km (0.3 mi)	1.2 km (0.8 mi)	200 m (600 ft)	2.6 km (1.6 mi)	4.5 km (2.8 mi)
2901	Bromine chloride	30 m (100 ft)	0.2 km (0.2 mi)	1.0 km (0.6 mi)	400 m (1250 ft)	2.4 km (1.5 mi)	6.5 km (4.0 mi)

TABLE 1 - INITIAL ISOLATION AND PROTECTIVE ACTION DISTANCES

ID No.	NAME OF MATERIAL	SMALL SPILLS (From a small package or small leak from a large package)						LARGE SPILLS (From a large package or from many small packages)					
		First ISOLATE in all Directions		Then PROTECT persons Downwind during-				First ISOLATE in all Directions		Then PROTECT persons Downwind during-			
				DAY		NIGHT				DAY		NIGHT	
		Meters	(Feet)	Kilometers	(Miles)	Kilometers	(Miles)	Meters	(Feet)	Kilometers	(Miles)	Kilometers	(Miles)
2927	Ethyl phosphonothioic dichloride, anhydrous	30 m	(100 ft)	0.1 km	(0.1 mi)	0.1 km	(0.1 mi)	30 m	(100 ft)	0.2 km	(0.1 mi)	0.2 km	(0.2 mi)
2927	Ethyl phosphorodichloridate	30 m	(100 ft)	0.1 km	(0.1 mi)	0.1 km	(0.1 mi)	30 m	(100 ft)	0.2 km	(0.2 mi)	0.3 km	(0.2 mi)
2927	Poisonous liquid, corrosive, n.o.s.												
2927	Poisonous liquid, corrosive, n.o.s. (Inhalation Hazard Zone A)	60 m	(200 ft)	0.8 km	(0.5 mi)	1.8 km	(1.1 mi)	300 m	(1000 ft)	2.9 km	(1.8 mi)	5.7 km	(3.6 mi)
2927	Poisonous liquid, corrosive, n.o.s. (Inhalation Hazard Zone B)	30 m	(100 ft)	0.1 km	(0.1 mi)	0.2 km	(0.1 mi)	60 m	(200 ft)	0.5 km	(0.3 mi)	0.8 km	(0.5 mi)
2927	Poisonous liquid, corrosive, organic, n.o.s.												
2927	Poisonous liquid, corrosive, organic, n.o.s. (Inhalation Hazard Zone A)	100 m	(300 ft)	1.2 km	(0.8 mi)	2.8 km	(1.8 mi)	600 m	(2000 ft)	7.8 km	(4.9 mi)	11.0+ km	(7.0+ mi)
2927	Poisonous liquid, corrosive, organic, n.o.s. (Inhalation Hazard Zone B)	30 m	(100 ft)	0.1 km	(0.1 mi)	0.2 km	(0.1 mi)	60 m	(200 ft)	0.5 km	(0.3 mi)	0.8 km	(0.5 mi)
2927	Toxic liquid, corrosive, n.o.s.												
2927	Toxic liquid, corrosive, n.o.s. (Inhalation Hazard Zone A)	60 m	(200 ft)	0.8 km	(0.5 mi)	1.8 km	(1.1 mi)	300 m	(1000 ft)	2.9 km	(1.8 mi)	5.7 km	(3.6 mi)
2927	Toxic liquid, corrosive, n.o.s. (Inhalation Hazard Zone B)	30 m	(100 ft)	0.1 km	(0.1 mi)	0.2 km	(0.1 mi)	60 m	(200 ft)	0.5 km	(0.3 mi)	0.8 km	(0.5 mi)
2927	Toxic liquid, corrosive, organic, n.o.s.												
2927	Toxic liquid, corrosive, organic, n.o.s. (Inhalation Hazard Zone A)	100 m	(300 ft)	1.2 km	(0.8 mi)	2.8 km	(1.8 mi)	600 m	(2000 ft)	7.8 km	(4.9 mi)	11.0+ km	(7.0+ mi)
2927	Toxic liquid, corrosive, organic, n.o.s. (Inhalation Hazard Zone B)	30 m	(100 ft)	0.1 km	(0.1 mi)	0.2 km	(0.1 mi)	60 m	(200 ft)	0.5 km	(0.3 mi)	0.8 km	(0.5 mi)

ID No.	Name of Material	Small Spills — First ISOLATE in all Directions	Small Spills — Then PROTECT persons Downwind during DAY	Small Spills — Then PROTECT persons Downwind during NIGHT	Large Spills — First ISOLATE in all Directions	Large Spills — Then PROTECT persons Downwind during DAY	Large Spills — Then PROTECT persons Downwind during NIGHT
2929	Poisonous liquid, flammable, n.o.s.	60 m (200 ft)	0.7 km (0.4 mi)	2.3 km (1.4 mi)	400 m (1250 ft)	4.6 km (2.9 mi)	8.9 km (5.5 mi)
2929	Poisonous liquid, flammable, n.o.s. (Inhalation Hazard Zone A)	30 m (100 ft)	0.1 km (0.1 mi)	0.2 km (0.1 mi)	60 m (200 ft)	0.5 km (0.3 mi)	0.8 km (0.5 mi)
2929	Poisonous liquid, flammable, n.o.s. (Inhalation Hazard Zone B)	100 m (300 ft)	1.1 km (0.7 mi)	2.6 km (1.6 mi)	600 m (2000 ft)	7.8 km (4.9 mi)	11.0+ km (7.0+ mi)
2929	Poisonous liquid, flammable, organic, n.o.s.; Poisonous liquid, flammable, organic, n.o.s. (Inhalation Hazard Zone A); Poisonous liquid, flammable, organic, n.o.s. (Inhalation Hazard Zone B)	30 m (100 ft)	0.1 km (0.1 mi)	0.2 km (0.1 mi)	60 m (200 ft)	0.5 km (0.3 mi)	0.8 km (0.5 mi)
2929	Toxic liquid, flammable, n.o.s.	60 m (200 ft)	0.7 km (0.4 mi)	2.3 km (1.4 mi)	400 m (1250 ft)	4.6 km (2.9 mi)	8.9 km (5.5 mi)
2929	Toxic liquid, flammable, n.o.s. (Inhalation Hazard Zone A)	30 m (100 ft)	0.1 km (0.1 mi)	0.2 km (0.1 mi)	60 m (200 ft)	0.5 km (0.3 mi)	0.8 km (0.5 mi)
2929	Toxic liquid, flammable, n.o.s. (Inhalation Hazard Zone B)	100 m (300 ft)	1.1 km (0.7 mi)	2.6 km (1.6 mi)	600 m (2000 ft)	7.8 km (4.9 mi)	11.0+ km (7.0+ mi)
2929	Toxic liquid, flammable, organic, n.o.s.; Toxic liquid, flammable, organic, n.o.s. (Inhalation Hazard Zone A); Toxic liquid, flammable, organic, n.o.s. (Inhalation Hazard Zone B)	30 m (100 ft)	0.1 km (0.1 mi)	0.4 km (0.2 mi)	60 m (200 ft)	0.5 km (0.3 mi)	2.3 km (1.4 mi)
2977	Radioactive material, Uranium hexafluoride, fissile **(when spilled in water)**; Uranium hexafluoride, fissile containing more than 1% Uranium-235 **(when spilled in water)**						

TABLE 1 - INITIAL ISOLATION AND PROTECTIVE ACTION DISTANCES

ID No.	NAME OF MATERIAL	SMALL SPILLS (From a small package or small leak from a large package)			LARGE SPILLS (From a large package or from many small packages)			
		First ISOLATE in all Directions	Then PROTECT persons Downwind during-		First ISOLATE in all Directions	Then PROTECT persons Downwind during-		
			DAY	NIGHT		DAY		NIGHT
		Meters (Feet)	Kilometers (Miles)	Kilometers (Miles)	Meters (Feet)	Kilometers (Miles)		Kilometers (Miles)
2978	Radioactive material, Uranium hexafluoride **(when spilled in water)**	30 m (100 ft)	0.1 km (0.1 mi)	0.4 km (0.2 mi)	60 m (200 ft)	0.5 km (0.3 mi)		2.2 km (1.4 mi)
2978	Uranium hexafluoride **(when spilled in water)**							
2978	Uranium hexafluoride, non-fissile **(when spilled in water)**							
2985	Chlorosilanes, flammable, corrosive, n.o.s. **(when spilled in water)**	30 m (100 ft)	0.1 km (0.1 mi)	0.2 km (0.1 mi)	100 m (300 ft)	0.5 km (0.3 mi)		1.6 km (1.0 mi)
2985	Chlorosilanes, n.o.s. **(when spilled in water)**							
2986	Chlorosilanes, corrosive, flammable, n.o.s. **(when spilled in water)**	30 m (100 ft)	0.1 km (0.1 mi)	0.2 km (0.1 mi)	100 m (300 ft)	0.5 km (0.3 mi)		1.6 km (1.0 mi)
2986	Chlorosilanes, n.o.s. **(when spilled in water)**							
2987	Chlorosilanes, corrosive, n.o.s. **(when spilled in water)**	30 m (100 ft)	0.1 km (0.1 mi)	0.2 km (0.1 mi)	100 m (300 ft)	0.5 km (0.3 mi)		1.6 km (1.0 mi)
2987	Chlorosilanes, n.o.s. **(when spilled in water)**							
2988	Chlorosilanes, n.o.s. **(when spilled in water)**	30 m (100 ft)	0.1 km (0.1 mi)	0.2 km (0.1 mi)	100 m (300 ft)	0.5 km (0.3 mi)		1.6 km (1.0 mi)
2988	Chlorosilanes, water-reactive, flammable, corrosive, n.o.s. **(when spilled in water)**							
3023	2-Methyl-2-heptanethiol	30 m (100 ft)	0.1 km (0.1 mi)	0.2 km (0.1 mi)	60 m (200 ft)	0.5 km (0.3 mi)		0.7 km (0.5 mi)
3023	tert-Octyl mercaptan							
3048	Aluminum phosphide pesticide **(when spilled in water)**	60 m (200 ft)	0.5 km (0.3 mi)	1.9 km (1.2 mi)	600 m (2000 ft)	5.8 km (3.6 mi)		11.0+ km (7.0+ mi)

ID No.	Name of Material	SMALL SPILLS First ISOLATE in all Directions	Then PROTECT persons Downwind during DAY	Then PROTECT persons Downwind during NIGHT	LARGE SPILLS First ISOLATE in all Directions	Then PROTECT persons Downwind during DAY	Then PROTECT persons Downwind during NIGHT
3049	Metal alkyl halides, n.o.s. **(when spilled in water)**	30 m (100 ft)	0.1 km (0.1 mi)	0.2 km (0.1 mi)	60 m (200 ft)	0.4 km (0.3 mi)	1.3 km (0.8 mi)
3049	Metal alkyl halides, water-reactive, n.o.s. **(when spilled in water)**						
3049	Metal aryl halides, n.o.s. **(when spilled in water)**						
3049	Metal aryl halides, water-reactive, n.o.s. **(when spilled in water)**						
3052	Aluminum alkyl halides **(when spilled in water)**	30 m (100 ft)	0.1 km (0.1 mi)	0.2 km (0.1 mi)	60 m (200 ft)	0.4 km (0.3 mi)	1.3 km (0.8 mi)
3052	Aluminum alkyl halides, liquid **(when spilled in water)**						
3052	Aluminum alkyl halides, solid **(when spilled in water)**						
3057	Trifluoroacetyl chloride	30 m (100 ft)	0.2 km (0.2 mi)	1.0 km (0.7 mi)	800 m (2500 ft)	4.6 km (2.9 mi)	11.0+ km (7.0+ mi)
3079	Methacrylonitrile, stabilized	30 m (100 ft)	0.1 km (0.1 mi)	0.2 km (0.1 mi)	60 m (200 ft)	0.5 km (0.3 mi)	0.9 km (0.5 mi)
3083	Perchloryl fluoride	30 m (100 ft)	0.2 km (0.1 mi)	0.7 km (0.4 mi)	500 m (1500 ft)	3.1 km (2.0 mi)	8.4 km (5.2 mi)
3122	Poisonous liquid, oxidizing, n.o.s.	60 m (200 ft)	0.8 km (0.5 mi)	1.8 km (1.1 mi)	300 m (1000 ft)	2.9 km (1.8 mi)	5.7 km (3.6 mi)
3122	Poisonous liquid, oxidizing, n.o.s. (Inhalation Hazard Zone A)	30 m (100 ft)	0.1 km (0.1 mi)	0.3 km (0.2 mi)	60 m (200 ft)	0.6 km (0.4 mi)	1.0 km (0.6 mi)
3122	Poisonous liquid, oxidizing, n.o.s. (Inhalation Hazard Zone B)	60 m (200 ft)	0.8 km (0.5 mi)	1.8 km (1.1 mi)	300 m (1000 ft)	2.9 km (1.8 mi)	5.7 km (3.6 mi)
3122 3122	Toxic liquid, oxidizing, n.o.s. Toxic liquid, oxidizing, n.o.s. (Inhalation Hazard Zone A)	60 m (200 ft)	0.8 km (0.5 mi)	1.8 km (1.1 mi)	300 m (1000 ft)	2.9 km (1.8 mi)	5.7 km (3.6 mi)
3122	Toxic liquid, oxidizing, n.o.s. (Inhalation Hazard Zone B)	30 m (100 ft)	0.1 km (0.1 mi)	0.3 km (0.2 mi)	60 m (200 ft)	0.6 km (0.4 mi)	1.0 km (0.6 mi)
3123 3123	Poisonous liquid, water-reactive, n.o.s. Poisonous liquid, water-reactive, n.o.s. (Inhalation Hazard Zone A)	60 m (200 ft)	0.8 km (0.5 mi)	1.8 km (1.1 mi)	300 m (1000 ft)	2.9 km (1.8 mi)	5.7 km (3.6 mi)

TABLE 1 - INITIAL ISOLATION AND PROTECTIVE ACTION DISTANCES

ID No.	NAME OF MATERIAL	SMALL SPILLS (From a small package or small leak from a large package)			LARGE SPILLS (From a large package or from many small packages)		
		First ISOLATE in all Directions — Meters (Feet)	Then PROTECT persons Downwind during— DAY Kilometers (Miles)	NIGHT Kilometers (Miles)	First ISOLATE in all Directions — Meters (Feet)	Then PROTECT persons Downwind during— DAY Kilometers (Miles)	NIGHT Kilometers (Miles)
3123	Poisonous liquid, water-reactive, n.o.s. (Inhalation Hazard Zone B)	30 m (100 ft)	0.1 km (0.1 mi)	0.2 km (0.1 mi)	60 m (200 ft)	0.5 km (0.3 mi)	0.8 km (0.5 mi)
3123	Poisonous liquid, which in contact with water emits flammable gases, n.o.s.	30 m (100 ft)	0.1 km (0.1 mi)	0.2 km (0.1 mi)	60 m (200 ft)	0.5 km (0.3 mi)	0.8 km (0.5 mi)
3123	Poisonous liquid, which in contact with water emits flammable gases, n.o.s. (Inhalation Hazard Zone A)	60 m (200 ft)	0.8 km (0.5 mi)	1.8 km (1.1 mi)	300 m (1000 ft)	2.9 km (1.8 mi)	5.7 km (3.6 mi)
3123	Poisonous liquid, which in contact with water emits flammable gases, n.o.s. (Inhalation Hazard Zone B)	30 m (100 ft)	0.1 km (0.1 mi)	0.2 km (0.1 mi)	60 m (200 ft)	0.5 km (0.3 mi)	0.8 km (0.5 mi)
3123	Toxic liquid, water-reactive, n.o.s.	30 m (100 ft)	0.1 km (0.1 mi)	0.2 km (0.1 mi)	60 m (200 ft)	0.5 km (0.3 mi)	0.8 km (0.5 mi)
3123	Toxic liquid, water-reactive, n.o.s. (Inhalation Hazard Zone A)	60 m (200 ft)	0.8 km (0.5 mi)	1.8 km (1.1 mi)	300 m (1000 ft)	2.9 km (1.8 mi)	5.7 km (3.6 mi)
3123	Toxic liquid, water-reactive, n.o.s. (Inhalation Hazard Zone B)	30 m (100 ft)	0.1 km (0.1 mi)	0.2 km (0.1 mi)	60 m (200 ft)	0.5 km (0.3 mi)	0.8 km (0.5 mi)
3123	Toxic liquid, which in contact with water emits flammable gases, n.o.s.	30 m (100 ft)	0.1 km (0.1 mi)	0.2 km (0.1 mi)	60 m (200 ft)	0.5 km (0.3 mi)	0.8 km (0.5 mi)
3123	Toxic liquid, which in contact with water emits flammable gases, n.o.s. (Inhalation Hazard Zone A)	60 m (200 ft)	0.8 km (0.5 mi)	1.8 km (1.1 mi)	300 m (1000 ft)	2.9 km (1.8 mi)	5.7 km (3.6 mi)
3123	Toxic liquid, which in contact with water emits flammable gases, n.o.s. (Inhalation Hazard Zone B)	30 m (100 ft)	0.1 km (0.1 mi)	0.2 km (0.1 mi)	60 m (200 ft)	0.5 km (0.3 mi)	0.8 km (0.5 mi)

ID No.	Name of Material	SMALL SPILLS First ISOLATE in all Directions	SMALL SPILLS Then PROTECT persons downwind during DAY	SMALL SPILLS Then PROTECT persons downwind during NIGHT	LARGE SPILLS First ISOLATE in all Directions	LARGE SPILLS Then PROTECT persons downwind during DAY	LARGE SPILLS Then PROTECT persons downwind during NIGHT
3160 3160	Liquefied gas, poisonous, flammable, n.o.s. Liquefied gas, poisonous, flammable, n.o.s. (Inhalation Hazard Zone A)	100 m (300 ft)	0.6 km (0.4 mi)	2.5 km (1.5 mi)	800 m (2500 ft)	4.4 km (2.7 mi)	8.9 km (5.6 mi)
3160	Liquefied gas, poisonous, flammable, n.o.s. (Inhalation Hazard Zone B)	30 m (100 ft)	0.2 km (0.1 mi)	0.8 km (0.5 mi)	400 m (1250 ft)	1.9 km (1.2 mi)	4.8 km (3.0 mi)
3160	Liquefied gas, poisonous, flammable, n.o.s. (Inhalation Hazard Zone C)	30 m (100 ft)	0.1 km (0.1 mi)	0.3 km (0.2 mi)	300 m (1000 ft)	1.3 km (0.8 mi)	4.1 km (2.6 mi)
3160	Liquefied gas, poisonous, flammable, n.o.s. (Inhalation Hazard Zone D)	30 m (100 ft)	0.1 km (0.1 mi)	0.2 km (0.1 mi)	150 m (500 ft)	0.7 km (0.5 mi)	2.7 km (1.7 mi)
3160 3160	Liquefied gas, toxic, flammable, n.o.s. Liquefied gas, toxic, flammable, n.o.s. (Inhalation Hazard Zone A)	100 m (300 ft)	0.6 km (0.4 mi)	2.5 km (1.5 mi)	800 m (2500 ft)	4.4 km (2.7 mi)	8.9 km (5.6 mi)
3160	Liquefied gas, toxic, flammable, n.o.s. (Inhalation Hazard Zone B)	30 m (100 ft)	0.2 km (0.1 mi)	0.8 km (0.5 mi)	400 m (1250 ft)	1.9 km (1.2 mi)	4.8 km (3.0 mi)
3160	Liquefied gas, toxic, flammable, n.o.s. (Inhalation Hazard Zone C)	30 m (100 ft)	0.1 km (0.1 mi)	0.3 km (0.2 mi)	300 m (1000 ft)	1.3 km (0.8 mi)	4.1 km (2.6 mi)
3160	Liquefied gas, toxic, flammable, n.o.s. (Inhalation Hazard Zone D)	30 m (100 ft)	0.1 km (0.1 mi)	0.2 km (0.1 mi)	150 m (500 ft)	0.7 km (0.5 mi)	2.7 km (1.7 mi)
3162 3162	Liquefied gas, poisonous, n.o.s. Liquefied gas, poisonous, n.o.s. (Inhalation Hazard Zone A)	100 m (300 ft)	0.5 km (0.3 mi)	2.1 km (1.3 mi)	800 m (2500 ft)	4.4 km (2.7 mi)	8.9 km (5.6 mi)
3162	Liquefied gas, poisonous, n.o.s. (Inhalation Hazard Zone B)	30 m (100 ft)	0.2 km (0.1 mi)	0.8 km (0.5 mi)	400 m (1250 ft)	1.9 km (1.2 mi)	4.8 km (3.0 mi)
3162	Liquefied gas, poisonous, n.o.s. (Inhalation Hazard Zone C)	30 m (100 ft)	0.1 km (0.1 mi)	0.4 km (0.2 mi)	200 m (600 ft)	1.0 km (0.6 mi)	3.2 km (2.0 mi)

TABLE 1 - INITIAL ISOLATION AND PROTECTIVE ACTION DISTANCES

ID No.	NAME OF MATERIAL	SMALL SPILLS (From a small package or small leak from a large package) First ISOLATE in all Directions Meters (Feet)	SMALL SPILLS Then PROTECT persons Downwind during- DAY Kilometers (Miles)	SMALL SPILLS Then PROTECT persons Downwind during- NIGHT Kilometers (Miles)	LARGE SPILLS (From a large package or from many small packages) First ISOLATE in all Directions Meters (Feet)	LARGE SPILLS Then PROTECT persons Downwind during- DAY Kilometers (Miles)	LARGE SPILLS Then PROTECT persons Downwind during- NIGHT Kilometers (Miles)
3162	Liquefied gas, poisonous, n.o.s. (Inhalation Hazard Zone D)	30 m (100 ft)	0.1 km (0.1 mi)	0.2 km (0.1 mi)	150 m (500 ft)	0.7 km (0.5 mi)	2.7 km (1.7 mi)
3162 3162	Liquefied gas, toxic, n.o.s. Liquefied gas, toxic, n.o.s. (Inhalation Hazard Zone A)	100 m (300 ft)	0.5 km (0.3 mi)	2.1 km (1.3 mi)	800 m (2500 ft)	4.4 km (2.7 mi)	8.9 km (5.6 mi)
3162	Liquefied gas, toxic, n.o.s. (Inhalation Hazard Zone B)	30 m (100 ft)	0.2 km (0.1 mi)	0.8 km (0.5 mi)	400 m (1250 ft)	1.9 km (1.2 mi)	4.8 km (3.0 mi)
3162	Liquefied gas, toxic, n.o.s. (Inhalation Hazard Zone C)	30 m (100 ft)	0.1 km (0.1 mi)	0.4 km (0.2 mi)	200 m (600 ft)	1.0 km (0.6 mi)	3.2 km (2.0 mi)
3162	Liquefied gas, toxic, n.o.s. (Inhalation Hazard Zone D)	30 m (100 ft)	0.1 km (0.1 mi)	0.2 km (0.1 mi)	150 m (500 ft)	0.7 km (0.5 mi)	2.7 km (1.7 mi)
3246 3246	Methanesulfonyl chloride Methanesulphonyl chloride	30 m (100 ft)	0.1 km (0.1 mi)	0.1 km (0.1 mi)	30 m (100 ft)	0.2 km (0.1 mi)	0.2 km (0.2 mi)
3275 3275	Nitriles, poisonous, flammable, n.o.s. Nitriles, toxic, flammable, n.o.s.	30 m (100 ft)	0.1 km (0.1 mi)	0.2 km (0.1 mi)	60 m (200 ft)	0.5 km (0.3 mi)	0.9 km (0.5 mi)
3276 3276 3276 3276	Nitriles, poisonous, liquid, n.o.s. Nitriles, poisonous, n.o.s. Nitriles, toxic, liquid, n.o.s. Nitriles, toxic, n.o.s.	30 m (100 ft)	0.1 km (0.1 mi)	0.2 km (0.1 mi)	60 m (200 ft)	0.5 km (0.3 mi)	0.9 km (0.5 mi)
3278 3278 3278 3278	Organophosphorus compound, poisonous, liquid, n.o.s. Organophosphorus compound, poisonous, n.o.s. Organophosphorus compound, toxic, liquid, n.o.s. Organophosphorus compound, toxic, n.o.s.	30 m (100 ft)	0.4 km (0.3 mi)	1.2 km (0.8 mi)	200 m (600 ft)	2.6 km (1.6 mi)	4.5 km (2.8 mi)

ID No.	Name of Material	SMALL SPILLS — First ISOLATE	SMALL SPILLS — Then PROTECT DAY	SMALL SPILLS — Then PROTECT NIGHT	LARGE SPILLS — First ISOLATE	LARGE SPILLS — Then PROTECT DAY	LARGE SPILLS — Then PROTECT NIGHT
3279	Organophosphorus compound, poisonous, flammable, n.o.s.	30 m (100 ft)	0.4 km (0.3 mi)	1.2 km (0.8 mi)	200 m (600 ft)	2.6 km (1.6 mi)	4.5 km (2.8 mi)
3279	Organophosphorus compound, toxic, flammable, n.o.s.	30 m (100 ft)	0.2 km (0.1 mi)	0.8 km (0.5 mi)	150 m (500 ft)	2.0 km (1.3 mi)	4.8 km (3.0 mi)
3280	Organoarsenic compound, liquid, n.o.s.	150 m (500 ft)	1.4 km (0.9 mi)	4.9 km (3.1 mi)	1000 m (3000 ft)	11.0+ km (7.0+ mi)	11.0+ km (7.0+ mi)
3280	Organoarsenic compound, n.o.s.						
3281	Metal carbonyls, liquid, n.o.s.	60 m (200 ft)	0.8 km (0.5 mi)	1.8 km (1.1 mi)	300 m (1000 ft)	2.9 km (1.8 mi)	5.7 km (3.6 mi)
3281	Metal carbonyls, n.o.s.						
3287	Poisonous liquid, inorganic, n.o.s.	30 m (100 ft)	0.2 km (0.1 mi)	0.3 km (0.2 mi)	150 m (500 ft)	0.6 km (0.4 mi)	1.1 km (0.7 mi)
3287	Poisonous liquid, inorganic, n.o.s. (Inhalation Hazard Zone A)	60 m (200 ft)	0.8 km (0.5 mi)	1.8 km (1.1 mi)	300 m (1000 ft)	2.9 km (1.8 mi)	5.7 km (3.6 mi)
3287	Poisonous liquid, inorganic, n.o.s. (Inhalation Hazard Zone B)	30 m (100 ft)	0.2 km (0.1 mi)	0.3 km (0.2 mi)	150 m (500 ft)	0.6 km (0.4 mi)	1.1 km (0.7 mi)
3287	Toxic liquid, inorganic, n.o.s.	60 m (200 ft)	0.8 km (0.5 mi)	1.8 km (1.1 mi)	300 m (1000 ft)	2.9 km (1.8 mi)	5.7 km (3.6 mi)
3287	Toxic liquid, inorganic, n.o.s. (Inhalation Hazard Zone A)						
3287	Toxic liquid, inorganic, n.o.s. (Inhalation Hazard Zone B)	30 m (100 ft)	0.2 km (0.1 mi)	0.3 km (0.2 mi)	150 m (500 ft)	0.6 km (0.4 mi)	1.1 km (0.7 mi)
3289	Poisonous liquid, corrosive, inorganic, n.o.s.	60 m (200 ft)	0.8 km (0.5 mi)	1.8 km (1.1 mi)	300 m (1000 ft)	2.9 km (1.8 mi)	5.7 km (3.6 mi)
3289	Poisonous liquid, corrosive, inorganic, n.o.s. (Inhalation Hazard Zone A)						
3289	Poisonous liquid, corrosive, inorganic, n.o.s. (Inhalation Hazard Zone B)	30 m (100 ft)	0.2 km (0.1 mi)	0.3 km (0.2 mi)	60 m (200 ft)	0.7 km (0.5 mi)	1.2 km (0.8 mi)
3289	Toxic liquid, corrosive, inorganic, n.o.s.	60 m (200 ft)	0.8 km (0.5 mi)	1.8 km (1.1 mi)	300 m (1000 ft)	2.9 km (1.8 mi)	5.7 km (3.6 mi)
3289	Toxic liquid, corrosive, inorganic, n.o.s. (Inhalation Hazard Zone A)						

TABLE 1 - INITIAL ISOLATION AND PROTECTIVE ACTION DISTANCES

ID No.	NAME OF MATERIAL	SMALL SPILLS (From a small package or small leak from a large package)			LARGE SPILLS (From a large package or from many small packages)			
		First ISOLATE in all Directions	Then PROTECT persons Downwind during-		First ISOLATE in all Directions	Then PROTECT persons Downwind during-		
			DAY	NIGHT		DAY	NIGHT	
		Meters (Feet)	Kilometers (Miles)	Kilometers (Miles)	Meters (Feet)	Kilometers (Miles)	Kilometers (Miles)	
3289	Toxic liquid, corrosive, inorganic, n.o.s. (Inhalation Hazard Zone B)	30 m (100 ft)	0.2 km (0.1 mi)	0.3 km (0.2 mi)	60 m (200 ft)	0.7 km (0.5 mi)	1.2 km (0.8 mi)	
3294	Hydrogen cyanide, solution in alcohol, with not more than 45% Hydrogen cyanide	30 m (100 ft)	0.1 km (0.1 mi)	0.3 km (0.2 mi)	200 m (600 ft)	0.5 km (0.3 mi)	1.9 km (1.2 mi)	
3300	Carbon dioxide and Ethylene oxide mixture, with more than 87% Ethylene oxide	30 m (100 ft)	0.1 km (0.1 mi)	0.2 km (0.1 mi)	150 m (500 ft)	0.8 km (0.5 mi)	2.5 km (1.6 mi)	
3300	Ethylene oxide and Carbon dioxide mixture, with more than 87% Ethylene oxide							
3303	Compressed gas, poisonous, oxidizing, n.o.s.	100 m (300 ft)	0.5 km (0.3 mi)	2.1 km (1.3 mi)	800 m (2500 ft)	4.4 km (2.7 mi)	8.9 km (5.6 mi)	
3303	Compressed gas, poisonous, oxidizing, n.o.s. (Inhalation Hazard Zone A)							
3303	Compressed gas, poisonous, oxidizing, n.o.s. (Inhalation Hazard Zone B)	60 m (200 ft)	0.2 km (0.2 mi)	1.0 km (0.6 mi)	500 m (1500 ft)	2.7 km (1.7 mi)	7.2 km (4.5 mi)	
3303	Compressed gas, poisonous, oxidizing, n.o.s. (Inhalation Hazard Zone C)	30 m (100 ft)	0.1 km (0.1 mi)	0.3 km (0.2 mi)	300 m (1000 ft)	1.3 km (0.8 mi)	4.1 km (2.6 mi)	
3303	Compressed gas, poisonous, oxidizing, n.o.s. (Inhalation Hazard Zone D)	30 m (100 ft)	0.1 km (0.1 mi)	0.2 km (0.1 mi)	150 m (500 ft)	0.7 km (0.5 mi)	2.7 km (1.7 mi)	

ID No.	Name of Material	SMALL SPILLS First ISOLATE in all Directions	SMALL SPILLS Then PROTECT persons Downwind DAY	SMALL SPILLS Then PROTECT persons Downwind NIGHT	LARGE SPILLS First ISOLATE in all Directions	LARGE SPILLS Then PROTECT persons Downwind DAY	LARGE SPILLS Then PROTECT persons Downwind NIGHT
3303 3303	Compressed gas, toxic, oxidizing, n.o.s. Compressed gas, toxic, oxidizing, n.o.s. (Inhalation Hazard Zone A)	100 m (300 ft)	0.5 km (0.3 mi)	2.1 km (1.3 mi)	800 m (2500 ft)	4.4 km (2.7 mi)	8.9 km (5.6 mi)
3303	Compressed gas, toxic, oxidizing, n.o.s. (Inhalation Hazard Zone B)	60 m (200 ft)	0.2 km (0.2 mi)	1.0 km (0.6 mi)	500 m (1500 ft)	2.7 km (1.7 mi)	7.2 km (4.5 mi)
3303	Compressed gas, toxic, oxidizing, n.o.s. (Inhalation Hazard Zone C)	30 m (100 ft)	0.1 km (0.1 mi)	0.3 km (0.2 mi)	300 m (1000 ft)	1.3 km (0.8 mi)	4.1 km (2.6 mi)
3303	Compressed gas, toxic, oxidizing, n.o.s. (Inhalation Hazard Zone D)	30 m (100 ft)	0.1 km (0.1 mi)	0.2 km (0.1 mi)	150 m (500 ft)	0.7 km (0.5 mi)	2.7 km (1.7 mi)
3304 3304	Compressed gas, poisonous, corrosive, n.o.s. Compressed gas, poisonous, corrosive, n.o.s. (Inhalation Hazard Zone A)	150 m (500 ft)	0.7 km (0.4 mi)	2.5 km (1.6 mi)	800 m (2500 ft)	4.7 km (2.9 mi)	10.3 km (6.4 mi)
3304	Compressed gas, poisonous, corrosive, n.o.s. (Inhalation Hazard Zone B)	30 m (100 ft)	0.2 km (0.1 mi)	1.0 km (0.6 mi)	400 m (1250 ft)	2.4 km (1.5 mi)	6.5 km (4.0 mi)
3304	Compressed gas, poisonous, corrosive, n.o.s. (Inhalation Hazard Zone C)	30 m (100 ft)	0.1 km (0.1 mi)	0.4 km (0.3 mi)	300 m (1000 ft)	1.7 km (1.1 mi)	3.6 km (2.2 mi)
3304	Compressed gas, poisonous, corrosive, n.o.s. (Inhalation Hazard Zone D)	30 m (100 ft)	0.1 km (0.1 mi)	0.2 km (0.1 mi)	150 m (500 ft)	0.7 km (0.5 mi)	2.7 km (1.7 mi)
3304 3304	Compressed gas, toxic, corrosive, n.o.s. Compressed gas, toxic, corrosive, n.o.s. (Inhalation Hazard Zone A)	150 m (500 ft)	0.7 km (0.4 mi)	2.5 km (1.6 mi)	800 m (2500 ft)	4.7 km (2.9 mi)	10.3 km (6.4 mi)

TABLE 1 - INITIAL ISOLATION AND PROTECTIVE ACTION DISTANCES

ID No.	NAME OF MATERIAL	SMALL SPILLS (From a small package or small leak from a large package)				LARGE SPILLS (From a large package or from many small packages)			
		First ISOLATE in all Directions		Then PROTECT persons Downwind during-		First ISOLATE in all Directions		Then PROTECT persons Downwind during-	
				DAY	NIGHT			DAY	NIGHT
		Meters (Feet)		Kilometers (Miles)	Kilometers (Miles)	Meters (Feet)		Kilometers (Miles)	Kilometers (Miles)
3304	Compressed gas, toxic, corrosive, n.o.s. (Inhalation Hazard Zone B)	30 m	(100 ft)	0.2 km (0.1 mi)	1.0 km (0.6 mi)	400 m	(1250 ft)	2.4 km (1.5 mi)	6.5 km (4.0 mi)
3304	Compressed gas, toxic, corrosive, n.o.s. (Inhalation Hazard Zone C)	30 m	(100 ft)	0.1 km (0.1 mi)	0.4 km (0.3 mi)	300 m	(1000 ft)	1.7 km (1.1 mi)	3.6 km (2.2 mi)
3304	Compressed gas, toxic, corrosive, n.o.s. (Inhalation Hazard Zone D)	30 m	(100 ft)	0.1 km (0.1 mi)	0.2 km (0.1 mi)	150 m	(500 ft)	0.7 km (0.5 mi)	2.7 km (1.7 mi)
3305	Compressed gas, poisonous, flammable, corrosive, n.o.s.	100 m	(300 ft)	0.7 km (0.4 mi)	2.5 km (1.6 mi)	800 m	(2500 ft)	4.7 km (2.9 mi)	10.3 km (6.4 mi)
3305	Compressed gas, poisonous, flammable, corrosive, n.o.s. (Inhalation Hazard Zone A)								
3305	Compressed gas, poisonous, flammable, corrosive, n.o.s. (Inhalation Hazard Zone B)	30 m	(100 ft)	0.2 km (0.1 mi)	1.0 km (0.6 mi)	800 m	(2500 ft)	4.2 km (2.6 mi)	10.3 km (6.4 mi)
3305	Compressed gas, poisonous, flammable, corrosive, n.o.s. (Inhalation Hazard Zone C)	30 m	(100 ft)	0.1 km (0.1 mi)	0.3 km (0.2 mi)	300 m	(1000 ft)	1.3 km (0.8 mi)	4.1 km (2.6 mi)
3305	Compressed gas, poisonous, flammable, corrosive, n.o.s. (Inhalation Hazard Zone D)	30 m	(100 ft)	0.1 km (0.1 mi)	0.2 km (0.1 mi)	150 m	(500 ft)	0.7 km (0.5 mi)	2.7 km (1.7 mi)
3305	Compressed gas, toxic, flammable, corrosive, n.o.s.	100 m	(300 ft)	0.7 km (0.4 mi)	2.5 km (1.6 mi)	800 m	(2500 ft)	4.7 km (2.9 mi)	10.3 km (6.4 mi)
3305	Compressed gas, toxic, flammable, corrosive, n.o.s. (Inhalation Hazard Zone A)								

ID No.	Name of Material	SMALL SPILLS First ISOLATE in all Directions	Then PROTECT persons Downwind during DAY	Then PROTECT persons Downwind during NIGHT	LARGE SPILLS First ISOLATE in all Directions	Then PROTECT persons Downwind during DAY	Then PROTECT persons Downwind during NIGHT
3305	Compressed gas, toxic, flammable, corrosive, n.o.s. (Inhalation Hazard Zone B)	30 m (100 ft)	0.2 km (0.1 mi)	1.0 km (0.6 mi)	800 m (2500 ft)	4.2 km (2.6 mi)	10.3 km (6.4 mi)
3305	Compressed gas, toxic, flammable, corrosive, n.o.s. (Inhalation Hazard Zone C)	30 m (100 ft)	0.1 km (0.1 mi)	0.3 km (0.2 mi)	300 m (1000 ft)	1.3 km (0.8 mi)	4.1 km (2.6 mi)
3305	Compressed gas, toxic, flammable, corrosive, n.o.s. (Inhalation Hazard Zone D)	30 m (100 ft)	0.1 km (0.1 mi)	0.2 km (0.1 mi)	150 m (500 ft)	0.7 km (0.5 mi)	2.7 km (1.7 mi)
3306	Compressed gas, poisonous, oxidizing, n.o.s. Compressed gas, poisonous, oxidizing, corrosive, n.o.s. (Inhalation Hazard Zone A)	100 m (300 ft)	0.6 km (0.4 mi)	2.5 km (1.5 mi)	800 m (2500 ft)	4.4 km (2.7 mi)	8.9 km (5.6 mi)
3306	Compressed gas, poisonous, oxidizing, corrosive, n.o.s. (Inhalation Hazard Zone B)	60 m (200 ft)	0.2 km (0.2 mi)	1.0 km (0.6 mi)	500 m (1500 ft)	2.7 km (1.7 mi)	7.2 km (4.5 mi)
3306	Compressed gas, poisonous, oxidizing, corrosive, n.o.s. (Inhalation Hazard Zone C)	30 m (100 ft)	0.1 km (0.1 mi)	0.3 km (0.2 mi)	300 m (1000 ft)	1.3 km (0.8 mi)	4.1 km (2.6 mi)
3306	Compressed gas, poisonous, oxidizing, corrosive, n.o.s. (Inhalation Hazard Zone D)	30 m (100 ft)	0.1 km (0.1 mi)	0.2 km (0.1 mi)	150 m (500 ft)	0.7 km (0.5 mi)	2.7 km (1.7 mi)
3306	Compressed gas, toxic, oxidizing, corrosive, n.o.s. Compressed gas, toxic, oxidizing, corrosive, n.o.s. (Inhalation Hazard Zone A)	100 m (300 ft)	0.6 km (0.4 mi)	2.5 km (1.5 mi)	800 m (2500 ft)	4.4 km (2.7 mi)	8.9 km (5.6 mi)
3306	Compressed gas, toxic, oxidizing, corrosive, n.o.s. (Inhalation Hazard Zone B)	60 m (200 ft)	0.2 km (0.2 mi)	1.0 km (0.6 mi)	500 m (1500 ft)	2.7 km (1.7 mi)	7.2 km (4.5 mi)

TABLE 1 - INITIAL ISOLATION AND PROTECTIVE ACTION DISTANCES

ID No.	NAME OF MATERIAL	SMALL SPILLS (From a small package or small leak from a large package)						LARGE SPILLS (From a large package or from many small packages)					
		First ISOLATE in all Directions		Then PROTECT persons Downwind during-				First ISOLATE in all Directions		Then PROTECT persons Downwind during-			
				DAY		NIGHT				DAY		NIGHT	
		Meters	(Feet)	Kilometers	(Miles)	Kilometers	(Miles)	Meters	(Feet)	Kilometers	(Miles)	Kilometers	(Miles)
3306	Compressed gas, toxic, oxidizing, corrosive, n.o.s. (Inhalation Hazard Zone C)	30 m	(100 ft)	0.1 km	(0.1 mi)	0.3 km	(0.2 mi)	300 m	(1000 ft)	1.3 km	(0.8 mi)	4.1 km	(2.6 mi)
3306	Compressed gas, toxic, oxidizing, corrosive, n.o.s. (Inhalation Hazard Zone D)	30 m	(100 ft)	0.1 km	(0.1 mi)	0.2 km	(0.1 mi)	150 m	(500 ft)	0.7 km	(0.5 mi)	2.7 km	(1.7 mi)
3307	Liquefied gas, poisonous, oxidizing, n.o.s.	100 m	(300 ft)	0.5 km	(0.3 mi)	2.1 km	(1.3 mi)	800 m	(2500 ft)	4.4 km	(2.7 mi)	8.9 km	(5.6 mi)
3307	Liquefied gas, poisonous, oxidizing, n.o.s. (Inhalation Hazard Zone A)												
3307	Liquefied gas, poisonous, oxidizing, n.o.s. (Inhalation Hazard Zone B)	60 m	(200 ft)	0.2 km	(0.2 mi)	1.0 km	(0.6 mi)	500 m	(1500 ft)	2.7 km	(1.7 mi)	7.2 km	(4.5 mi)
3307	Liquefied gas, poisonous, oxidizing, n.o.s. (Inhalation Hazard Zone C)	30 m	(100 ft)	0.1 km	(0.1 mi)	0.3 km	(0.2 mi)	300 m	(1000 ft)	1.3 km	(0.8 mi)	4.1 km	(2.6 mi)
3307	Liquefied gas, poisonous, oxidizing, n.o.s. (Inhalation Hazard Zone D)	30 m	(100 ft)	0.1 km	(0.1 mi)	0.2 km	(0.1 mi)	150 m	(500 ft)	0.7 km	(0.5 mi)	2.7 km	(1.7 mi)
3307	Liquefied gas, toxic, oxidizing, n.o.s.	100 m	(300 ft)	0.5 km	(0.3 mi)	2.1 km	(1.3 mi)	800 m	(2500 ft)	4.4 km	(2.7 mi)	8.9 km	(5.6 mi)
3307	Liquefied gas, toxic, oxidizing, n.o.s. (Inhalation Hazard Zone A)												
3307	Liquefied gas, toxic, oxidizing, n.o.s. (Inhalation Hazard Zone B)	60 m	(200 ft)	0.2 km	(0.2 mi)	1.0 km	(0.6 mi)	500 m	(1500 ft)	2.7 km	(1.7 mi)	7.2 km	(4.5 mi)
3307	Liquefied gas, toxic, oxidizing, n.o.s. (Inhalation Hazard Zone C)	30 m	(100 ft)	0.1 km	(0.1 mi)	0.3 km	(0.2 mi)	300 m	(1000 ft)	1.3 km	(0.8 mi)	4.1 km	(2.6 mi)

ID No.	NAME OF MATERIAL	SMALL SPILLS First ISOLATE (meters/feet)	SMALL SPILLS Then PROTECT DAY (km/mi)	SMALL SPILLS Then PROTECT NIGHT (km/mi)	LARGE SPILLS First ISOLATE (meters/feet)	LARGE SPILLS Then PROTECT DAY (km/mi)	LARGE SPILLS Then PROTECT NIGHT (km/mi)
3307	Liquefied gas, toxic, oxidizing, n.o.s. (Inhalation Hazard Zone D)	30 m (100 ft)	0.1 km (0.1 mi)	0.2 km (0.1 mi)	150 m (500 ft)	0.7 km (0.5 mi)	2.7 km (1.7 mi)
3308 3308	Liquefied gas, poisonous, corrosive, n.o.s. Liquefied gas, poisonous, corrosive, n.o.s. (Inhalation Hazard Zone A)	150 m (500 ft)	0.7 km (0.4 mi)	2.5 km (1.6 mi)	800 m (2500 ft)	4.7 km (2.9 mi)	10.3 km (6.4 mi)
3308	Liquefied gas, poisonous, corrosive, n.o.s. (Inhalation Hazard Zone B)	30 m (100 ft)	0.2 km (0.1 mi)	1.0 km (0.6 mi)	400 m (1250 ft)	2.4 km (1.5 mi)	6.5 km (4.0 mi)
3308	Liquefied gas, poisonous, corrosive, n.o.s. (Inhalation Hazard Zone C)	30 m (100 ft)	0.1 km (0.1 mi)	0.4 km (0.3 mi)	300 m (1000 ft)	1.7 km (1.1 mi)	3.6 km (2.2 mi)
3308	Liquefied gas, poisonous, corrosive, n.o.s. (Inhalation Hazard Zone D)	30 m (100 ft)	0.1 km (0.1 mi)	0.2 km (0.1 mi)	150 m (500 ft)	0.7 km (0.5 mi)	2.7 km (1.7 mi)
3308 3308	Liquefied gas, toxic, corrosive, n.o.s. Liquefied gas, toxic, corrosive, n.o.s. (Inhalation Hazard Zone A)	150 m (500 ft)	0.7 km (0.4 mi)	2.5 km (1.6 mi)	800 m (2500 ft)	4.7 km (2.9 mi)	10.3 km (6.4 mi)
3308	Liquefied gas, toxic, corrosive, n.o.s. (Inhalation Hazard Zone B)	30 m (100 ft)	0.2 km (0.1 mi)	1.0 km (0.6 mi)	400 m (1250 ft)	2.4 km (1.5 mi)	6.5 km (4.0 mi)
3308	Liquefied gas, toxic, corrosive, n.o.s. (Inhalation Hazard Zone C)	30 m (100 ft)	0.1 km (0.1 mi)	0.4 km (0.3 mi)	300 m (1000 ft)	1.7 km (1.1 mi)	3.6 km (2.2 mi)
3308	Liquefied gas, toxic, corrosive, n.o.s. (Inhalation Hazard Zone D)	30 m (100 ft)	0.1 km (0.1 mi)	0.2 km (0.1 mi)	150 m (500 ft)	0.7 km (0.5 mi)	2.7 km (1.7 mi)
3309 3309	Liquefied gas, poisonous, flammable, corrosive, n.o.s. Liquefied gas, poisonous, flammable, corrosive, n.o.s. (Inhalation Hazard Zone A)	100 m (300 ft)	0.7 km (0.4 mi)	2.5 km (1.6 mi)	800 m (2500 ft)	4.7 km (2.9 mi)	10.3 km (6.4 mi)
3309	Liquefied gas, poisonous, flammable, corrosive, n.o.s. (Inhalation Hazard Zone B)	30 m (100 ft)	0.2 km (0.1 mi)	1.0 km (0.6 mi)	800 m (2500 ft)	4.2 km (2.6 mi)	10.3 km (6.4 mi)

TABLE 1 - INITIAL ISOLATION AND PROTECTIVE ACTION DISTANCES

ID No.	NAME OF MATERIAL	SMALL SPILLS (From a small package or small leak from a large package)				LARGE SPILLS (From a large package or from many small packages)				
		First ISOLATE in all Directions	Then PROTECT persons Downwind during-			First ISOLATE in all Directions	Then PROTECT persons Downwind during-			
				DAY	NIGHT			DAY	NIGHT	
		Meters (Feet)		Kilometers (Miles)	Kilometers (Miles)	Meters (Feet)		Kilometers (Miles)	Kilometers (Miles)	
3309	Liquefied gas, poisonous, flammable, corrosive, n.o.s. (Inhalation Hazard Zone C)	30 m	(100 ft)	0.1 km (0.1 mi)	0.3 km (0.2 mi)	300 m	(1000 ft)	1.3 km (0.8 mi)	4.1 km (2.6 mi)	
3309	Liquefied gas, poisonous, flammable, corrosive, n.o.s. (Inhalation Hazard Zone D)	30 m	(100 ft)	0.1 km (0.1 mi)	0.2 km (0.1 mi)	150 m	(500 ft)	0.7 km (0.5 mi)	2.7 km (1.7 mi)	
3309	Liquefied gas, toxic, flammable, corrosive, n.o.s.	100 m	(300 ft)	0.7 km (0.4 mi)	2.5 km (1.6 mi)	800 m	(2500 ft)	4.7 km (2.9 mi)	10.3 km (6.4 mi)	
3309	Liquefied gas, toxic, flammable, corrosive, n.o.s. (Inhalation Hazard Zone A)	100 m	(300 ft)	0.7 km (0.4 mi)	2.5 km (1.6 mi)	800 m	(2500 ft)	4.7 km (2.9 mi)	10.3 km (6.4 mi)	
3309	Liquefied gas, toxic, flammable, corrosive, n.o.s. (Inhalation Hazard Zone B)	30 m	(100 ft)	0.2 km (0.1 mi)	1.0 km (0.6 mi)	800 m	(2500 ft)	4.2 km (2.6 mi)	10.3 km (6.4 mi)	
3309	Liquefied gas, toxic, flammable, corrosive, n.o.s. (Inhalation Hazard Zone C)	30 m	(100 ft)	0.1 km (0.1 mi)	0.3 km (0.2 mi)	300 m	(1000 ft)	1.3 km (0.8 mi)	4.1 km (2.6 mi)	
3309	Liquefied gas, toxic, flammable, corrosive, n.o.s. (Inhalation Hazard Zone D)	30 m	(100 ft)	0.1 km (0.1 mi)	0.2 km (0.1 mi)	150 m	(500 ft)	0.7 km (0.5 mi)	2.7 km (1.7 mi)	
3310	Liquefied gas, poisonous, oxidizing, corrosive, n.o.s.	100 m	(300 ft)	0.6 km (0.4 mi)	2.5 km (1.5 mi)	800 m	(2500 ft)	4.4 km (2.7 mi)	8.9 km (5.6 mi)	
3310	Liquefied gas, poisonous, oxidizing, corrosive, n.o.s. (Inhalation Hazard Zone A)	100 m	(300 ft)	0.6 km (0.4 mi)	2.5 km (1.5 mi)	800 m	(2500 ft)	4.4 km (2.7 mi)	8.9 km (5.6 mi)	
3310	Liquefied gas, poisonous, oxidizing, corrosive, n.o.s. (Inhalation Hazard Zone B)	60 m	(200 ft)	0.2 km (0.2 mi)	1.0 km (0.6 mi)	500 m	(1500 ft)	2.7 km (1.7 mi)	7.2 km (4.5 mi)	

ID No.	Name of Material	SMALL SPILLS — First ISOLATE (Meters / Feet)	SMALL SPILLS — Then PROTECT persons Downwind during DAY	SMALL SPILLS — Then PROTECT persons Downwind during NIGHT	LARGE SPILLS — First ISOLATE (Meters / Feet)	LARGE SPILLS — Then PROTECT persons Downwind during DAY	LARGE SPILLS — Then PROTECT persons Downwind during NIGHT
3310	Liquefied gas, poisonous, oxidizing, corrosive, n.o.s. (Inhalation Hazard Zone C)	30 m (100 ft)	0.1 km (0.1 mi)	0.3 km (0.2 mi)	300 m (1000 ft)	1.3 km (0.8 mi)	4.1 km (2.6 mi)
3310	Liquefied gas, poisonous, oxidizing, corrosive, n.o.s. (Inhalation Hazard Zone D)	30 m (100 ft)	0.1 km (0.1 mi)	0.2 km (0.1 mi)	150 m (500 ft)	0.7 km (0.5 mi)	2.7 km (1.7 mi)
3310	Liquefied gas, toxic, oxidizing, corrosive, n.o.s.						
3310	Liquefied gas, toxic, oxidizing, corrosive, n.o.s. (Inhalation Hazard Zone A)	100 m (300 ft)	0.6 km (0.4 mi)	2.5 km (1.5 mi)	800 m (2500 ft)	4.4 km (2.7 mi)	8.9 km (5.6 mi)
3310	Liquefied gas, toxic, oxidizing, corrosive, n.o.s. (Inhalation Hazard Zone B)	60 m (200 ft)	0.2 km (0.2 mi)	1.0 km (0.6 mi)	500 m (1500 ft)	2.7 km (1.7 mi)	7.2 km (4.5 mi)
3310	Liquefied gas, toxic, oxidizing, corrosive, n.o.s. (Inhalation Hazard Zone C)	30 m (100 ft)	0.1 km (0.1 mi)	0.3 km (0.2 mi)	300 m (1000 ft)	1.3 km (0.8 mi)	4.1 km (2.6 mi)
3310	Liquefied gas, toxic, oxidizing, corrosive, n.o.s. (Inhalation Hazard Zone D)	30 m (100 ft)	0.1 km (0.1 mi)	0.2 km (0.1 mi)	150 m (500 ft)	0.7 km (0.5 mi)	2.7 km (1.7 mi)
3318	Ammonia solution, with more than 50% Ammonia	30 m (100 ft)	0.1 km (0.1 mi)	0.2 km (0.1 mi)	150 m (500 ft)	0.8 km (0.5 mi)	2.3 km (1.4 mi)
3355	Insecticide gas, poisonous, flammable, n.o.s.						
3355	Insecticide gas, poisonous, flammable, n.o.s. (Inhalation Hazard Zone A)	100 m (300 ft)	0.6 km (0.4 mi)	2.5 km (1.5 mi)	800 m (2500 ft)	4.4 km (2.7 mi)	8.9 km (5.6 mi)
3355	Insecticide gas, poisonous, flammable, n.o.s. (Inhalation Hazard Zone B)	30 m (100 ft)	0.2 km (0.1 mi)	0.8 km (0.5 mi)	400 m (1250 ft)	1.9 km (1.2 mi)	4.8 km (3.0 mi)

TABLE 1 - INITIAL ISOLATION AND PROTECTIVE ACTION DISTANCES

ID No.	NAME OF MATERIAL	SMALL SPILLS (From a small package or small leak from a large package)			LARGE SPILLS (From a large package or from many small packages)			
		First ISOLATE in all Directions	Then PROTECT persons Downwind during-		First ISOLATE in all Directions	Then PROTECT persons Downwind during-		
		Meters (Feet)	DAY Kilometers (Miles)	NIGHT Kilometers (Miles)	Meters (Feet)	DAY Kilometers (Miles)	NIGHT Kilometers (Miles)	
3355	Insecticide gas, poisonous, flammable, n.o.s. (Inhalation Hazard Zone C)	30 m (100 ft)	0.1 km (0.1 mi)	0.3 km (0.2 mi)	300 m (1000 ft)	1.3 km (0.8 mi)	4.1 km (2.6 mi)	
3355	Insecticide gas, poisonous, flammable, n.o.s. (Inhalation Hazard Zone D)	30 m (100 ft)	0.1 km (0.1 mi)	0.2 km (0.1 mi)	150 m (500 ft)	0.7 km (0.5 mi)	2.7 km (1.7 mi)	
3355	Insecticide gas, toxic, flammable, n.o.s. (Inhalation Hazard Zone A)	100 m (300 ft)	0.6 km (0.4 mi)	2.5 km (1.5 mi)	800 m (2500 ft)	4.4 km (2.7 mi)	8.9 km (5.6 mi)	
3355	Insecticide gas, toxic, flammable, n.o.s. (Inhalation Hazard Zone B)	30 m (100 ft)	0.2 km (0.1 mi)	0.8 km (0.5 mi)	400 m (1250 ft)	1.9 km (1.2 mi)	4.8 km (3.0 mi)	
3355	Insecticide gas, toxic, flammable, n.o.s. (Inhalation Hazard Zone C)	30 m (100 ft)	0.1 km (0.1 mi)	0.3 km (0.2 mi)	300 m (1000 ft)	1.3 km (0.8 mi)	4.1 km (2.6 mi)	
3355	Insecticide gas, toxic, flammable, n.o.s. (Inhalation Hazard Zone D)	30 m (100 ft)	0.1 km (0.1 mi)	0.2 km (0.1 mi)	150 m (500 ft)	0.7 km (0.5 mi)	2.7 km (1.7 mi)	
3361	Chlorosilanes, poisonous, corrosive, n.o.s. (when spilled in water)	30 m (100 ft)	0.1 km (0.1 mi)	0.2 km (0.1 mi)	100 m (300 ft)	0.5 km (0.3 mi)	1.6 km (1.0 mi)	
3361	Chlorosilanes, toxic, corrosive, n.o.s. (when spilled in water)							
3362	Chlorosilanes, poisonous, corrosive, flammable, n.o.s. (when spilled in water)	30 m (100 ft)	0.1 km (0.1 mi)	0.2 km (0.1 mi)	100 m (300 ft)	0.5 km (0.3 mi)	1.6 km (1.0 mi)	
3362	Chlorosilanes, toxic, corrosive, flammable, n.o.s. (when spilled in water)							

ID No.	Name of Material	SMALL SPILLS First ISOLATE in all Directions	SMALL SPILLS Then PROTECT persons Downwind during DAY	SMALL SPILLS Then PROTECT persons Downwind during NIGHT	LARGE SPILLS First ISOLATE in all Directions	LARGE SPILLS Then PROTECT persons Downwind during DAY	LARGE SPILLS Then PROTECT persons Downwind during NIGHT
3381	Poisonous by inhalation liquid, n.o.s. (Inhalation Hazard Zone A)	60 m (200 ft)	0.8 km (0.5 mi)	1.8 km (1.1 mi)	300 m (1000 ft)	2.9 km (1.8 mi)	5.7 km (3.6 mi)
3381	Toxic by inhalation liquid, n.o.s. (Inhalation Hazard Zone A)						
3382	Poisonous by inhalation liquid, n.o.s. (Inhalation Hazard Zone B)	30 m (100 ft)	0.1 km (0.1 mi)	0.2 km (0.1 mi)	60 m (200 ft)	0.5 km (0.3 mi)	0.8 km (0.5 mi)
3382	Toxic by inhalation liquid, n.o.s. (Inhalation Hazard Zone B)						
3383	Poisonous by inhalation liquid, flammable, n.o.s. (Inhalation Hazard Zone A)	60 m (200 ft)	0.7 km (0.4 mi)	2.3 km (1.4 mi)	400 m (1250 ft)	4.6 km (2.9 mi)	8.9 km (5.5 mi)
3383	Toxic by inhalation liquid, flammable, n.o.s. (Inhalation Hazard Zone A)						
3384	Poisonous by inhalation liquid, flammable, n.o.s. (Inhalation Hazard Zone B)	30 m (100 ft)	0.1 km (0.1 mi)	0.2 km (0.1 mi)	60 m (200 ft)	0.5 km (0.3 mi)	0.8 km (0.5 mi)
3384	Toxic by inhalation liquid, flammable, n.o.s. (Inhalation Hazard Zone B)						
3385	Poisonous by inhalation liquid, water-reactive, n.o.s. (Inhalation Hazard Zone A)	60 m (200 ft)	0.8 km (0.5 mi)	1.8 km (1.1 mi)	300 m (1000 ft)	2.9 km (1.8 mi)	5.7 km (3.6 mi)
3385	Toxic by inhalation liquid, water-reactive, n.o.s. (Inhalation Hazard Zone A)						
3386	Poisonous by inhalation liquid, water-reactive, n.o.s. (Inhalation Hazard Zone B)	30 m (100 ft)	0.1 km (0.1 mi)	0.2 km (0.1 mi)	60 m (200 ft)	0.5 km (0.3 mi)	0.8 km (0.5 mi)
3386	Toxic by inhalation liquid, water-reactive, n.o.s. (Inhalation Hazard Zone B)						

TABLE 1 - INITIAL ISOLATION AND PROTECTIVE ACTION DISTANCES

ID No.	NAME OF MATERIAL	SMALL SPILLS (From a small package or small leak from a large package) First ISOLATE in all Directions Meters (Feet)	Then PROTECT persons Downwind during- DAY Kilometers (Miles)	NIGHT Kilometers (Miles)	LARGE SPILLS (From a large package or from many small packages) First ISOLATE in all Directions Meters (Feet)	Then PROTECT persons Downwind during- DAY Kilometers (Miles)	NIGHT Kilometers (Miles)
3387	Poisonous by inhalation liquid, oxidizing, n.o.s. (Inhalation Hazard Zone A)	60 m (200 ft)	0.8 km (0.5 mi)	1.8 km (1.1 mi)	300 m (1000 ft)	2.9 km (1.8 mi)	5.7 km (3.6 mi)
3387	Toxic by inhalation liquid, oxidizing, n.o.s. (Inhalation Hazard Zone A)						
3388	Poisonous by inhalation liquid, oxidizing, n.o.s. (Inhalation Hazard Zone B)	30 m (100 ft)	0.1 km (0.1 mi)	0.3 km (0.2 mi)	60 m (200 ft)	0.6 km (0.4 mi)	1.0 km (0.6 mi)
3388	Toxic by inhalation liquid, oxidizing, n.o.s. (Inhalation Hazard Zone B)						
3389	Poisonous by inhalation liquid, corrosive, n.o.s. (Inhalation Hazard Zone A)	60 m (200 ft)	0.8 km (0.5 mi)	1.8 km (1.1 mi)	300 m (1000 ft)	2.9 km (1.8 mi)	5.7 km (3.6 mi)
3389	Toxic by inhalation liquid, corrosive, n.o.s. (Inhalation Hazard Zone A)						
3390	Poisonous by inhalation liquid, corrosive, n.o.s. (Inhalation Hazard Zone B)	30 m (100 ft)	0.1 km (0.1 mi)	0.2 km (0.1 mi)	60 m (200 ft)	0.5 km (0.3 mi)	0.8 km (0.5 mi)
3390	Toxic by inhalation liquid, corrosive, n.o.s. (Inhalation Hazard Zone B)						
3456	Nitrosylsulfuric acid, solid (when spilled in water) Nitrosylsulphuric acid, solid (when spilled in water)	30 m (100 ft)	0.1 km (0.1 mi)	0.5 km (0.3 mi)	200 m (600 ft)	0.7 km (0.5 mi)	2.5 km (1.6 mi)
3461	Aluminum alkyl halides, solid (when spilled in water)	30 m (100 ft)	0.1 km (0.1 mi)	0.2 km (0.1 mi)	60 m (200 ft)	0.4 km (0.3 mi)	1.3 km (0.8 mi)
9191	Chlorine dioxide, hydrate, frozen	30 m (100 ft)	0.1 km (0.1 mi)	0.1 km (0.1 mi)	30 m (100 ft)	0.2 km (0.2 mi)	0.6 km (0.4 mi)

ID No.	Name of Material	Small Spills — Isolate	Small Spills — Day	Small Spills — Night	Large Spills — Isolate	Large Spills — Day	Large Spills — Night
9192	Fluorine, refrigerated liquid (cryogenic liquid)	30 m (100 ft)	0.1 km (0.1 mi)	0.3 km (0.2 mi)	150 m (500 ft)	0.8 km (0.5 mi)	3.1 km (1.9 mi)
9202	Carbon monoxide, refrigerated liquid (cryogenic liquid)	30 m (100 ft)	0.1 km (0.1 mi)	0.1 km (0.1 mi)	150 m (500 ft)	0.7 km (0.5 mi)	2.7 km (1.7 mi)
9206	Methyl phosphonic dichloride	30 m (100 ft)	0.1 km (0.1 mi)	0.2 km (0.1 mi)	60 m (200 ft)	0.5 km (0.3 mi)	0.7 km (0.4 mi)
9263	Chloropivaloyl chloride	30 m (100 ft)	0.1 km (0.1 mi)	0.1 km (0.1 mi)	30 m (100 ft)	0.3 km (0.2 mi)	0.4 km (0.2 mi)
9264	3,5-Dichloro-2,4,6-trifluoropyridine	30 m (100 ft)	0.1 km (0.1 mi)	0.1 km (0.1 mi)	30 m (100 ft)	0.3 km (0.2 mi)	0.3 km (0.2 mi)
9269	Trimethoxysilane	30 m (100 ft)	0.2 km (0.1 mi)	0.5 km (0.3 mi)	150 m (500 ft)	1.0 km (0.7 mi)	2.0 km (1.3 mi)

See Next Page for Table of Water-Reactive Materials Which Produce Toxic Gases

TABLE 2 - WATER-REACTIVE MATERIALS WHICH PRODUCE TOXIC GASES

Materials Which Produce Large Amounts of Toxic-by-Inhalation (TIH) Gas(es) *When Spilled in Water*

ID No.	Guide No.	Name of Material	TIH Gas(es) Produced	
1162	155	Dimethyldichlorosilane	HCl	
1183	139	Ethyldichlorosilane	HCl	
1196	155	Ethyltrichlorosilane	HCl	
1242	139	Methyldichlorosilane	HCl	
1250	155	Methyltrichlorosilane	HCl	
1295	139	Trichlorosilane	HCl	
1298	155	Trimethylchlorosilane	HCl	
1305	155P	Vinyltrichlorosilane	HCl	
1305	155P	Vinyltrichlorosilane, stabilized	HCl	
1340	139	Phosphorus pentasulfide, free from yellow and white Phosphorus	H_2S	
1340	139	Phosphorus pentasulphide, free from yellow and white Phosphorus	H_2S	
1360	139	Calcium phosphide	PH_3	
1384	135	Sodium dithionite	H_2S	SO_2
1384	135	Sodium hydrosulfite	H_2S	SO_2
1384	135	Sodium hydrosulphite	H_2S	SO_2
1397	139	Aluminum phosphide	PH_3	
1412	139	Lithium amide	NH_3	
1419	139	Magnesium aluminum phosphide	PH_3	
1432	139	Sodium phosphide	PH_3	
1541	155	Acetone cyanohydrin, stabilized	HCN	
1680	157	Potassium cyanide	HCN	
1680	157	Potassium cyanide, solid	HCN	
1689	157	Sodium cyanide	HCN	
1689	157	Sodium cyanide, solid	HCN	

Chemical Symbols for TIH Gases:

Br_2	Bromine	HF	Hydrogen fluoride	PH_3	Phosphine
Cl_2	Chlorine	HI	Hydrogen iodide	NO_2	Nitrogen dioxide
HBr	Hydrogen bromide	H_2S	Hydrogen sulfide	SO_2	Sulfur dioxide
HCl	Hydrogen chloride	H_2S	Hydrogen sulphide	SO_2	Sulphur dioxide
HCN	Hydrogen cyanide	NH_3	Ammonia		

Use this list only when material is spilled in water.

TABLE 2 - WATER-REACTIVE MATERIALS WHICH PRODUCE TOXIC GASES

Materials Which Produce Large Amounts of Toxic-by-Inhalation (TIH) Gas(es)
When Spilled in Water

ID No.	Guide No.	Name of Material	TIH Gas(es) Produced	
1716	156	Acetyl bromide	HBr	
1717	155	Acetyl chloride	HCl	
1724	155	Allyltrichlorosilane, stabilized	HCl	
1725	137	Aluminum bromide, anhydrous	HBr	
1726	137	Aluminum chloride, anhydrous	HCl	
1728	155	Amyltrichlorosilane	HCl	
1732	157	Antimony pentafluoride	HF	
1741	125	Boron trichloride	HCl	
1745	144	Bromine pentafluoride	HF	Br_2
1746	144	Bromine trifluoride	HF	Br_2
1747	155	Butyltrichlorosilane	HCl	
1752	156	Chloroacetyl chloride	HCl	
1753	156	Chlorophenyltrichlorosilane	HCl	
1754	137	Chlorosulfonic acid	HCl	
1754	137	Chlorosulfonic acid and Sulfur trioxide mixture	HCl	
1754	137	Chlorosulphonic acid	HCl	
1754	137	Chlorosulphonic acid and Sulphur trioxide mixture	HCl	
1754	137	Sulfur trioxide and Chlorosulfonic acid	HCl	
1754	137	Sulphur trioxide and Chlorosulphonic acid	HCl	
1758	137	Chromium oxychloride	HCl	
1762	156	Cyclohexenyltrichlorosilane	HCl	
1763	156	Cyclohexyltrichlorosilane	HCl	
1765	156	Dichloroacetyl chloride	HCl	
1766	156	Dichlorophenyltrichlorosilane	HCl	

Chemical Symbols for TIH Gases:

Br_2	Bromine	HF	Hydrogen fluoride	PH_3	Phosphine
Cl_2	Chlorine	HI	Hydrogen iodide	NO_2	Nitrogen dioxide
HBr	Hydrogen bromide	H_2S	Hydrogen sulfide	SO_2	Sulfur dioxide
HCl	Hydrogen chloride	H_2S	Hydrogen sulphide	SO_2	Sulphur dioxide
HCN	Hydrogen cyanide	NH_3	Ammonia		

TABLE 2 - WATER-REACTIVE MATERIALS WHICH PRODUCE TOXIC GASES

Materials Which Produce Large Amounts of Toxic-by-Inhalation (TIH) Gas(es) *When Spilled in Water*

ID No.	Guide No.	Name of Material	TIH Gas(es) Produced		
1767	155	Diethyldichlorosilane	HCl		
1769	156	Diphenyldichlorosilane	HCl		
1771	156	Dodecyltrichlorosilane	HCl		
1777	137	Fluorosulfonic acid	HF		
1777	137	Fluorosulphonic acid	HF		
1781	156	Hexadecyltrichlorosilane	HCl		
1784	156	Hexyltrichlorosilane	HCl		
1799	156	Nonyltrichlorosilane	HCl		
1800	156	Octadecyltrichlorosilane	HCl		
1801	156	Octyltrichlorosilane	HCl		
1804	156	Phenyltrichlorosilane	HCl		
1806	137	Phosphorus pentachloride	HCl		
1808	137	Phosphorus tribromide	HBr		
1809	137	Phosphorus trichloride	HCl		
1810	137	Phosphorus oxychloride	HCl		
1815	132	Propionyl chloride	HCl		
1816	155	Propyltrichlorosilane	HCl		
1818	157	Silicon tetrachloride	HCl		
1828	137	Sulfur chlorides	HCl	SO_2	H_2S
1828	137	Sulphur chlorides	HCl	SO_2	H_2S
1834	137	Sulfuryl chloride	HCl		
1834	137	Sulphuryl chloride	HCl		
1836	137	Thionyl chloride	HCl	SO_2	
1838	137	Titanium tetrachloride	HCl		

Chemical Symbols for TIH Gases:

Br_2	Bromine	HF	Hydrogen fluoride	PH_3	Phosphine
Cl_2	Chlorine	HI	Hydrogen iodide	NO_2	Nitrogen dioxide
HBr	Hydrogen bromide	H_2S	Hydrogen sulfide	SO_2	Sulfur dioxide
HCl	Hydrogen chloride	H_2S	Hydrogen sulphide	SO_2	Sulphur dioxide
HCN	Hydrogen cyanide	NH_3	Ammonia		

Use this list only when material is spilled in water.

TABLE 2 - WATER-REACTIVE MATERIALS WHICH PRODUCE TOXIC GASES

Materials Which Produce Large Amounts of Toxic-by-Inhalation (TIH) Gas(es) *When Spilled in Water*

ID No.	Guide No.	Name of Material	TIH Gas(es) Produced	
1898	156	Acetyl iodide	HI	
1923	135	Calcium dithionite	H_2S	SO_2
1923	135	Calcium hydrosulfite	H_2S	SO_2
1923	135	Calcium hydrosulphite	H_2S	SO_2
1929	135	Potassium dithionite	H_2S	SO_2
1929	135	Potassium hydrosulfite	H_2S	SO_2
1929	135	Potassium hydrosulphite	H_2S	SO_2
1931	171	Zinc dithionite	H_2S	SO_2
1931	171	Zinc hydrosulfite	H_2S	SO_2
1931	171	Zinc hydrosulphite	H_2S	SO_2
2004	135	Magnesium diamide	NH_3	
2011	139	Magnesium phosphide	PH_3	
2012	139	Potassium phosphide	PH_3	
2013	139	Strontium phosphide	PH_3	
2308	157	Nitrosylsulfuric acid	NO_2	
2308	157	Nitrosylsulfuric acid, liquid	NO_2	
2308	157	Nitrosylsulfuric acid, solid	NO_2	
2308	157	Nitrosylsulphuric acid	NO_2	
2308	157	Nitrosylsulphuric acid, liquid	NO_2	
2308	157	Nitrosylsulphuric acid, solid	NO_2	
2353	132	Butyryl chloride	HCl	
2395	132	Isobutyryl chloride	HCl	
2434	156	Dibenzyldichlorosilane	HCl	
2435	156	Ethylphenyldichlorosilane	HCl	

Chemical Symbols for TIH Gases:

Br_2	Bromine	HF	Hydrogen fluoride	PH_3	Phosphine
Cl_2	Chlorine	HI	Hydrogen iodide	NO_2	Nitrogen dioxide
HBr	Hydrogen bromide	H_2S	Hydrogen sulfide	SO_2	Sulfur dioxide
HCl	Hydrogen chloride	H_2S	Hydrogen sulphide	SO_2	Sulphur dioxide
HCN	Hydrogen cyanide	NH_3	Ammonia		

Use this list only when material is spilled in water.

TABLE 2 - WATER-REACTIVE MATERIALS WHICH PRODUCE TOXIC GASES

Materials Which Produce Large Amounts of Toxic-by-Inhalation (TIH) Gas(es)
When Spilled in Water

ID No.	Guide No.	Name of Material	TIH Gas(es) Produced
2437	156	Methylphenyldichlorosilane	HCl
2495	144	Iodine pentafluoride	HF
2691	137	Phosphorus pentabromide	HBr
2692	157	Boron tribromide	HBr
2806	138	Lithium nitride	NH_3
2977	166	Radioactive material, Uranium hexafluoride, fissile	HF
2977	166	Uranium hexafluoride, fissile containing more than 1% Uranium-235	HF
2978	166	Radioactive material, Uranium hexafluoride	HF
2978	166	Uranium hexafluoride	HF
2978	166	Uranium hexafluoride non fissile or fissile-excepted	HF
2985	155	Chlorosilanes, flammable, corrosive, n.o.s.	HCl
2985	155	Chlorosilanes, n.o.s.	HCl
2986	155	Chlorosilanes, corrosive, flammable, n.o.s.	HCl
2986	155	Chlorosilanes, n.o.s.	HCl
2987	156	Chlorosilanes, corrosive, n.o.s.	HCl
2987	156	Chlorosilanes, n.o.s.	HCl
2988	139	Chlorosilanes, n.o.s.	HCl
2988	139	Chlorosilanes, water-reactive, flammable, corrosive, n.o.s.	HCl
3048	157	Aluminum phosphide pesticide	PH_3
3049	138	Metal alkyl halides, n.o.s.	HCl
3049	138	Metal alkyl halides, water-reactive, n.o.s.	HCl
3049	138	Metal aryl halides, n.o.s.	HCl
3049	138	Metal aryl halides, water-reactive, n.o.s.	HCl

Chemical Symbols for TIH Gases:

Br_2	Bromine	HF	Hydrogen fluoride	PH_3	Phosphine
Cl_2	Chlorine	HI	Hydrogen iodide	NO_2	Nitrogen dioxide
HBr	Hydrogen bromide	H_2S	Hydrogen sulfide	SO_2	Sulfur dioxide
HCl	Hydrogen chloride	H_2S	Hydrogen sulphide	SO_2	Sulphur dioxide
HCN	Hydrogen cyanide	NH_3	Ammonia		

Use this list only when material is spilled in water.

TABLE 2 - WATER-REACTIVE MATERIALS WHICH PRODUCE TOXIC GASES

Materials Which Produce Large Amounts of Toxic-by-Inhalation (TIH) Gas(es) *When Spilled in Water*

ID No.	Guide No.	Name of Material	TIH Gas(es) Produced
3052	135	Aluminum alkyl halides	HCl
3052	135	Aluminum alkyl halides, liquid	HCl
3052	135	Aluminum alkyl halides, solid	HCl
3361	156	Chlorosilanes, poisonous, corrosive, n.o.s.	HCl
3361	156	Chlorosilanes, toxic, corrosive, n.o.s.	HCl
3362	155	Chlorosilanes, poisonous, corrosive, flammable, n.o.s.	HCl
3362	155	Chlorosilanes, toxic, corrosive, flammable, n.o.s.	HCl
3456	157	Nitrosylsulfuric acid, solid	NO_2
3456	157	Nitrosylsulphuric acid, solid	NO_2
3461	135	Aluminum alkyl halides, solid	HCl
9191	143	Chlorine dioxide, hydrate, frozen	Cl_2

Chemical Symbols for TIH Gases:

Br_2	Bromine	HF	Hydrogen fluoride	PH_3	Phosphine
Cl_2	Chlorine	HI	Hydrogen iodide	NO_2	Nitrogen dioxide
HBr	Hydrogen bromide	H_2S	Hydrogen sulfide	SO_2	Sulfur dioxide
HCl	Hydrogen chloride	H_2S	Hydrogen sulphide	SO_2	Sulphur dioxide
HCN	Hydrogen cyanide	NH_3	Ammonia		

Use this list only when material is spilled in water.

PROTECTIVE CLOTHING

Street Clothing and Work Uniforms. These garments, such as uniforms worn by police and emergency medical services personnel, provide almost no protection from the harmful effects of dangerous goods.

Structural Fire Fighters' Protective Clothing (SFPC). This category of clothing, often called turnout or bunker gear, means the protective clothing normally worn by fire fighters during structural fire fighting operations. It includes a helmet, coat, pants, boots, gloves and a hood to cover parts of the head not protected by the helmet and facepiece. This clothing must be used with full-facepiece positive pressure self-contained breathing apparatus (SCBA). This protective clothing should, at a minimum, meet the OSHA Fire Brigades Standard (29 CFR 1910.156). Structural fire fighters' protective clothing provides limited protection from heat and cold, but may not provide adequate protection from the harmful vapors or liquids that are encountered during dangerous goods incidents. Each guide includes a statement about the use of SFPC in incidents involving those materials referenced by that guide. Some guides state that SFPC provides limited protection. In those cases, the responder wearing SFPC and SCBA may be able to perform an expedient, that is quick "in-and-out", operation. However, this type of operation can place the responder at risk of exposure, injury or death. The incident commander makes the decision to perform this operation only if an overriding benefit can be gained (i.e., perform an immediate rescue, turn off a valve to control a leak, etc.). The coverall-type protective clothing customarily worn to fight fires in forests or wildlands is **not** SFPC and is not recommended nor referred to elsewhere in this guidebook.

Positive Pressure Self-Contained Breathing Apparatus (SCBA). This apparatus provides a constant, positive pressure flow of air within the facepiece, even if one inhales deeply while doing heavy work. Use apparatus certified by NIOSH and the Department of Labor/Mine Safety and Health Administration in accordance with 42 CFR Part 84. Use it in accordance with the requirements for respiratory protection specified in OSHA 29 CFR 1910.134 (Respiratory Protection) and/or 29 CFR 1910.156 (f) (Fire Brigades Standard). Chemical-cartridge respirators or other filtering masks are not acceptable substitutes for positive pressure self-contained breathing apparatus. Demand-type SCBA does not meet the OSHA 29 CFR 1910.156 (f)(1)(i) of the Fire Brigades Standard. If it is suspected that a Chemical Warfare Agent (CW) is involved, the use of NIOSH-certified respirators with CBRN protection are highly recommended.

Chemical Protective Clothing and Equipment. Safe use of this type of protective clothing and equipment requires specific skills developed through training and experience. It is generally not available to, or used by, first responders. This type of special clothing may protect against one chemical, yet be readily permeated by chemicals for which it was not designed. Therefore, protective clothing should not be used unless it is compatible with the released material. This type of special clothing offers little or no protection against heat and/ or cold. Examples of this type of equipment have been described as (1) Vapor Protective

Suits (NFPA 1991), also known as Totally-Encapsulating Chemical Protective (TECP) Suits or Level A* protection (OSHA 29 CFR 1910.120, Appendix A & B), and (2) Liquid-Splash Protective Suits (NFPA 1992 & 1993), also known as Level B* or C* protection (OSHA 29 CFR 1910.120, Appendix A & B) or suits for chemical/biological terrorism incidents (NFPA 1994), class 1, 2 or 3 Ensembles. No single protective clothing material will protect you from all dangerous goods. Do not assume any protective clothing is resistant to cold and/or heat or flame exposure unless it is so certified by the manufacturer. (NFPA 1991 5-3 Flammability Resistance Test and 5-6 Cold Temperature Performance Test)

* Consult glossary for additional protection levels under the heading "Protective Clothing".

FIRE AND SPILL CONTROL

FIRE CONTROL

Water is the most common and generally most available fire extinguishing agent. Exercise caution in selecting a fire extinguishing method since there are many factors to be considered in an incident. Water may be ineffective in fighting fires involving some materials; its effectiveness depends greatly on the method of application.

Fires involving a spill of flammable liquids are generally controlled by applying a fire fighting foam to the surface of the burning material. Fighting flammable liquid fires requires foam concentrate which is <u>chemically compatible</u> with the burning material, <u>correct mixing</u> of the foam concentrate with water and air, and <u>careful application and maintenance</u> of the foam blanket. There are two general types of fire fighting foam: regular and alcohol-resistant. Examples of regular foam are protein-base, fluoroprotein, and aqueous film forming foam (AFFF). Some flammable liquids, including many petroleum products, can be controlled by applying regular foam. Other flammable liquids, including polar solvents (flammable liquids which are water soluble) such as alcohols and ketones, have different chemical properties. A fire involving these materials cannot be easily controlled with regular foam and requires application of alcohol-resistant foam. Polar-solvent fires may be difficult to control and require a higher foam application rate than other flammable liquid fires (see NFPA/ANSI Standards 11 and 11A for further information). Refer to the appropriate guide to determine which type of foam is recommended. Although it is impossible to make specific recommendations for flammable liquids which have subsidiary corrosive or toxic hazards, alcohol-resistant foam may be effective for many of these materials. The emergency response telephone number on the shipping document, or the appropriate emergency response agency, should be contacted as soon as possible for guidance on the proper fire extinguishing agent to use. The final selection of the agent and method depends on many factors such as incident location, exposure hazards, size of the fire, environmental concerns, as well as the availability of extinguishing agents and equipment at the scene.

WATER REACTIVE MATERIALS

Water is sometimes used to flush spills and to reduce or direct vapors in spill situations. Some of the materials covered by the guidebook can react violently or even explosively with water. In these cases, consider letting the fire burn or leaving the spill alone (except to prevent its spreading by diking) until additional technical advice can be obtained. The applicable guides clearly warn you of these potentially dangerous reactions. These materials require technical advice since

    (1)   water getting inside a ruptured or leaking container may cause an explosion;

    (2)   water may be needed to cool adjoining containers to prevent their rupturing (exploding) or further spread of the fires;

    (3)   water may be effective in mitigating an incident involving a water-reactive material only if it can be applied at a sufficient flooding rate for an extended period; and

(4)   the products from the reaction with water may be more toxic, corrosive, or otherwise more undesirable than the product of the fire without water applied. When responding to an incident involving water-reactive materials, take into account the existing conditions such as wind, precipitation, location and accessibility to the incident, as well as the availability of the agents to control the fire or spill. Because there are variables to consider, the decision to use water on fires or spills involving water-reactive materials should be based on information from an authoritative source; for example, a producer of the material, who can be contacted through the emergency response telephone number or the appropriate emergency response agency.

VAPOR CONTROL

Limiting the amount of vapor released from a pool of flammable or corrosive liquids is an operational concern. It requires the use of proper protective clothing, specialized equipment, appropriate chemical agents, and skilled personnel. Before engaging in vapor control, get advice from an authoritative source as to the proper tactics.

There are several ways to minimize the amount of vapors escaping from pools of spilled liquids, such as special foams, adsorbing agents, absorbing agents, and neutralizing agents. To be effective, these vapor control methods must be selected for the specific material involved and performed in a manner that will mitigate, not worsen, the incident.

Where specific materials are known, such as at manufacturing or storage facilities, it is desirable for the dangerous goods response team to prearrange with the facility operators to select and stockpile these control agents in advance of a spill. In the field, first responders may not have the most effective vapor control agent for the material available. They are likely to have only water and only one type of fire fighting foam on their vehicles. If the available foam is inappropriate for use, they are likely to use water spray. Because the water is being used to form a vapor seal, care must be taken not to churn or further spread the spill during application. Vapors that do not react with water may be directed away from the site using the air currents surrounding the water spray. Before using water spray or other methods to safely control vapor emission or to suppress ignition, obtain technical advice, based on specific chemical name identification.

CRIMINAL/TERRORIST USE OF CHEMICAL/BIOLOGICAL/RADIOLOGICAL AGENTS

The following is intended to supply information to first responders for use in making a preliminary assessment of a situation that they suspect involves criminal/terrorist use of chemical, biological agents and/or radioactive materials (CBRN). To aid in the assessment, a list of observable indicators of the use and/or presence of a CB agent or radioactive material is provided in the following paragraphs.

DIFFERENCES BETWEEN A CHEMICAL, BIOLOGICAL AND RADIOLOGICAL AGENT

Chemical and biological agents as well as radioactive materials can be dispersed in the air we breathe, the water we drink, or on surfaces we physically contact. Dispersion methods may be as simple as opening a container, using conventional (garden) spray devices, or as elaborate as detonating an improvised explosive device.

Chemical Incidents are characterized by the rapid onset of medical symptoms (minutes to hours) and easily observed signatures (colored residue, dead foliage, pungent odor, dead insects and animals).

Biological Incidents are characterized by the onset of symptoms in hours to days. Typically, there will be no characteristic signatures because biological agents are usually odorless and colorless. Because of the delayed onset of symptoms in a biological incident, the area affected may be greater due to the movement of infected individuals.

Radiological Incidents are characterized by the onset of symptoms, if any, in days to weeks or longer. Typically, there will be no characteristic signatures because radioactive materials are usually odorless and colorless. Specialized equipment is required to determine the size of the affected area, and whether the level of radioactivity presents an immediate or long-term health hazard. Because radioactivity is not detectable without special equipment, the affected area may be greater due to the migration of contaminated individuals.

At the levels created by most probable sources, not enough radiation would be generated to kill people or cause severe illness. In a radiological incident generated by a "dirty bomb", or Radiological Dispersal Device (RDD), in which a conventional explosive is detonated to spread radioactive contamination, the primary hazard is from the explosion. However, certain radioactive materials dispersed in the air could contaminate up to several city blocks, creating fear and possibly panic, and requiring potentially costly cleanup.

INDICATORS OF A POSSIBLE CHEMICAL INCIDENT

Dead animals/birds/fish   Not just an occasional road kill, but numerous animals (wild and domestic, small and large), birds, and fish in the same area.

INDICATORS OF A POSSIBLE CHEMICAL INCIDENT (Continued)

Lack of insect life
If normal insect activity (ground, air, and/or water) is missing, check the ground/water surface/shore line for dead insects. If near water, check for dead fish/aquatic birds.

Unexplained odors
Smells may range from fruity to flowery to sharp/pungent to garlic/ horseradish-like to bitter almonds/peach kernels to new mown hay. It is important to note that the particular odor is completely out of character with its surroundings.

Unusual numbers of dying or sick people (mass casualties)
Health problems including nausea, disorientation, difficulty in breathing, convulsions, localized sweating, conjunctivitis (reddening of eyes/nerve agent symptoms), erythema (reddening of skin/vesicant symptoms) and death.

Pattern of casualties
Casualties will likely be distributed downwind, or if indoors, by the air ventilation system.

Blisters/rashes
Numerous individuals experiencing unexplained water-like blisters, weals (like bee stings), and/or rashes.

Illness in confined area
Different casualty rates for people working indoors versus outdoors dependent on where the agent was released.

Unusual liquid droplets
Numerous surfaces exhibit oily droplets/film; numerous water surfaces have an oily film. (No recent rain.)

Different looking areas
Not just a patch of dead weeds, but trees, shrubs, bushes, food crops, and/or lawns that are dead, discolored, or withered. (No current drought.)

Low-lying clouds
Low-lying cloud/fog-like condition that is not consistent with its surroundings.

Unusual metal debris
Unexplained bomb/munitions-like material, especially if it contains a liquid.

INDICATORS OF A POSSIBLE BIOLOGICAL INCIDENT

Unusual numbers of sick or dying people or animals
Any number of symptoms may occur. Casualties may occur hours to days after an incident has occurred. The time required before symptoms are observed is dependent on the agent used.

Unscheduled and unusual spray being disseminated
Especially if outdoors during periods of darkness.

Abandoned spray devices
Devices may not have distinct odors.

INDICATORS OF A POSSIBLE RADIOLOGICAL INCIDENT

Radiation Symbols   Containers may display a "propeller" radiation symbol.

Unusual metal debris   Unexplained bomb/munitions-like material.

Heat-emitting material   Material that is hot or seems to emit heat without any sign of an external heat source.

Glowing material   Strongly radioactive material may emit or cause radioluminescence.

Sick people/animals   In very improbable scenarios there may be unusual numbers of sick or dying people or animals. Casualties may occur hours to days or weeks after an incident has occurred. The time required before symptoms are observed is dependent on the radioactive material used, and the dose received. Possible symptoms include skin reddening or vomiting.

PERSONAL SAFETY CONSIDERATIONS

When approaching a scene that may involve CB agents or radioactive materials, the most critical consideration is the safety of oneself and other responders. Protective clothing and respiratory protection of appropriate level of safety must be used. In incidents where it is suspected that CBRN materials have been used as weapons, NIOSH-certified respirators with CBRN protection are highly recommended. Be aware that the presence and identification of CB agents or radioactive materials may not be verifiable, especially in the case of biological or radiological agents. The following actions/measures to be considered are applicable to either a chemical, biological or radiological incident. The guidance is general in nature, not all encompassing, and its applicability should be evaluated on a case-by-case basis.

Approach and response strategies. Protect yourself and use a safe approach (minimize any exposure time, maximize the distance between you and the item that is likely to harm you, use cover as protection and wear appropriate personal protective equipment and respiratory protection). Identify and estimate the hazard by using indicators as provided above. Isolate the area and secure the scene; potentially contaminated people should be isolated and decontaminated as soon as possible. To the extent possible, take measures to limit the spread of contamination. In the event of a chemical incident, the fading of chemical odors is not necessarily an indication of reduced vapor concentrations. Some chemicals deaden the senses giving the false perception that the chemical is no longer present.

If there is any indication that an area may be contaminated with radioactive materials, including the site of any non-accidental explosion, responder personnel should be equipped with radiation detection equipment that would alert them if they are entering a radiologically compromised environment, and should have received adequate training in its use. This equipment should be designed in such a way that it can also alert the responders when an unacceptable ambient dose rate or ambient dose has been reached.

Initial actions to consider in a potential CBRN/Hazmat Terrorism Event:

- Avoid using cell phones, radios, etc. within 100 meters (300 feet) of a suspect device.
- NOTIFY your local police by calling 911.
- Set up Incident command upwind and uphill of the area.
- Do NOT touch or move suspicious packages/containers.
- Be cautious regarding potential presence of secondary devices (e.g. Improvised Explosive Devices, IEDs).
- Avoid contamination.
- Limit access to only those responsible for rescue of victims or assessment of unknown materials or devices.
- Evacuate and isolate individuals potentially exposed to dangerous goods/ hazardous materials.
- Isolate contaminated areas and secure the scene for analysis of material.

Decontamination measures. Emergency responders should follow standard decontamination procedures (flush-strip-flush). Mass casualty decontamination should begin as soon as possible by stripping (all clothing) and flushing (soap and water). If biological agents are involved or suspected, careful washing and use of a brush are more effective. If chemical agents are suspected, the most important and effective decontamination will be that done within the first one or two minutes. If possible, further decontamination should be performed using a 0.5% hypochlorite solution (1 part household bleach mixed with 9 parts water). If biological agents are suspected, a contact time of 10 to 15 minutes should be allowed before rinsing. The solution can be used on soft tissue wounds, but must not be used in eyes or open wounds of the abdomen, chest, head, or spine. For further information contact the agencies listed in this guidebook.

For persons contaminated with radioactive material, remove them to a low radiation area if necessary. Remove their clothing and place it in a clearly marked sealed receptacle, such as a plastic bag, for later testing. Use decontamination methods described above, but avoid breaking the skin, e.g., from shaving, or overly vigorous brushing. External radiological contamination on intact skin surface rarely causes a high enough dose to be a hazard to either the contaminated person or the first responders. For this reason, except in very unusual circumstances, an injured person who is also radiologically contaminated should be medically stabilized, taking care to minimize the spread of the contamination to the extent possible, before decontamination measures are initiated.

NOTE: The above information was developed in part by the Department of National Defence (Canada), the U.S. Department of the Army, Aberdeen Proving Ground and the Federal Bureau of Investigation (FBI).

Glossary

AEGL(s)   Acute Exposure Guideline Level(s), AEGLs represent threshold exposure limits for the general public and are applicable to emergency exposure periods ranging from 10 minutes to 8 hours. Three levels AEGL-1, AEGL-2 and AEGL-3 are developed for each of five exposure periods (10 and 30 minutes, 1 hour, 4 hours, and 8 hours) and are distinguished by varying degrees of severity of toxic effects; see AEGL-1, AEGL-2 and AEGL-3.

AEGL-1   AEGL-1 is the airborne concentration (expressed as parts per million or milligrams per cubic meter [ppm or mg/m^3]) of a substance above which it is predicted that the general population, including susceptible individuals, could experience notable discomfort, irritation, or certain asymptomatic, non-sensory effects. However, the effects are not disabling and are transient and reversible upon cessation of exposure.

AEGL-2   AEGL-2 is the airborne concentration (expressed as ppm or mg/m^3) of a substance above which it is predicted that the general population, including susceptible individuals, could experience irreversible or other serious, long-lasting adverse health effects or an impaired ability to escape.

AEGL-3   AEGL-3 is the airborne concentration (expressed as ppm or mg/m^3) of a substance above which it is predicted that the general population, including susceptible individuals, could experience life-threatening health effects or death.

Alcohol resistant foam   A foam that is resistant to "polar" chemicals such as ketones and esters which may break down other types of foam.

Biological agents   Living organisms that cause disease, sickness and mortality in humans. Anthrax and Ebola are examples of biological agents. **Refer to GUIDE 158**.

Blister agents (vesicants) Substances that cause blistering of the skin. Exposure is through liquid or vapor contact with any exposed tissue (eyes, skin, lungs). Mustard (H), Distilled Mustard (HD), Nitrogen Mustard (HN) and Lewisite (L) are blister agents.

Symptoms: Red eyes, skin irritation, burning of skin, blisters, upper respiratory damage, cough, hoarseness.

Glossary

Blood agents Substances that injure a person by interfering with cell respiration (the exchange of oxygen and carbon dioxide between blood and tissues). Hydrogen cyanide (AC) and Cyanogen chloride (CK) are blood agents.

Symptoms: Respiratory distress, headache, unresponsiveness, seizures, coma.

Burn Refers to either a chemical or thermal burn, the former may be caused by corrosive substances and the latter by liquefied cryogenic gases, hot molten substances, or flames.

CBRN Chemical, biological, radiological or nuclear warfare agent.

Choking agents Substances that cause physical injury to the lungs. Exposure is through inhalation. In extreme cases, membranes swell and lungs become filled with liquid (pulmonary edema). Death results from lack of oxygen; hence, the victim is "choked". Phosgene (CG) is a choking agent.

Symptoms: Irritation to eyes/nose/throat, respiratory distress, nausea and vomiting, burning of exposed skin.

CO_2 Carbon dioxide gas.

Cold zone Area where the command post and support functions that are necessary to control the incident are located. This is also referred to as the clean zone, green zone or support zone in other documents. (EPA Standard Operating Safety Guidelines, OSHA 29 CFR 1910.120, NFPA 472)

Combustible liquid Liquids which have a flash point greater than 60.5°C (141°F) and below 93°C (200°F). U.S. regulations permit a flammable liquid with a flash point between 38°C (100°F) and 60.5°C (141°F) to be reclassed as a combustible liquid.

Compatibility Group Letters identify explosives that are deemed to be compatible. Class 1 materials are considered to be "compatible" if they can be transported together without significantly increasing either the probability of an incident or, for a given quantity, the magnitude of the effects of such an incident.

A   Substances which are expected to mass detonate very soon after fire reaches them.

Glossary

B   Articles which are expected to mass detonate very soon after fire reaches them.

C   Substances or articles which may be readily ignited and burn violently without necessarily exploding.

D   Substances or articles which may mass detonate (with blast and/or fragment hazard) when exposed to fire.

E&F Articles which may mass detonate in a fire.

G   Substances and articles which may mass explode and give off smoke or toxic gases.

H   Articles which in a fire may eject hazardous projectiles and dense white smoke.

J   Articles which may mass explode.

K   Articles which in a fire may eject hazardous projectiles and toxic gases.

L   Substances and articles which present a special risk and could be activated by exposure to air or water.

N   Articles which contain only extremely insensitive detonating substances and demonstrate a negligible probability of accidental ignition or propagation.

S   Packaged substances or articles which, if accidentally initiated, produce effects that are usually confined to the immediate vicinity.

Control zones   Designated areas at dangerous goods incidents, based on safety and the degree of hazard. Many terms are used to describe control zones; however, in this guidebook, these zones are defined as the hot/exclusion/red/restricted zone, warm/contamination reduction/yellow/limited access zone, and cold/support/green/clean zone. (EPA Standard Operating Safety Guidelines, OSHA 29 CFR 1910.120, NFPA 472)

Cryogenic liquid   A refrigerated, liquefied gas that has a boiling point colder than -90°C (-130°F) at atmospheric pressure.

Dangerous Water Reactive Material   Produces significant toxic gas when it comes in contact with water.

Glossary

Decomposition products Products of a chemical or thermal break-down of a substance.

Decontamination The removal of dangerous goods from personnel and equipment to the extent necessary to prevent potential adverse health effects. Always avoid direct or indirect contact with dangerous goods; however, if contact occurs, personnel should be decontaminated as soon as possible. Since the methods used to decontaminate personnel and equipment differ from one chemical to another, contact the chemical manufacturer, through the agencies listed on the inside back cover, to determine the appropriate procedure. Contaminated clothing and equipment should be removed after use and stored in a controlled area (warm/contamination reduction/limited access zone) until cleanup procedures can be initiated. In some cases, protective clothing and equipment cannot be decontaminated and must be disposed of in a proper manner.

Dry chemical A preparation designed for fighting fires involving flammable liquids, pyrophoric substances and electrical equipment. Common types contain sodium bicarbonate or potassium bicarbonate.

Edema The accumulation of an excessive amount of watery fluid in cells and tissues. Pulmonary edema is an excessive buildup of water in the lungs, for instance, after inhalation of a gas that is corrosive to lung tissue.

ERPG(s) Emergency Response Planning Guideline(s). Values intended to provide estimates of concentration ranges above which one could reasonably anticipate observing adverse health effects; see ERPG-1, ERPG-2 and ERPG-3.

ERPG-1 The maximum airborne concentration below which it is believed nearly all individuals could be exposed for up to 1 hour without experiencing more than mild, transient adverse health effects or without perceiving a clearly defined objectionable odor.

ERPG-2 The maximum airborne concentration below which it is believed nearly all individuals could be exposed for up to 1 hour without experiencing or developing irreversible or other serious health effects or symptoms that could impair an individual's ability to take protective action.

Glossary

ERPG-3

The maximum airborne concentration below which it is believed nearly all individuals could be exposed for up to 1 hour without experiencing or developing life-threatening health effects.

Flammable liquid

A liquid that has a flash point of 60.5°C (141°F) or lower.

Flash point

Lowest temperature at which a liquid or solid gives off vapor in such a concentration that, when the vapor combines with air near the surface of the liquid or solid, a flammable mixture is formed. Hence, the lower the flash point, the more flammable the material.

Hazard zones (Inhalation Hazard Zones)

HAZARD ZONE A: Gases: LC50 of less than or equal to 200 ppm,
Liquids: V equal to or greater than 500 LC50 and LC50 less than or equal to 200 ppm,

HAZARD ZONE B: Gases: LC50 greater than 200 ppm and less than or equal to 1000 ppm,
Liquids: V equal to or greater than 10 LC50; LC50 less than or equal to 1000 ppm and criteria for Hazard Zone A are not met.

HAZARD ZONE C: LC50 greater than 1000 ppm and less than or equal to 3000 ppm,

HAZARD ZONE D: LC50 greater than 3000 ppm and less than or equal to 5000 ppm.

Hot zone

Area immediately surrounding a dangerous goods incident which extends far enough to prevent adverse effects from released dangerous goods to personnel outside the zone. This zone is also referred to as exclusion zone, red zone or restricted zone in other documents. (EPA Standard Operating Safety Guidelines, OSHA 29 CFR 1910.120, NFPA 472)

IED

See "Improvised Explosive Device".

Immiscible

In this guidebook, means that a material does not mix readily with water.

Improvised Explosive Device

A bomb that is manufactured from commercial, military or homemade explosives.

Large spill

A spill that involves quantities that are greater than 200 liters for liquids and greater than 300 kilograms for solids.

Glossary

LC50

Lethal concentration 50. The concentration of a material administered by inhalation that is expected to cause the death of 50% of an experimental animal population within a specified time. (Concentration is reported in either ppm or mg/m^3)

Mass explosion

Explosion which affects almost the entire load virtually instantaneously.

mg/m^3

Milligrams of a material per cubic meter of air.

Miscible

In this guidebook, means that a material mixes readily with water.

mL/m^3

Milliliters of a material per cubic meter of air. (1 mL/m^3 equals 1 ppm)

Nerve agents

Substances that interfere with the central nervous system. Exposure is primarily through contact with the liquid (via skin and eyes) and secondarily through inhalation of the vapor. Tabun (GA), Sarin (GB), Soman (GD) and VX are nerve agents.

Symptoms: Pinpoint pupils, extreme headache, severe tightness in the chest, dyspnea, runny nose, coughing, salivation, unresponsiveness, seizures.

Non-polar

See "Immiscible".

n.o.s.

These letters refer to "not otherwise specified". The entries which use this description are generic names such as "Corrosive liquid, n.o.s." This means that the actual chemical name for that corrosive liquid is not listed in the regulations; therefore, a generic name must be used to describe it on shipping papers.

Noxious

In this guidebook, means that a material may be harmful or injurious to health or physical well-being.

Oxidizer

A chemical which supplies its own oxygen and which helps other combustible material burn more readily.

P

The letter "P" following a guide number in the yellow-bordered and blue-bordered pages identifies a material which may polymerize violently under high temperature conditions or contamination with other products. This polymerization will produce heat and high pressure buildup in containers which may explode or rupture. (See polymerization below)

Glossary

Packing Group

The Packing Group (PG) is assigned based on the degree of danger presented by the hazardous material:

PG I : Great danger
PG II : Medium danger
PG III : Minor danger

PG

See Packing Group

pH

pH is a value that represents the acidity or alkalinity of a water solution. Pure water has a pH of 7. A pH value below 7 indicates an acid solution (a pH of 1 is extremely acidic). A pH above 7 indicates an alkaline solution (a pH of 14 is extremely alkaline). Acids and alkalies (bases) are commonly referred to as corrosive materials.

PIH

Poison Inhalation Hazard. Term used to describe gases and volatile liquids that are toxic when inhaled. (Same as TIH)

Polar

See "Miscible".

Polymerization

This term describes a chemical reaction which is generally associated with the production of plastic substances. Basically, the individual molecules of the chemical (liquid or gas) react with each other to produce what can be described as a long chain. These chains can be formed in many useful applications. A well known example is the styrofoam (polystyrene) coffee cup which is formed when liquid molecules of styrene react with each other or polymerize forming a solid, therefore changing the name from styrene to polystyrene (poly means many).

ppm

Parts per million. (1 ppm equals 1 mL/m^3)

Protective clothing

Includes both respiratory and physical protection. One cannot assign a level of protection to clothing or respiratory devices separately. These levels were accepted and defined by response organizations such as U.S. Coast Guard, NIOSH, and U.S. EPA.

Level A: SCBA plus totally encapsulating chemical resistant clothing (permeation resistant).

Level B: SCBA plus hooded chemical resistant clothing (splash suit).

Level C: Full or half-face respirator plus hooded chemical resistant clothing (splash suit).

Level D: Coverall with no respiratory protection.

Glossary

Pyrophoric   A material which ignites spontaneously upon exposure to air (or oxygen).

Radiation Authority   As referred to in GUIDES 161 through 166 for radioactive materials, the Radiation Authority is either a Federal, state/ provincial agency or state/province designated official. The responsibilities of this authority include evaluating radiological hazard conditions during normal operations and during emergencies. If the identity and telephone number of the authority are not known by emergency responders, or included in the local response plan, the information can be obtained from the agencies listed on the inside back cover. They maintain a periodically updated list of radiation authorities.

Radioactivity   The property of some substances to emit invisible and potentially harmful radiation.

Refrigerated liquid   See "Cryogenic liquid".

Small spill   A spill that involves quantities that are less than 200 liters for liquids and less than 300 kilograms for solids.

Straight (solid) stream   Method used to apply or distribute water from the end of a hose. The water is delivered under pressure for penetration. In an efficient straight (solid) stream, approximately 90% of the water passes through an imaginary circle 38 cm (15 inches) in diameter at the breaking point. Hose (solid or straight) streams are frequently used to cool tanks and other equipment exposed to flammable liquid fires, or for washing burning spills away from danger points. However, straight streams will cause a spill fire to spread if improperly used or when directed into open containers of flammable and combustible liquids.

TIH   Toxic Inhalation Hazard. Term used to describe gases and volatile liquids that are toxic when inhaled. (Same as PIH)

V   Saturated vapor concentration in air of a material in mL/m^3 (volatility) at 20°C and standard atmospheric pressure.

Vapor density   Weight of a volume of pure vapor or gas (with no air present) compared to the weight of an equal volume of dry air at the same temperature and pressure. A vapor density less than 1 (one) indicates that the vapor is lighter than air and will tend to rise. A vapor density greater than 1 (one) indicates that the vapor is heavier than air and may travel along the ground.

Glossary

Vapor pressure

Pressure at which a liquid and its vapor are in equilibrium at a given temperature. Liquids with high vapor pressures evaporate rapidly.

Viscosity

Measure of a liquid's internal resistance to flow. This property is important because it indicates how fast a material will leak out through holes in containers or tanks.

Warm zone

Area between Hot and Cold zones where personnel and equipment decontamination and hot zone support take place. It includes control points for the access corridor and thus assists in reducing the spread of contamination. Also referred to as the contamination reduction corridor (CRC), contamination reduction zone (CRZ), yellow zone or limited access zone in other documents. (EPA Standard Operating Safety Guidelines, OSHA 29 CFR 1910.120, NFPA 472)

Water-sensitive

Substances which may produce flammable and/or toxic decomposition products upon contact with water.

Water spray (fog)

Method or way to apply or distribute water. The water is finely divided to provide for high heat absorption. Water spray patterns can range from about 10 to 90 degrees. Water spray streams can be used to extinguish or control the burning of a fire or to provide exposure protection for personnel, equipment, buildings, etc. **(This method can be used to absorb vapors, knock-down vapors or disperse vapors. Direct a water spray (fog), rather than a straight (solid) stream, into the vapor cloud to accomplish any of the above).**

Water spray is particularly effective on fires of flammable liquids and volatile solids having flash points above 37.8°C (100°F).

Regardless of the above, water spray can be used successfully on flammable liquids with low flash points. The effectiveness depends particularly on the method of application. With proper nozzles, even gasoline spill fires of some types have been extinguished when coordinated hose lines were used to sweep the flames off the surface of the liquid. Furthermore, water spray carefully applied has frequently been used with success in extinguishing fires involving flammable liquids with high flash points (or any viscous liquids) by causing frothing to occur only on the surface, and this foaming action blankets and extinguishes the fire.

PUBLICATION DATA

The 2008 Emergency Response Guidebook (ERG2008) was prepared by the staff of Transport Canada, the U.S. Department of Transportation, and the Secretariat of Communications and Transport of Mexico with the assistance of many interested parties from government and industry including the collaboration of CIQUIME of Argentina. The principal authors of the ERG are Transport Canada's Michel Cloutier and U.S. DOT's George Cushmac. Printing and publication services are provided through U.S. DOT's Pipeline and Hazardous Materials Safety Administration, (PHMSA) Office of Hazardous Materials Initiatives and Training.

ERG2008 is based on earlier Transport Canada, U.S. DOT, and Secretariat of Communications and Transport emergency response guidebooks. ERG2008 is published in three languages: English, French and Spanish. The Emergency Response Guidebook has been translated and printed in other languages, including Chinese, German, Hebrew, Japanese, Portuguese, Korean, Hungarian, Polish, Turkish and Thai.

We encourage countries that wish to participate in future editions of the Guidebook to provide their emergency response center information for inclusion. Please contact any of the websites or telephone numbers in the paragraph below.

DISTRIBUTION OF THIS GUIDEBOOK

The primary objective is to place one copy of the ERG2008 in each publicly owned emergency service vehicle through distribution to Federal, state, provincial and local public safety authorities. The distribution of this guidebook is being accomplished through the voluntary cooperation of a network of key agencies. Emergency service organizations that have not yet received copies of ERG2008 should contact the respective distribution center in their country, state or province. In the U.S., information about the distribution center for your location may be obtained from the Office of Hazardous Materials Safety web site at http://hazmat.dot.gov or call 202-366-4900. In Canada, contact CANUTEC at 613-992-4624 or via the web site at http://www.canutec.gc.ca for information. In Mexico, call SCT at 52-55-5684-1275 or 684-0188 or via email at iflores@sct.gob.mx. In Argentina, call CIQUIME at 011-4613-1100, or via the web site at http://www.ciquime.org.ar, or via email at gre2008@ciquime.org.ar

REPRODUCTION and RESALE

Copies of this document which are provided free of charge to fire, police and other emergency services may not be resold. ERG2008 (PHH50-ERG2008) may be reproduced without further permission subject to the following:

The names and the seals of the participating governments may not be reproduced on a copy of this document unless that copy accurately reproduces the entire content (text, format, and coloration) of this document without modification. In addition, the publisher's full name and address must be displayed on the outside back cover of each copy, replacing the wording placed on the center of the back cover.

Constructive comments concerning ERG2008 are solicited; in particular, comments concerning its use in handling incidents involving dangerous goods. Comments should be addressed to:

In Canada:

Director, CANUTEC
Transport Dangerous Goods
Transport Canada
Ottawa, Ontario
Canada K1A 0N5

Phone: 613-992-4624 (information)
Fax: 613-954-5101
Email: canutec@tc.gc.ca

In the U.S.:

U. S. Department of Transportation
Pipeline and Hazardous Materials Safety Administration
Office of Hazardous Materials Initiatives and Training (PHH-50)
Washington, DC 20590-0001

Phone: 202-366-4900
Fax: 202-366-7342
Email: ERG2008@dot.gov

In Mexico:

Secretariat for Communications and Transport
Land Transport Directorate
Hazardous Materials and Wastes Directorate
Calz. de las Bombas No. 411-9 piso
Col. San Bartolo Coapa
Coyoacan 04800, D.F.
Mexico

Phone and Fax: +52-55-5684-1275 and 684-0188

In Argentina:

Chemistry Information Center for Emergencies (CIQUIME)
Juan Bautista Alberdi 2986
C1406GSS Buenos Aires, Argentina
Tel. +54-11-4613-1100   Fax (011) 4613-3707
Email: gre2008@ciquime.org.ar

NOTES

NOTES

NOTES

NOTES

The Emergency Response Guidebook is normally revised and reissued every four years. However, in the event of a significant mistake, omission or change in the state of knowledge, special instructions to change the guidebook (in pen-and-ink, with paste-over stickers, or with a supplement) may be issued.

Users of this guidebook should check periodically (about every 6 months) to make sure their version is current. Changes should be annotated below. Contact:

DOT/PHMSA
http://hazmat.dot.gov/pubs/erg/guidebook.htm

TRANSPORT CANADA
http://www.tc.gc.ca/canutec/en/guide/guide.htm

CIQUIME
http://www.ciquime.org.ar

This guidebook incorporates changes dated:

_____

_____

_____

EMERGENCY RESPONSE TELEPHONE NUMBERS

MEXICO

1. **SETIQ**

01-800-00-214-00 in the Mexican Republic
For calls originating in Mexico City and the Metropolitan Area
5559-1588
For calls originating elsewhere, call
+52-55-5559-1588

2. **CENACOM**

01-800-00-413-00 in the Mexican Republic
For calls originating in Mexico City and the Metropolitan Area
5128-0000 exts. 11470, 11471, 11472, 11473, 11474, 11475, 11476 and 11477
For calls originating elsewhere, call
+52-55-5128-0000 exts. 11470, 11471, 11472, 11474, 11475 and 11476

ARGENTINA

1. **CIQUIME**

0-800-222-2933 in the Republic of Argentina
For calls originating elsewhere, call
+54-11-4613-1100

BRAZIL

1. **PRÓ-QUÍMICA**

0-800-118270
(Toll-free in Brazil)
For calls originating elsewhere, call
+55-11-232-1144
(Collect calls are accepted)

COLOMBIA

1. **CISPROQUIM**

01-800-091-6012 in Colombia
For calls originating in Bogotá, Colombia call
288-6012
For calls originating elsewhere call
+57-1-288-6012

For additional details see the section entiitled **"WHO TO CALL FOR ASSISTANCE"**.